DUE DATE	RETURN DATE	DUE DATE	RETURN DATE
JAN 6 1991			
DEC 17 1990			

The Physiological Basis of
Hearing

A Review

Wolf D. Keidel, M.D., F.A.S.A.
Director, Institute of Physiology and Biokybernetics
Erlangen-Nuernberg University

S. Kallert, M.D.
Institute of Physiology and Biokybernetics
Erlangen-Nuernberg University

M. Korth, M.D.
Institute of Physiology and Biokybernetics
Erlangen-Nuernberg University

Special Editor

Larry Humes, Ph.D.
Associate Director, Research and Training Program
Division of Hearing and Speech Science
Vanderbilt University School of Medicine
Nashville, Tennessee

1983
Thieme-Stratton Inc.
New York

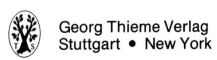

Georg Thieme Verlag
Stuttgart • New York

Publisher: Thieme-Stratton Inc.
381 Park Avenue South
New York, New York 10016

The Physiological Basis of Hearing (A Review)
Keidel • Kallert • Korth

TSI ISBN 0-86577-072-7
GTV ISBN 3-13-635801-5

Printed in the United States of America.

Last digit is print number 5 4 3 2 1

To all my American friends
to whom I am indebted so much.

Wolf D. Keidel

ACKNOWLEDGMENTS

The authors would like to thank all the staff members of the Institute für Physiologie und Biokybernetik, especially Dr. L.U.E. Kohllöffel, Dr. E. David, Dr. P. Finkenzeller, Dr. M. Spreng (formerly Dr. G. Stange), and especially Dr. Keidel's teacher, Professor Otto F. Ranke for valuable discussions and the introduction of fundamental ideas for this book. We are also deeply indebted to Mrs. Pfister for writing the manuscript, Mr. and Mrs. Burian for preparing the drawings and Mrs. Werner for essential help in obtaining the permission to reproduce most of the figures. Finally, we would like to thank Thieme-Stratton publishers for the effort that they put into publishing this monograph. Our most sincere thanks, however, is directed to Dr. Larry Humes for all his help with the English grammar and smoothing over the translation of the technical terminology.

CONTENTS

FOREWORD

Our knowledge of the physiology of the auditory system lags far behind that of the visual system. At present it is not possible even to fully describe the transformation (transduction) of mechanical sound waves into nervous excitation, let alone the basic and fundamental principles of operation of the remainder of the auditory system. For example, regarding the anatomical fine structure of the auditory nerve, very little is known about changes in tonotopic organization as the nerve progresses from the modiolus toward the cochlear nucleus, a gap which is of profound importance to the eventual clinical application of electrical stimulation of the VIIIth nerve in the near future. Similarly our understanding of the anatomical organization of the cochlear nucleus and higher relay stations of the so-called "specific" and "unspecific" pathways of the auditory system is limited.

Obviously, a complete summarizing description of the information processing conducted by the auditory system must be postponed until our knowledge of the physiology of the ear has sufficiently improved. This is especially true since, up to now, no logical description can be given and some details necessarily would appear incoherent. However, the purpose of a review is not to answer all questions about the topic of interest but to reproduce the present state of science in this topic area. In this sense, a review of the physiology of the ear may be justified as a kind of statement of account despite the restrictions just mentioned.*

Moreover, there are electrophysiological findings that can gain in clinical value before their physiological bases have been understood thoroughly. A recent example can be found in the simultaneous recording of acoustically evoked potentials from various parts of the auditory pathway,†

---

* Emphasis has been placed on the literature of the last ten years. More details can be found in "Handbook of Sensory Physiology," Vol. V, Parts 1, 2 and 3, Eds.: W.D. Keidel and W.D. Neff, Springer publishers, 1976.

† References 583, 596, 610.

the description of which should be available for the otologist. Improvements of this kind can lead to substantial progress in clinical diagnostics and thus may contribute indirectly to the understanding of the function of various parts of the auditory pathway.

INTRODUCTION

The Physiological Basis of Hearing (A Review) represents the most comprehensive and thorough review available on the topic of auditory physiology. The mechanical events within the cochlea preceding transduction by the hair cells are reviewed in detail. The focus of this book is clearly auditory electrophysiology—from the cochlea through the cortex. This has been sorely lacking in many other texts on auditory physiology that for various reasons have focused on the most peripheral portions of the auditory system.

The authors of this book have done a remarkable job of pulling together a diverse literature. The review of contemporary work includes appropriate references to data obtained from studies of single nerve fibers at various locations along the auditory pathway as well as frequent citations of investigations utilizing surface-recorded evoked potentials. Where possible, the authors attempt to incorporate existing knowledge of the response characteristics of auditory-nerve fibers from various centers along the auditory pathway into an information-processing scheme.

The focus on electrophysiology is indeed timely. The availability of this review should aid scientists and clinicians alike in further research and clinical assessment of cochlear implants. Furthermore, future use of auditory evoked potentials by the neurologist, otologist, and audiologist, whether used to assist in establishing the site of lesion or assessing the hearing of difficult-to-test patients, can benefit considerably from the availability of this thorough review. Finally, it is unquestionable that students of the various auditory disciplines—otology, audiology, psycho-acoustics, and physiological acoustics—will derive great benefit from this exhaustive compendium of contemporary auditory physiology.

In summary, clinicians, researchers, professors, and advanced students should all find this review of auditory physiology to be of assistance to them in their endeavors. *The Physiological Basis of Hearing (A Review)* provides a solid foundation formed from existing knowledge of the auditory system upon which future investigations and clinical practices can be built. As Disraeli once said, "The more extensive a man's knowledge of what has been done, the greater will be his power of knowing what to do."

Larry Humes, Ph.D.
Division of Hearing and Speech Sciences
School of Medicine
Vanderbilt University
Nashville, Tennessee

I. PHYSIOLOGY OF THE INNER EAR

A. The Adequate Stimulus*

The adequate stimulus of the ear is the sound wave. Sound waves are elastic waves in deformable media. In solid media they occur as longitudinal or transverse waves. In homogenous fluids and gases, however, there are only longitudinal waves. This results because the elastic shear forces necessary for the propagation of transverse movements are generally lacking in homogenous fluids and gases so that transverse waves occur only as surface waves on border areas. Whereas light propagates as electromagnetic wave also in the vacuum, sound waves, by nature, are only existent in matter. However, during sound propagation the transport of energy and impulse also takes place without transport of mass.

Only those elastic oscillations which normally lead to auditory sensations in humans are designated as sound. This applies to the frequency range between 20 Hz and 20 kHz approximately.† It is only within this frequency range that a clear-cut relation exists for humans between frequency and pitch, such that under otherwise constant conditions a pitch sensation can be ascribed to a certain frequency.‡ Lower frequencies (infrasound) are perceived as vibration, not as sound, while higher frequencies (ultrasonics) may possibly elicit sound sensations. The pitch sensation of the latter, however, corresponds, irrespective of stimulus frequency, with the highest perceivable tone of approximately 20 kHz.[608, 927] As a rule, for frequencies beyond the range of 20 Hz to 20 kHz hearing

---

* Regarding this topic, only enough detail will be provided as required for the later presentation. Comprehensive descriptions of the properties of sound are given in textbooks on acoustics (e.g., E. Skudrzyk [1040, 1041], F. Trendelenburg [1163], and W. Reichardt [946]).

† Many animals are able to hear ultrasonics.

‡ Of course this holds true only within the scope of pitch discrimination.

1

threshold matches tickle or pain threshold.[927] Therefore, these waves are not generally regarded as adequate sound stimuli.

The intensity of sound waves leading to auditory perception, the dynamic range of the ear, extends approximately from 10^{-16} W/cm^2 to 10^{-4} W/cm^2, with the lower intensity corresponding to auditory threshold and the higher intensity to tickle or pain threshold. Since threshold intensity depends upon the frequency of the test tone (Fig. 1) it can not be given by one single intensity value. As a rule, sound intensity is expressed in dB SPL.*

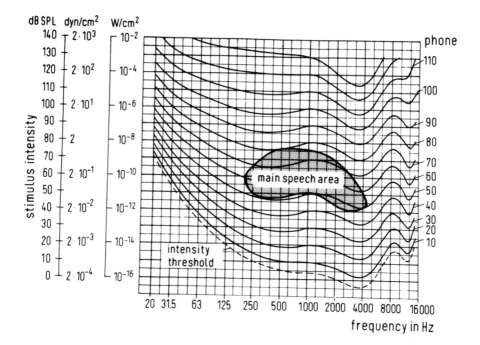

FIGURE 1. Curves of threshold sound intensity and equal loudness as a function of the frequency of the test tone according to measurements made by Fletcher and Munson (353) and Robinson and Dadson (962), from DIN 45630, sheet 2. The intensity threshold corresponds to a loudness of 4 phons and not to 0 phons.

---

* SPL = sound pressure level, i.e. referred to the internationally acknowledged standard value of 20 μPa = 20 μN/m^2 = 2 · 10^{-4} dyn/cm^2 corresponding with the threshold intensity at 4000 Hz (= minimum of hearing threshold curve). The intensity of any given sound in dB results from the computation of the value

$$20 \cdot \log \left(\frac{\text{effective sound pressure in } \mu\text{Pa}}{20 \, \mu\text{Pa}} \right)$$

All natural sounds are quite complex if sound pressure is represented as a function of time. Isolated pure tones or sinusoidal waves do not occur naturally. Even in the laboratory pure tones can be generated only with considerable technical effort. Yet the pure tone plays an important part in the physiology of the ear. Reasons for this are given by Jean Baptiste Fourier's enormous achievement of harmonic analysis. According to his idea, any given periodic oscillation can be regarded as the sum of a generally infinite number of harmonic subcomponents representing integer multiples of one fundamental frequency. The fundamental frequency is equal to the frequency of the non-harmonic oscillation. Even aperiodic events can be analyzed in this way if the integral is used instead of the sum. The result is that periodic oscillations are described by discrete spectra whereas non-periodic events can be described by continuous spectra.*

Ohm[864, 865] introduced the principle of Fourier's analysis into acoustics (Ohm's law of acoustics). Thus, any given sound (even a click) can be conceived of as being the sum or the integral of sine waves, that is, pure tones. Consequently, the pure tone appears to be the elementary unit of all sound. Therefore, it was only natural to wonder whether the ear might be capable of performing a Fourier-analysis of sound stimuli.

B. Origins of Modern Physiology of the Inner Ear

Adapting these ideas, von Helmholtz[479, 480] advanced a hypothesis accounting for the mechanism of Fourier's analysis within the ear. His hypothesis of resonance was based on the idea that after transfer of sound waves to the perilymph of the scala vestibuli of the inner ear the basilar membrane or portions of it would resonate, such that high frequencies lead to deformations close to the stapes and low frequencies lead to deformations close to the helicotrema. The site of resonance for the various frequencies was supposed to be arranged along the basilar membrane in such a way that sounds of decreasing frequencies would be patterned on to the basilar membrane by a maximum of deformation at increasing distance from the stapes.† Thus, any given frequency is associated with a certain site along the

---

* For further details see textbooks of mathematics and theoretical physics.
† This was attributed to the changing width of the basilar membrane. The width of the basilar membrane increases from the basal turn to the helicotrema. In the basal turn the width is approximately 100 μm; in the middle turn, 340 μm; and in the apical turn, 500 μm.

basilar membrane and vice versa (place theory). In a sense, von Helmholtz extended the law of the "specific nerve energies" layed down for the various sensory modalities by Müller.[830] According to this law, any sensation triggered by a stimulus depends on the excited nerve fiber only, not on the stimulus. In accordance with this principle von Helmholtz' theory maintained that those nerve fibers originating from a certain site of resonance would be responsible for a certain pitch perception.

A frequency analysis applying narrowly-tuned resonators is appealing due to its clarity. It would explain at once the ear's excellent ability (optimally 0.1%) to discriminate pitch (Fig. 2, Fig. 3).

Besides very fine frequency analysis, the auditory system is capable of performing excellent temporal resolutions. This has been examined extensively in modern times in connection with speech recognition,* but was already known to von Helmholtz from his studies of music. In order to explain the high temporal resolution a relatively strong damping of the resonators must be assumed (Fig. 4). Strong damping, however, results in poorer frequency analysis. This conflict was pointed out long ago by Wien.[1229] Von Helmholtz acknowledged that perception of the quaver effect in music required damping that would have to be so strong that the half-width of the resonance would amount to half a tone.

The conflict surrounding frequency versus temporal analysis of sound by the human auditory system has its origin in the classical experiments of Seebeck.[1025] His results were used by Ohm[864] to support his own ideas favoring frequency analysis, an interpretation opposed by Seebeck.[1026] In modern times the ideas of Seebeck favoring a temporal analysis have been further extended, particularly by Schouten,[1013-1017] Licklider[719, 720] and de Boer.[122, 123] A summarizing review is given by de Boer.[124] Also modern electrophysiological results support both place and time coding in the cochlea.[974]

There is no doubt that a relation exists between pitch sensation and the site of excitation within the inner ear. However, a relation exists also between pitch sensation and the periodicity of a sound stimulus, even though this is correct only for the low frequency range (missing fundamental, residue phenomenon, periodicity pitch). The latter phenomenon has also been demonstrated electrophysiologically. One example is the experiment carried out by Smith et al.[1047] They combined the frequencies 730, 1095, 1460, and 1825 Hz to form a complex sound. They then showed that not only an additional tone of the missing fundamental frequency of 365 Hz can be heard, but that the corresponding periodicity also occurs in the EEG (described by Marsh and Worden[746] as frequency following response =

---

* Regarding this topic consult the following recent literature: 2, 174, 197, 258, 324, 350, 373 504–507, 649, 650–652, 689, 727, 860, 861, 868, 869, 934, 1106, 1125.

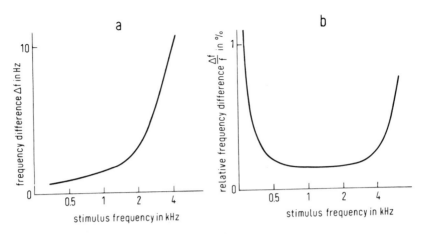

FIGURE 2. A, Frequency difference threshold = smallest frequency difference, Δf, perceivable as pitch difference, plotted as a function of the frequency of the test tone. B, Relative frequency difference Δf/f as a function of the frequency of the test tone. (According to Licklider [718]; Harris [453]; König [676]; from Kay [551]).

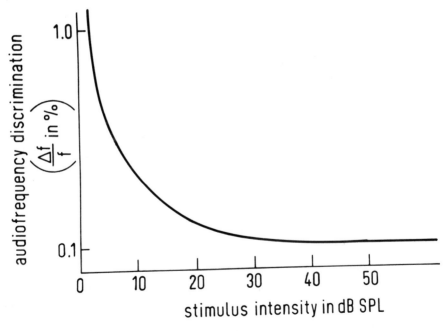

FIGURE 3. Relative frequency difference limen Δf/f as a function of intensity. Frequency of test tone 1 kHz. (According to Kay [551].)

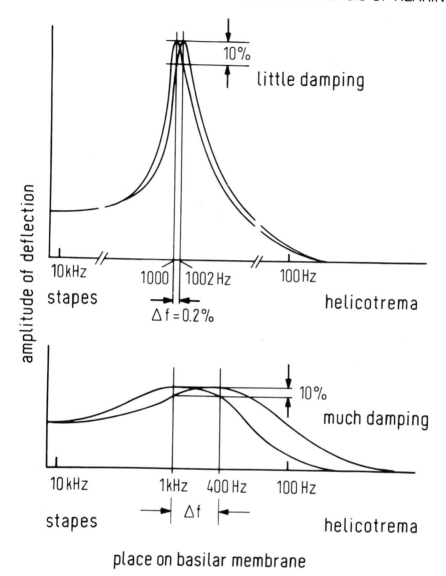

FIGURE 4. Effect of damping on frequency discrimination. It is assumed that for frequency discrimination a difference in the amplitude of deflection of 10% is necessary. Above: Little damping, good frequency discrimination, but long time delay for the oscillation to reach its maximum and then to disappear. Therefore poor temporal resolution. Below: Much damping, poor frequency discrimination, but short time delay for the oscillation to reach its maximum and then to disappear. Therefore good temporal resolution. (According to Keidel [599].)

FFR), just as if a sound stimulus of 365 Hz was present. However, whereas the FFR of a pure-tone stimulus of 365 Hz is reduced by a suitable narrow-band noise, it stays preserved after the complex stimulus was combined with a narrrow-band noise. This supports the view that the sensation of the pitch of the missing fundamental is based on the periodicity of the stimulus and not on a low frequency spectral component represented at a certain location within the inner ear.

Apart from the resonance hypothesis (von Helmholtz) and the travelling wave theory (von Békésy), as well as the well known telephone theory[999] and the sound image theory (Mehrorts- or Klangbildtheorie*), other attempts were made to explain the function of the inner ear. For a historical review the reader is referred to Bast and Anson[62] and to Wever.[1208]

C. Mechanics of the Inner Ear

The pioneering work of von Békésy[70-103] was a breakthrough in the field of experimental physiology of the inner ear; in the field of mathematics it was the work of Ranke.[922-930] Von Békésy observed the behavior of the basilar membrane directly in the opened cochlea as well as in suitable models. In doing so, he found a motion pattern of the basilar membrane known in the literature as the "travelling wave." It was described by him for the first time in 1928.[70] At about the same time, Ranke[922] gave the first mathematical description of the mechanics of the inner ear which, likewise, led to the "travelling waves."

The term "travelling wave" characterizes the following finding: sinusoidal movements of the stapes (as occurring upon stimulation with a continuous pure tone) give rise to a movement of the basilar membrane having all temporal and spatial properties of a transverse wave propagating from the stapes to the helicotrema. This wave has some characteristic features. With increasing distance from the stapes the amplitude of deflection increases slowly and, after having passed a maximum, drops to zero very rapidly (Fig. 5).

A change of frequency causes a shift of the amplitude maximum in the sense as predicted by von Helmholtz — with increasing frequency the maximum moves towards the stapes. Thus, the travelling wave leads to a relation between the frequency of the tone and the site of maximum amplitude in the sense of the place theory. The basic mechanism however, is not resonance as understood by von Helmholtz.†

---

* References 321, 322, 764.

† The basic mechanisms are energy transport (wave propagation) combined with energy absorption (resonance).

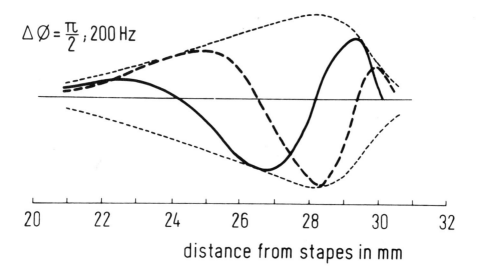

FIGURE 5. Two instantaneous pictures of the deflection of the basilar membrane displaced by a quarter of a period (solid line and heavy dashed line) and the envelope of these displacement patterns (thin dashed line) at 200 Hz from measurements on preparations of the petrous bone. (According to von Békésy [75].)

The frequency of the travelling wave along the basilar membrane remains equal to the frequency of the stapes oscillation. Travelling wave velocity, however, changes such that the velocity decreases steadily with increasing amplitude of the membrane's deflection (Fig. 6). Decreasing velocity dictates that the wavelength becomes shorter. The short wavelength range coincides with the highest amplitudes of deflection. Thereafter the wave decreases rapidly.

The decrease of the wavelength causes a considerable phase lag with respect to the movement of the stapes (Fig. 7). At very low stimulating frequencies (e.g. 50 Hz in Fig. 7) the whole membrane oscillates in phase. With increasing frequency noticeable phase differences occur; a wave develops having several cycles.

The properties of travelling waves can best be understood by experimentation with models. In doing so, any important parameter can be varied and the resulting changes of the wave can be studied. The ingenious modelmaker von Békésy[103] noted it would be a good principle to copy the original at first as accurately as possible and then to simplify the model step by step while the properties in question are tested by comparative examinations with the original. In this way it can be seen which qualities of the original system are important with respect to the properties to be tested and which can be left out for the sake of simplification of the model in order to end up with a parsimonious functional model. Fundamental and

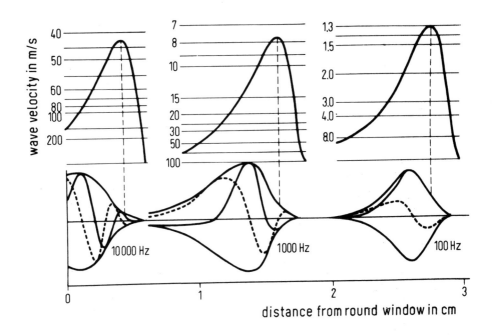

FIGURE 6. Dependency of the wave velocity and of the maxima of deflection of the basilar membrane on the space within the cochlea. (According to Ranke [925].)

progressive experiments with mechanical models* of the inner ear have been carried out by von Békésy,[70, 74, 80] Diestel,[269] Tonndorf,[1142–1155] Helle,[477] and Zwicker.[1259–1261]

First, von Békésy determined the elasticity of the basilar membrane in cadavers by measuring the shift of volume per millimeter length of membrane resulting from an increase in pressure on one side of the membrane (Fig. 8). Figure 9 shows the result. The volume shift is small close to the stapes and increases about 100 times towards the helicotrema.

---

* The most relevant references dealing with non-mechanical ear models:
1.—Mathematical models: 30, 352, 390, 445, 510, 577, 643, 714, 721, 885, 922–925, 958, 1036, 1103–1105, 1174, 1262–1264, 1266.
2.—Electronic models: 63, 125, 218, 346–348, 337, 378, 391, 492, 502, 597, 833, 1035, 1191.
3.—Electronic computer models: 337, 350, 348, 481, 597, 833.

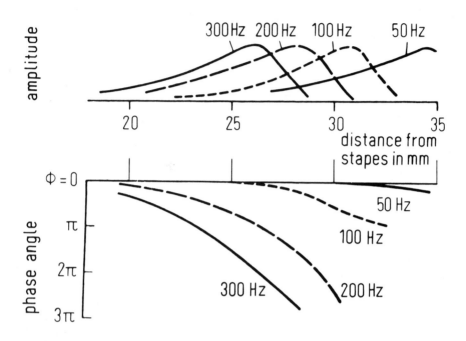

FIGURE 7. Envelopes of the deflection of the basilar membrane (above) and the phase difference between the oscillation at the respective place on the basilar membrane and the movement of the stapes (below). From measurements on preparation of the petrous bone. (According to von Békésy [75].)

Von Békésy demonstrated further that the basilar membrane is not firmly stretched. On the one side it is attached to the bony lamina spiralis, on the other side to the ligamentum spirale (a loose sponge-like tissue). Weakening the attachment of the ligamentum spirale to the surrounding bone or even lateral compression by means of a small object (Fig. 10) does not cause any change in the pattern of the travelling wave.

Removal of Reissner's membrane and of the organ of Corti does not change the pattern of the wave either. Thus, in a model the basilar membrane can be replaced by a rubber plate of suitable elasticity. This plate should not be stretched but be attached on either side (Fig. 11).

The width of the rubber membrane seems to be unimportant. Moreover, it can be arranged in a way opposite to the conditions found in the cochlea, that is the width may decrease from the stapes to the helicotrema provided that the elasticity is of the right value and that the change of elasticity has the proper amplitude and direction. This alone is

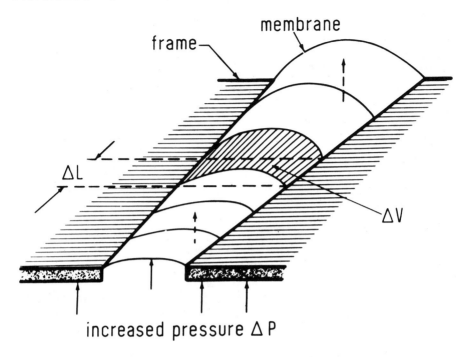

FIGURE 8. Diagram describing the volume displacement ΔV per membrane length ΔL upon action of a unilateral increase in pressure ΔP. (According to von Békésy [103].)

important. Figure 12 shows several changes of the model that had no effect on the travelling wave.*

By suspending aluminum-dust particles the movement of the perilymph can be studied in a model (Fig. 13). Near the stapes only longitudinal movements can be seen. With further advancement of the wave, however, depending on the extensability of the membrane, additional transverse movements occur as the pressure of the longitudinal wave proceeds. Thus, due to differences in the amplitude of movement and by virtue of the phase difference between the two directions of movement, elliptical and circular movements occur.

The transverse component can be observed only up to a certain depth of the channel but not near the wall opposite to the membrane. Therefore, the transverse waves are surface waves (see page 1).

Surface waves can be grouped into gravity waves and capillary waves according to the nature of the counteracting forces. Capillary waves are

---

* The high stability of the pattern of oscillations that is maintained even after changing the input impedance may account for the fact that frequency discrimination remains unchanged during the middle-ear infection when the tympanic cavity is filled with fluid.

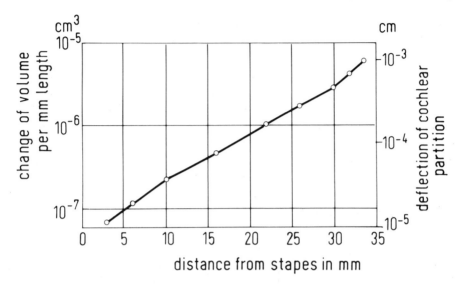

FIGURE 9. Change of volume per mm length of the cochlear canal and maximal deflection of the cochlear partition upon action of a unilateral increase in pressure of 1000 dyn/cm². (According to von Békésy [93].)

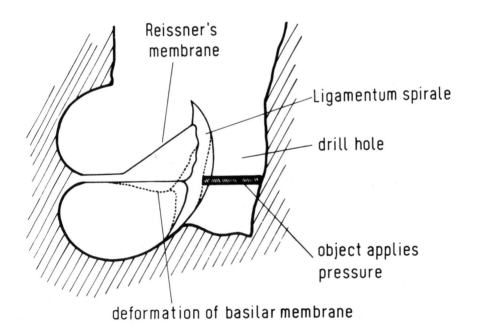

FIGURE 10. Loosening and compression of the basilar membrane. (According to von Békésy [103].)

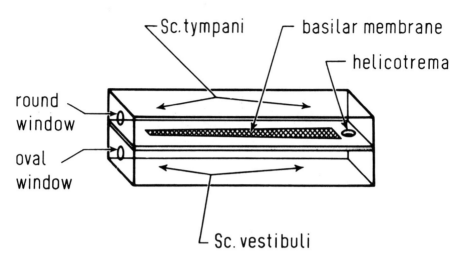

FIGURE 11. Model of the inner ear as used by Tonndorf. It corresponds very precisely with the original model of von Békésy. The walls are transparent. A mixture of glycerin and water of suitable viscosity is used as perilymph. (According to Tonndorf [1153].)

caused by virtue of surface tension at the border areas between liquid and gaseous media whereas gravity waves are caused by gravity. Gravity waves are the conspicuous large-scale water waves of common language use. Capillary waves are, for example, the ripples on a pond. Within the inner ear only capillary waves can be encountered for reasons of structural properties since the counteracting force is given by the membrane. Tonndorf[1146] proved the capillary character of the travelling wave by comparing group- and wave velocity. He concluded that the travelling wave is independent of gravity and consequently independent of the orientation of the ear in space.

Thus, the elasticity as well as the gradient of the membrane's elasticity are crucial factors for the pattern of the oscillation.* The velocity of propagation of the travelling wave is given by the elasticity. The velocity (c) changes as a function of elasticity (better: modulus of elasticity and compliance); it decreases with increasing distance from the stapes. Thus, the wavelength (λ) also decreases since the frequency (f) stays constant and the velocity is given by the equation:

$$c = f \cdot \lambda$$

---

* Von Békésy (85) demonstrated how the different patterns of oscillation could be obtained for the various hypotheses mentioned on page 7 only by varying the membrane elasticity of his model. Ranke (924, 925) came up with the same result mathematically by changing damping and the effective mass relations.

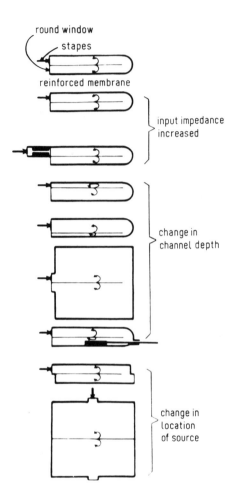

FIGURE 12. Study of the location of maximal membrane deflection for the same stimulus frequency following changes of the shape of the canal but not of the membrane properties. The location of maximal membrane deflection is marked by two circular arrows indicating that turbulences occuring at high stimulus intensities were used as criterion. Widening of the depth of one or of both canals from 1 to 30 mm, lengthening of one canal and change of the elasticity of the oval window are of no effect on the location of the turbulences. Only upon shortening the depth of the canal to about 0.3 mm, the shape of the turbulence changes and its location shifts towards the stapes. Of particular interest is the fact that the change in location of the stapes and of the round window (i.e. the change in location of the stimulus source) does not seem to affect the oscillation. (According to von Békésy [74].)

In contrast, the amplitude becomes larger since the compliance of the membrane increases with increasing distance from the stapes according to the change of elasticity.* This is counteracted by a decrease in amplitude caused by frictional losses. At first, however, the increase in amplitude dominates. Now, with respect to capillary waves, another effect comes into play to which Ranke[†] focussed his attention repeatedly. As long as the depth of the channel from the membrane to the opposite wall stays small in relation to the wavelength, the velocity of the wave is independent of frequency — it is of constant magnitude for all frequencies. As soon as the wavelength arrives at a value close to the product of 2π x depth of channel, the velocity of the wave becomes frequency-dependent and is smaller for higher than for lower frequencies (abnormal dispersion). This causes an additional decrease in velocity and consequently a shortening of wavelength for a narrow frequency range. If a constant velocity (c) of propagation is assumed for all frequencies (f), the wavelength is smallest for the high frequencies and increases with decreasing frequency since:

$$\lambda = \frac{c}{f}$$

Since, by virtue of elasticity changes of the membrane, a steady decrease of velocity takes place for all frequencies, the wavelengths of the highest frequencies are the first to approach the product 2π x channel depth. The wavelength of progressively deeper frequencies follow and, thus, the deepest arrive at the helicotrema. A shorter wavelength is equivalent to a larger number of oscillations per unit of length. This fact together with the large amplitudes cause high losses due to friction and, finally, a fading away of a wave having the proper frequency. Low-frequency components with longer wavelengths, however, are able to advance further. This led to the idea of regarding the mechanical function of the inner ear as that of a number of low-pass filters connected in series. Basically, electronic models are conceived in this way. Thus, the term filter is a common expression in modern language that is applicable to the mechanics of the inner ear. According to Kohllöffel[669] and Johnstone[1234] the minimal wavelength ranges between 0.75 and 2mm.

The oscillations of the basilar membrane have been studied with techniques other than modelling. Von Békésy[74] made the first direct

---

* It should be pointed out here that for the description of the mechanism of the inner ear the frequently false-mentioned notion of the "incompressibility" of the inner ear fluid should not be used. Moreover, it is justified to presume compressibility in order to understand the propagation of sound as longitudinal waves (e.g. at the stapes). This applies also to water. For propagation of waves, elasticity of the medium, i.e. compressibility, is necessary.

† References 924, 925, 927.

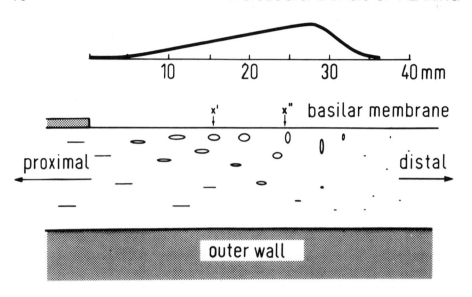

FIGURE 13. Movement of particles (aluminum dust) in the fluid of the scala vestibuli of the model upon stimulation with a 50 Hz pure-tone. For the sake of clarity, the amplitude of the movements is exaggerated. Above, the corresponding envelope of the membrane movement is shown. (According to Tonndorf [1144].)

observations with a light microscope under stroboscopic illumination. In order to obtain visible deflections (resolving power of the light microscope!) he had to apply stimuli of atypical magnitude. At 140 dB SPL he obtained amplitudes on the order of 1 μm. By extrapolation he estimated the absolute hearing threshold to be equivalent to a deflection of the basilar membrane of approximately 10^{-13} m = 0.001 Å (for comparison: the wavelength range of the visible light extends between 4000 and 7500 Å and the diameter of atoms ranges between 1 and 5 Å; thus, the deflection of the basilar membrane at hearing threshold would be smaller than 1% of the diameter of an atom).

By applying recent technical developments, measurements could be made using stimuli having intensities more representative of natural sounds. By use of the Mössbauer-effect, for example, the movements of the basilar membrane have been measured within an intensity range of 65 to 115 dB SPL.* With the aid of laser light and the criterion of "fuzziness," Kohllöffel[668-671] studied the oscillations of the basilar membrane for stimulus intensities between 90 and 130 dB. By use of capacitive probes, Wilson[1232, 1233] and Wilson and Johnstone[1234] were able to measure down to 40 dB at 100 dB SPL. The laser method introduced by Kohllöffel is the only

---

* References 522–524, 526, 948–953.

one, like the von Békésy-method, to make visible the spatial distribution of the amplitudes of deflection.

These recent measurements lead to substantially improved results. In addition, some data were gathered from living animals, eliminating potential postmortem changes that might affect the data. In general, these recent results agree with those of von Békésy's experiments in so far as the deflection amplitude extrapolated to hearing threshold amounts to approximately 10^{-3} Å.* More importantly, however, these recent data confirm that the mechanical tuning curve is much wider than the tuning curve of a single auditory nerve fiber (Fig. 14). A mechanical tuning curve demonstrates how much the stimulus intensity has to be changed as a function of frequency in order to produce a constant amplitude of deflection at a specific site on the basilar membrane. The tuning curve of an auditory-nerve fiber describes the threshold intensity as a function of frequency. If this threshold is passed, nervous excitation is triggered. In analogy to the mechanical tuning curve it can be stated: the neuronal tuning curve demonstrates how much the stimulus intensity has to be changed as a function of frequency in order to trigger the same event in a certain nerve fiber.

For each fiber a distinct frequency exists, for which the tuning curve has an absolute minimum. This frequency is called the best or characteristic frequency. Thus, stimulus intensities above this curve trigger action potentials in that particular fiber while intensities underneath the curve do not elicit any activity. Therefore, the area above the tuning curve is called the response area of the fiber. The neuronal and mechanical tuning curves shown in Figure 14 are chosen such that their respective characteristic frequencies are of equal value.

As can be seen, a striking discrepancy exists between the broad mechanical tuning curves and the corresponding sharply-tuned curves of the auditory-nerve fibers. The two neuronal curves having the higher optimal frequencies can be conceived of as being composed of two parts: a wide tuning curve with ascending slopes comparable to those of the corresponding mechanical tuning curves regarding steepness and intensity range, and an additional section noticed by a break in the slope on the low-frequency side, thereby increasing the steepness of the slope. Thus, the threshold is lowered by 40 to 60 dB for the neural tuning curve and the sharpness of neuronal tuning is increased.

The steepness of the slope on the low-frequency side of the neuronal tuning curves ranges between 5 and 25 dB/octave in the flat part and attains values of 100 to 600 dB/octave in the steep part. On the high-frequency side the gradient is smallest near the characteristic frequency and, with

---

* In Rhode's (950) opinion, the threshold is estimated too low because of non-linearities which he observed. He assumed the threshold for 7 kHz to be at 10^{-1} Å or even at 1 Å.

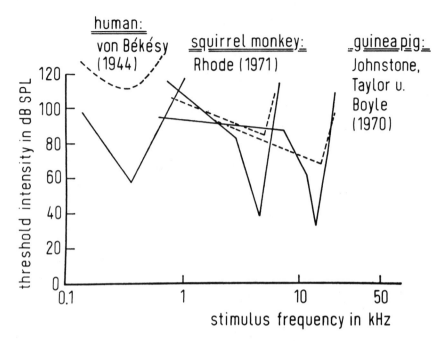

FIGURE 14. Comparison between mechanical tuning curves of the basilar membrane (dashed curves) and the corresponding tuning curves of single auditory-nerve fibers (smooth curve). The curves are shown in relation to the intensity range actually measured. (According to Kiang [631] and Evans [303], from Kay [551].)

increasing stimulus intensity, reaches values of 200 to 500 dB/octave[1236] or even 1000 dB/octave.[308, 309] A summary of those data is given by Møller[780] and Keidel and Kallert.[616]

According to the most recent measurements mentioned above, the slope of the mechanical tuning curves for characteristic frequencies above 3 kHz ranges between 7 and 12 dB/octave on the low-frequency side and between 100 and 130 dB/octave* on the high-frequency side. Moreover, there is a dependence on characteristic frequency such that at higher characteristic frequencies steeper slopes can be observed. In addition, Kohllöffel,[670] studying postmortem changes in the guinea pig during the first three days, observed a decrease of slope from 8 dB to 4.5 dB/octave and from 90 dB to 46 dB/octave, on the low-frequency and high-frequency sides, respectively.

By the use of the Mössbauer method and capacitive probes, a plateau could be observed on the high-frequency side about 30 to 40 dB above the minimum of the tuning curve. A corresponding behavior could not be found with the neuronal tuning curves.

---

* Up to 300 dB/octave at the most (Reference 952).

D. Electrical Potentials of the Inner Ear

Several clearly different electrical potentials can be recorded from the inner ear (Table 1). The endolymphatic potential (= endocochlear potential = EP) can be recorded without any stimulus acting upon the ear. It was described first by von Békésy[77-79] who, by slowly advancing a microelectrode, found the potential distribution shown in Table 1. This potential has been studied further by Tasaki et al.[1135] The endolymphatic space (Fig. 15) has a positive potential* (80 to 150 mV close to the round window, 50 to 80 mV in the higher turns) and is limited by Reissner's membrane, the stria vascularis and the lamina reticularis. The basilar membrane and the organ of Corti lie beyond the endolymphatic space.

The intracellular potential of the hair cells is -60 to -80 mV. Thus, at the apical surface of the hair cells a potential difference of approximately 140 mV exists.

According to the measurements of Lawrence,[702-704] Lawrence and Nuttall,[705] and Lawrence et al.[706] the potential of the tectorial membrane, of the subtectorial space, and of the sulcus spiralis internus is equal to the potential of the perilymph or somewhat more negative. Thus, the tectorial membrane represents the border of the endolymphatic space, not the lamina reticularis (Fig. 15 b). This is conceivable if the tectorial membrane, as described by Ross,[986] inserts at the lamina reticularis or, as observed by Hilding,[483] at Hensen's cells and at the inner border cells. No data are available on the chemical composition of the fluid of the inner tunnel, of Nuel's space and of the subtectorial space. Therefore, it should not be referred to as endolymph or perilymph but, for instance, as cortilymph[291] and subtectorial lymph.[941]. Other results, however, indicate that a connection exists between the subtectorial space and the endolymphatic space.[1129]

The borders of this space could be confirmed by the system's behavior against potassium ions. Whereas the perilymph contains much sodium (130 to 150 mval/1) and little potassium (4 to 5 mval/1), comparable to other extracelluar fluids, Smith et al.[1045] were the first to show that in the guinea pig† the endolymph contained a surprisingly high amount of potassium (140 to 160 mval/1) and only little sodium (12 to 16 mval/1). If potassium is injected into the scala tympani the cochlear microphonics as well as the

---

* References 107, 777, 882.

† Similar values have been found in the cat by Citron et al. (191) and in the human by Rauch and Köstlin (942). The total calcium concentration in the endolymph is $3 \cdot 10^{-5}$ mol/1, the total magnesium concentration is $1 \cdot 10^{-5}$ mol/1 (Reference 130).

Table 1.
Bio-potentials of the inner ear

Name	Recording	
Endocochlear potential (d.c. potential)	Microelectrode in the endolymph or within the cells of the organ of Corti. Reference electrode in the neck of the animal or in the perilymph. Order of magnitude 100 mV	Schematic results obtained from the cochlea of a guinea pig (according to von Békésy, [77]).
Cochlear microphonics (CM)	Recording as for the endocochlear potentials or with a macroelectrode from the cochlea. Order of magnitude 1mV	CM obtained from the 1st and 3rd turn of the cochlea of a guinea pig. The stimulus intensity is adjusted such that the amplitudes of the 1st turn are of equal magnitude (according to Davis, [228]).
Summating potential (SP)	Recording as for the cochlear microphonics Order of magnitude 1mV–10mV	Recorded from the round window of a guinea pig. Downward deflection = SP superimposed by CM and AP (recording by Pestalozza and Davis [884]).
Action potentials (AP)	Summed action potentials of the cochlear nerve as in the peripheral nerve. Recording with macroelectrodes from the base of the cochlear. Recording of single potentials of single fibers of the cochlear nerve with microelectrodes.	summed action pot. single actions pot.

(From Keidel [601]).

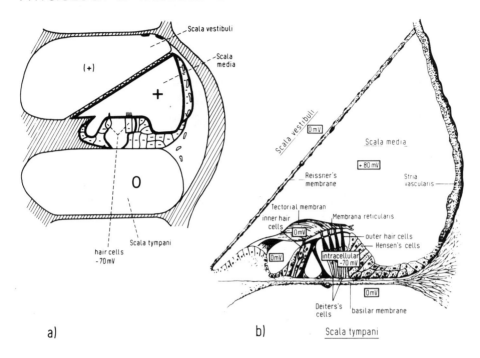

FIGURE 15. Borders of the endolymphatic space. (A, according to Tasaki et al. [1135] [tectorial membrane not shown]. B, according to Lawrence et al. [706].)

action potential[1132] disappear very rapidly. Thus, the basilar membrane is permeable for the potassium ions. The borders of the endolymphatic space, however, are not. The endolymphatic potential is hardly impaired by potassium injected into the scala tympani.[1145] Thus, it does not depend as much on the potassium concentration on either side of the limiting membrane but it is very sensitive to hypoxia.*

Bosher and Warren[128] and Mendelsohn and Konishi[756] found that during hypoxia the endocochlear potential changes much faster than the composition of ions. Bosher and Warren[129] also observed that the build-up of the normal gradient of ion concentration in the inner ear of newborn rats precedes the development of the endochochlear potential by days.

Tasaki and Spyropoulos[1133] proved that the endolymphatic potential is not generated by the hair cells since in the Waltzing-guinea pig (a guinea pig breed with degenerated outer hair cells) it is of normal magnitude. Finally they showed that in the normal guinea pig a positive potential remained in the area of the stria vascularis after removal of the endolymph (Fig. 16). From these findings and from results with other techniques, as with radioisotopes,[687] it can be concluded that K^+ must be transported actively

---

* References 249, 838, 1022.

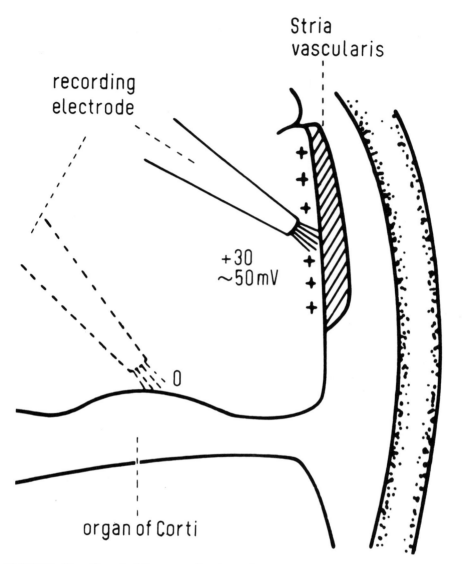

FIGURE 16. Proof of the contribution of the stria vascularis to the positive endolymphatic potential. (According to Tasaki and Spyropoulos [1133].)

into the scala media and that the stria vascularis contributes substantially to the build-up of the endolymphatic potential. Also, the experiments of Smith et al.[1046] and Gannon et al.[389] support this view since according to them the endolymphatic space of the vestibular system, that has no stria vascularis, does not have a positive endolymphatic potential (Fig. 17). From the different effects of anoxia and disturbed electrolyte concentration on the EP[682–686] Kuijpers and Bonting[697, 698] concluded that the EP is made out of two components, namely a positive one generated by a Ouabain-sensitive

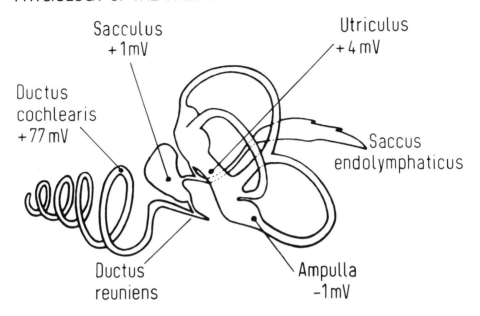

Sacculus
+1mV

Utriculus
+4mV

Ductus
cochlearis
+77mV

Saccus
endolymphaticus

Ductus
reuniens

Ampulla
-1mV

FIGURE 17. As a consequence of the action of the stria vascularis the endolymphatic potential of the cochlea has a positivity of +77 mV with reference to the perilymph. The magnitude of the endolymphatic potential of the vestibule however, does not deviate significantly from zero. Accordingly, an anatomical substratum comparable to the stria is lacking there. (According to Davis [228].)

electrically operated K-pump (stria vascularis) and a negative one, the K-diffusion potential.

The cochlear microphonics can be recorded from various places of the inner ear and also from close surrounding areas (e.g. the round window). With some qualifications, the cochlear microphonic can be used to describe the temporal course of the deflections of the basilar membrane. This potential was described first by Wever and Bray.[1209] Confirming their results, Adrian[9] showed that the cochlear microphonics are not identical with the action potential. Saul and Davis[1008] were able to separate the action potential of the nerve from the cochlear microphonics. They assumed the source of the cochlear microphonics to be in the cochlea. The cochlear microphonics are particularly large when recorded from the round window. Recording from the inside of the cochlea, however, naturally affords better insight into cochlear physiology.

Tasaki et al.[1134] recorded cochlear microphonics from the scala tympani of the different turns of the cochlea in the guinea pig. They were the first to demonstrate that the amplitude of the cochlear microphonics depended on the recording site since it could be related to the deflection of the basilar membrane (Fig. 18).

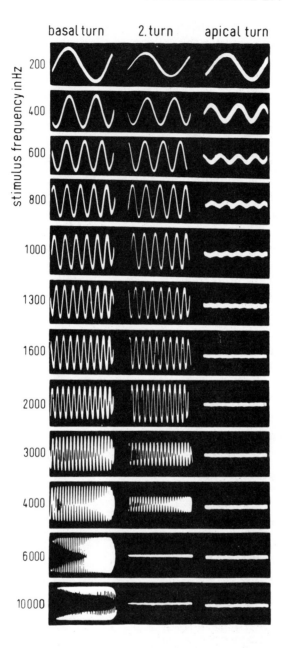

FIGURE 18. Oscillograms recorded simultaneously from the 1st, 2nd and 4th turns of the cochlea in the guinea pig. The amplification was adjusted such that at the lowest stimulus frequency the amplitude of the cochlear microphonics was of equal magnitude for the three locations of recording. The stimulus intensity was adjusted such that at all frequencies the amplitude of the cochlear microphonic was of equal magnitude in the basal turn. (According to Tasaki et al. [1134].)

Recall that for the mechanical travelling wave a frequency-dependent phase shift was noticed between the movement of the basilar membrane at a certain place and the movement of the stapes. A similar phase lag has also been observed for the cochlear microphonic (Fig. 19).

Ample data have been collected by Honrubia and Ward,[495] by Weiss et al.[1192] and Sohmer et al.[1057] Figure 20 shows the distribution of the amplitude of the cochlear microphonics along the cochlear partition for different stimulus frequencies and intensities.

Figure 21 shows tuning curves of the cochlear microphonics. They demonstrate (in manners analogous to the mechanical tuning curves, see page 18) how the stimulus intensity has to be changed for differing stimulus frequencies in order to obtain a constant amplitude at a certain place within the cochlea.

There is no intensity threshold for the cochlear microphonics.[569] The dynamic range of the intensity function (= amplitude as function of stimulus intensity at constant stimulus frequency) is linear over a wide range before running through a maximum (Fig. 22). The deviation from linearity has not yet been explained adequately. A limiting mechanism is unlikely to be active especially since the cochlear microphonics do not change their shape even at high intensities (sinusoid stays sinusoid, see Fig. 22). Whitfield and Ross[1219] assume a superimposition of out-of-phase potentials generated by sources distant from the recording site. Ranke et al.[932] regarded the cochlear microphonics recorded from a specific site as an integral vector of the activity of the whole cochlea. This would account for the small amplitude of the cochlear microphonics in humans recorded from the round window. Karlan et al.[543] suppose that the cochlear microphonics are composed of activities contributed by the inner and outer hair cells. From their assumption of a phase shift between the components coming from the inner and outer hair cells and of a different slope of the respective intensity functions they reason that the relative contribution of both changes as a function of intensity. After elimination of the outer hair cell activity with Kanamycin, Dallos[214] in fact described a remaining component with a phase shift of $\pi/2$.

For a long time the hair cells have been regarded as being the source of the cochlear microphonics. Damage to the hair cells by streptomycin[251] or noise, for example, changes the cochlear microphonics and they are missing completely in animals with a congenital absence of hair cells.[225] If a microelectrode is advanced from the scala tympani through the basilar membrane and the organ of Corti into the scala media, the cochlear microphonics stay unchanged until the tip of the electrode is pushed through the lamina recticularis. There an abrupt phase shift of 180° takes place.[225, 1135] This is shown schematically in Figure 23. Thus, in general, the lamina reticularis is regarded as being the locus for the generation of the cochlear microphonics even though Fex[335] points out that after critical examination this is by no means conclusive.

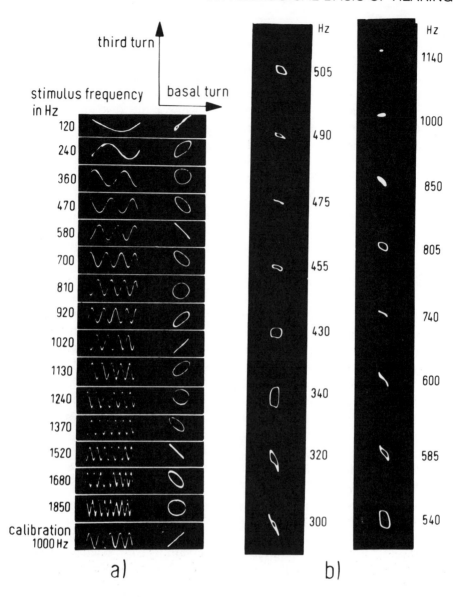

FIGURE 19. A, Left: Cochlear microphonics for different stimulus frequencies recorded from the first cochlear turn (guinea pig). Right: Lissajous figures that are obtained when the horizontal and the vertical deflection of the oscilloscope beam are driven by synchronous recordings from the 1st and 3rd turn. (According to Tasaki et al. [1134].) B, Lissajous figures of the cochlear microphonics recorded for stimulus frequencies at 300 to 1140 Hz. With increasing frequency, several transitions of phase are noticed. (According to Ranke et al. [932].)

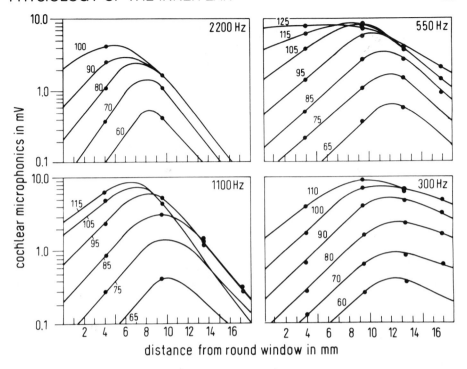

distance from round window in mm

FIGURE 20. Distribution of the amplitude of the cochlear microphonics along the cochlea of the guinea pig. The recording was done from the scala media. The parameter is the stimulus intensity in dB SPL. (According to Honrubia and Ward [496].)

When cochlear microphonics are recorded from one of the scalae the potential at the recording site receives its input from a large source area (Fig. 24). Consequently, the cochlear microphonics recorded with one electrode represent the sum of the activity of all hair cells.

The contribution of each hair cell, however, is weighted differently according to its position relative to the electrode. With the use of a multi-electrode array (12 stainless steel electrodes, diameter 50 μm, distance between electrodes 150 to 180 μm) Kohllöffel[667] was able to subject these recording conditions of the cochlear microphonic to a closer examination in the guinea pig. He showed that, upon computation of the components contributed by the different source locations, frequency response curves resulted in a slope of 9.3 dB/octave on the low frequency side and a slope of 109 dB/octave on the high frequency side (Fig. 25). Thus, his results are in very good agreement with the most recent measurements of the deflection of the basilar membrane (see pages 16–18).

It is generally believed that the cochlear microphonics arise from bending the cilia of the hair cells. This has been concluded from studies of the behavior of sensory cells closely resembling in structure the hair cells of

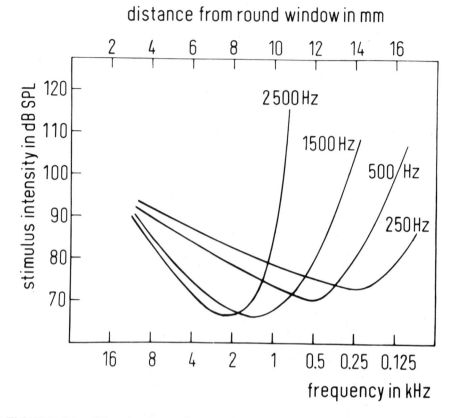

FIGURE 21. Stimulus intensity in dB SPL required to produce a constant amplitude of the cochlear microphonics (0.56 mV) as a function of the stimulus frequency for four different recording locations within the scala media (tuning curves of the cochlear microphonics). (According to Honrubia and Ward [495].)

the cochlea such as the cells of the vestibular system and of the lateral-line system in fish and amphibians.

With the use of stroboscopic techniques or direct coupling of the stimulus to the cupula the relation between the mechanical movement of the cupula and the electrical response of the cell could be observed in the lateral-line organ.* The change of the electrical potential was generally found to be directly proportional to the deflection of the cupula. Alkon and Bak,[28] on the other hand, found a logarithmic relation between the amplitude of deflection and the magnitude of the receptor potential of hair cells analogous to the cochlear microphonic in the statocysts of molluscs. They also found, however, a linear relation between the amplitude of the receptor potential and the temporal density of action potentials in the afferent nerve fiber.

* References 354, 362, 449, 451, 520, 699.

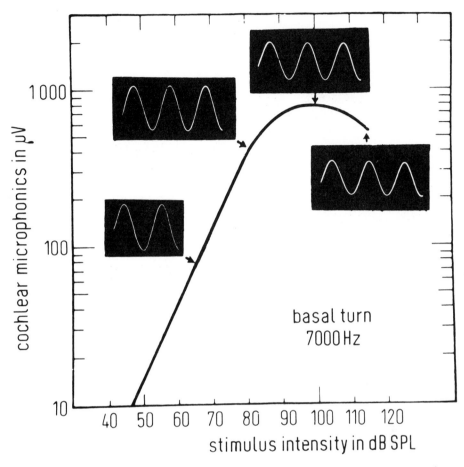

FIGURE 22. Intensity function of cochlear microphonics recorded from the first cochlear turn in the guinea pig. (According to Davis and Eldredge [243].)

Von Békésy[79] conducted an experiment in which he mechanically deflected the basilar membrane with a fine needle. Thereby he was able to compare the mechanical energy of the needle with the released electrical energy (that results from the cochlear microphonic and the electrical current thus generated). If the cochlear microphonic arose in a way similar to the piezoelectric effect, simply by moving charges, then the electrical energy could not be larger than the mechanical energy of the stimulus. After a single deflection of the membrane no further mechanical energy will be conveyed. Yet, von Békésy observed that the potential change caused by a single deflection of the membrane stays constant as long as the deflection continues. Therefore, the electrical energy is not limited by the mechanical energy of the stimulus. This means that the mechanical movement modulates the energy flow of a different source but does not provide the energy itself.

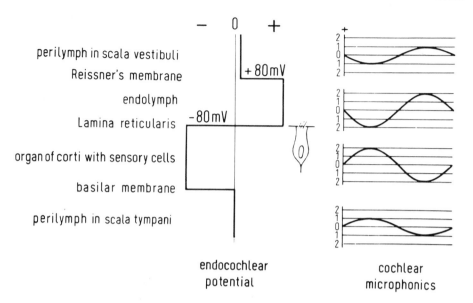

FIGURE 23. Potential shift of the endocochlear potential and phase shift of the cochlear microphonics at the lamina reticularis. (According to Keidel, W.D. Physiologie des Hörens. Klinische Wochenschrift 37, 1205-1217 [1959].)

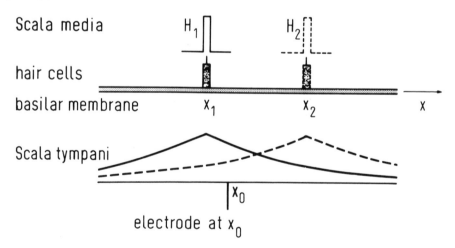

FIGURE 24. Schematic description of the potential composed of components originating from different sources at different distances from the recording electrode. X_1 and X_2 are two hair cells generating the potentials H_1 and H_2, respectively. The smooth and the dashed curves represent the respective decrease of the potential as a function of distance from the source. With a recording electrode at X_0 the sum of the potential components is recorded. For periodic potential changes the phase difference between H_1 and H_2 has to be taken into consideration. (According to Kohllöffel [667].)

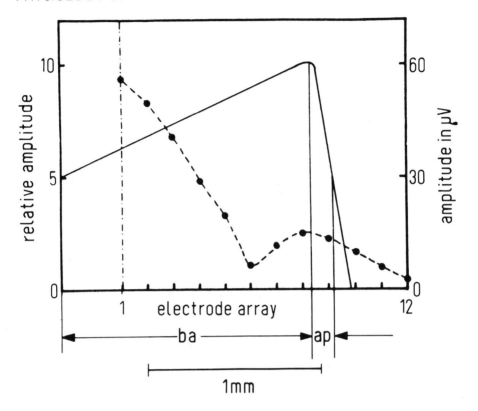

FIGURE 25. Smooth curve = function H$_{(x)}$ upon action of a 13.5 kHz tone computed from the measurements of the cochlear microphonics (dashed curve). H$_{(x)}$ is the source strength as a function of space on the basilar membrane. The solid circles connected by the dashed line represent the actual cochlear microphonic amplitudes recorded with the twelve-element multi-electrode array. (According to Kohllöffel [667].)

In these experiments von Békésy[79] further proved that the deflection itself acts as stimulus, not the velocity of the deflection.* The movement of the needle and therefore of the deflection also had the shape of a trapezoid (Fig. 26a). If the cochlear microphonics are determined by the deflection, they should resemble the trapezoid (Fig. 26b). If they are determined by the velocity of the deflection, however, they should correspond to the first derivative of the trapezoid (Fig. 26c). A combined dependency on deflection and velocity would result in the sum of both (Fig. 26d). In fact, the trapezoid was observed (Fig. 26e).

Although the hair cells of the vestibular system and of the lateral-line organ resemble that of the cochlea in many respects they have, in addition to

---

* In the meantime Sellick and Russell (1029) and Nuttall et al. (862) could find inner hair cell responses to both the displacement and to the velocity of the basilar membrane motion (see also page 69).

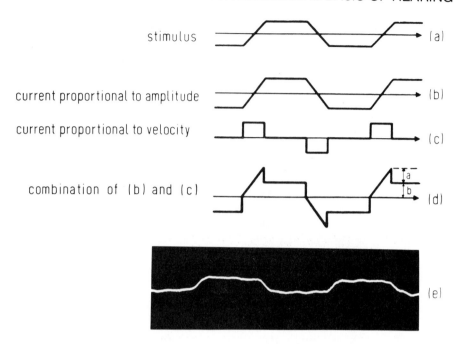

FIGURE 26. A, Shape of stimulus. B to D, Corresponding conceivable cochlear microphonics. E, Actually recorded cochlear microphonics. (According to von Békésy [78].)

a larger number of stereocilia, one hair of a special structure, the kinocilium. In general, it holds true that the deflection of the hair towards the kinocilium has an excitatory effect whereas a deflection in the opposite direction has an inhibitory effect, that is to say that the receptor potential undergoes a change towards depolarization and hyperpolarization, respectively.* Thus, a directional selectivity exists for the positive and negative extent of the cell potential. Deflections in other directions have an effect determined by the extent their components point in the preferred direction; thus deflections vertical to the preferred direction have no effect on the potential.

The hair cells of the adult mammalian cochlea are lacking the kinocilia,[295, 361] they disappear during maturation of the organ of Corti.[644, 722] Only the basal body of the kinocilium is preserved. According to Engström et al.[295] this structure is supposed to determine the directional selectivity of excitation.† The hairs of the cochlear hair cells show a quite regular arrangement (Fig. 27). The hairs or cilia of the outer hair cells are arranged in a W-shape (about 150 hairs per cell) while those of the inner hair cells form straight lines (about 50 hairs per cell) parallel to the longitudinal

---

* References 356, 358, 734, 1164, 1165, 1203.
† In the cat, Spoendlin (1063) was unable to find even the basal bodies.

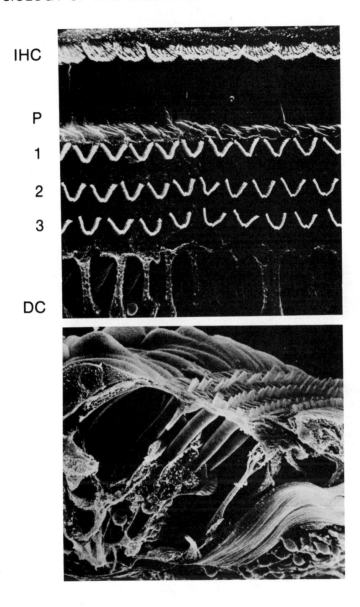

IHC

P

1

2

3

DC

FIGURE 27. (Above) Scanning micrograph of the surface of the organ of Corti in the cat. The inner hair cells (IHC), the heads of the pillar cells (P) and three rows of outer hair cells (1, 2, 3) are shown. The processus phalangeales of the third row of Deiter's cells (DC) can also be seen since Hensen's cells were removed. (According to Bredberg et al.[142].) (Below) Scanning micrograph of a cross section of the organ of Corti. The surface is formed by the lamina reticularis to which the ends of the outer hair cells carrying the hairs are attached. The cell bodies of the outer hair cells rest on Deiter's supporting cells. To the left of the outer hair cells, the outer tunnel is shown; to the right, Nuel's space. (According to Bredberg [139].)

direction of the basilar membrane.[476] The basal body is located on the side of the cell opposite the modiolus, on the outer side of the cell.

By stimulating the tectorial membrane with a fine vibrating needle von Békésy[81] observed that close to the outer edge of the tectorial membrane radial vibration causes the largest cochlear microphonics. This is consistent with the directioned sensitivity of the hair cells described above.

The inner edge of the tectorial membrane close to the modiolus showed maximal excitability with longitudinal vibration, but the radial component was still effective to a lower degree with a polarization opposite to the outer edge. However, one has to take into account that the inner hair cells are not located underneath the inner edge of the tectorial membrane and that the tectorial membrane is attached to the modiolus but is only loosely attached to the outer edge. Thus, the mechanical stimulating conditions are different as discussed by von Békésy.

The relation between the different electrical potentials of the inner ear and the mechanism for their generation might be understood from their dependence on metabolic processes.[1022] Necker[838] for example, was able to demonstrate that anoxia (in the pigeon) lasting for a short time does not affect the positive component of the cochlear microphonics (CM^+), whereas the negative component (CM^-) disappears completely, but reversibly. This is in agreement with the idea that hyperpolarizing membrane processes consume energy whereas depolarizing processes, being diffusion processes, can take place for a limited amount of time without energy consumption. (For example, after poisoning the Na-K-pump of a nerve fiber many action potentials can be elicited as long as the difference in concentration of the ions in question between the intra- and extracellular space is large enough). In addition, it was found that the endocochlear potential (in the starling) and the action potential (in the kaiman) showed a behavior similar to the negative component of the cochlear microphonics. These results are in good agreement with those found in the mammalian cochlea.[697, 698]

The summating potential was described first by Davis et al.[248] It is defined as a d.c.-potential recorded from the cochlea that persists for the duration of the sound stimulus. In general, it is positive in the scala tympani, but negative in the scala media and the scala vestibuli. Under certain conditions (e.g., low stimulus intensity, anoxia, increased pressure in the scala tympani), however, it changes its polarity.[250] Thus, two separate components with different polarity were assumed.[251] Konishi and Yasuno[681] and Necker and Schwartzkopff[839] were able to show that the summating potential changes its polarity at the lamina reticularis as do the cochlear microphonics. The generation of the summating potentials could be explained by the assymmetry of the cochlear microphonics,[1219] but they do not show this asymmetry. In addition, the amplitude of the cochlear microphonics can be exceeded by the amplitude of the summating potential, such as at high frequencies and at high stimulus intensities.[1212] Thus, Butler,[162] and Johnstone and Johnstone[527] and Engebretson and Eldredge[288] tried to attribute the summating potential to asymmetric deflections of the basilar membrane.

Depending on the method of recording, Dallos[213-216] defined two components of the summating potential: (1) the potential difference between scala vestibuli and scala tympani was named DIF* SP; and (2) the sum of the potentials of the two scalae with reference to ground potential was named AVE† SP. For these components Dallos obtained a clear relation with the mechanical travelling wave (Fig. 28). The DIF-component reaches its maximum negativity in the range of resonance, but at the same location the AVE-component has its maximum positivity. The amplitude of the summating potentials depends on stimulus duration as well as on stimulus intensity (Fig. 29). For stimulus durations longer than 50 ms after-effects have been described.‡ If the potential is negative during the stimulus, a positive after-effect can be found the size of which is dependent on the stimulus duration. The amplitude of the summating potential as well as of the cochlear microphonics can be changed by a polarizing current flowing from the scala vestibuli to the scala tympani.[228]

The origin and significance of the summating potential are unknown. Davis[232] regards them as being a by-product of the asymmetries of those mechanisms leading to the cochlear microphonics. Honrubia and Ward,[496] however, consider the summating potentials to be a generator potential. The deflection of the basilar membrane proximal to the site of resonance is of higher amplitude towards the scala tympani, distal to the site of resonance it is of higher amplitude towards the scala vestibuli.[93, 1147] Likewise, the summating potential of the scala media (referenced to zero potential, e.g. the neck of the animal) is of positive polarity distal to the site of resonance, proximally it is negative.§ This corresponds with von Békésy's[77] experimental finding according to which an upward deflection of the basilar membrane (towards scala media) leads to a relative negativity of the scala media with respect to the scala tympani.

The action potential (Table 1, page 20) can be recorded from the base of the cochlea as a compound action potential or, with the aid of microelectrodes, as a single-fiber action potential from single fibers of the auditory nerve. The action potential is the actual excitatory output to the inner ear. The single-fiber action potentials are dealt with more extensively in the section on the cochlear nerve (page 79).

Action potentials of single fibers obey the all-or-nothing law, show a refractive period, and follow all other properties of action potentials encountered in other myelinated nerve fibers. Naturally, the shape of the compound action potential depends on the localization of the electrodes and on the method of recording. With the usual electrode arrangement (e.g.,

---

* DIF = Differential recording
† AVE = Averaged recording (arithmetic mean)
‡ References 879, 1108, 1213.
§ References 164, 496, 1135, 1136.

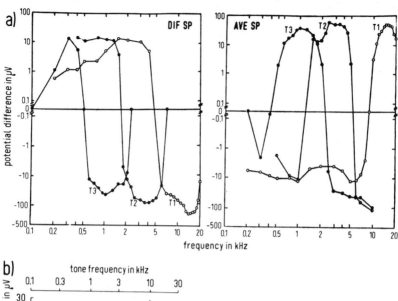

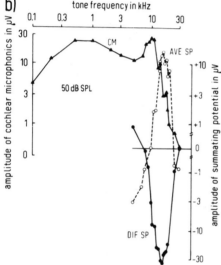

FIGURE 28. A, DIF SP and AVE SP recorded from three different turns of the cochlea as a function of the stimulus frequency for a constant deflection of the stapes of 1 nm. (According to Dallos [215].) B, Comparison between cochlear microphonics, DIF SP, and AVE SP recorded from the basal turn (guinea pig) at 50 dB SPL. (According to Dallos [214].)

round window with the neck muscles as reference) a multiphasic compound action potential can be recorded following stimulation with a click. The negative portions of the potential with respect to their temporal sequence are named N_1, N_2 and N_3. After the cochlear nerve has been inactivated in the internal meatus the compound action potential recorded from the cochlea (in the guinea pig) becomes monophasic and varies monotonically with intensity.[708] With pure tones of low frequency (up to 3 kHz

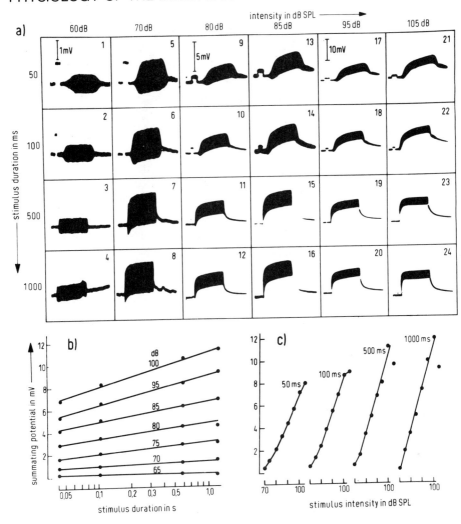

FIGURE 29. A, Summating potentials (with superimposed cochlear microphonics) of the first turn of the cochlea of the guinea pig for different intensities and stimulus duration of a 3.4 kHz tone burst. The recording was done with glass microelectrodes. B, and C, Relations obtained from A between magnitude of summating potential and stimulus intensity and stimulus duration respectively. (According to Honrubia and Ward [496].)

approximately) the periodicity of the stimulus is reflected also in the compound action potential. Using these low frequencies, the temporal relation between the cochlear microphonics and the action potential has been studied with intracochlear electrodes. According to Deatherage et al.[256] the action potential appears whenever the scala vestibuli become negative with respect to the scala tympani.

The compound action potential shows latencies that are measured as the difference between the beginning of the cochlear microphonics and the beginning of the compound action potential.* This latency is at least 0.6 to 1 ms and depends systematically on the stimulus intensity.[884]

The compound action potential also shows adaptation while the cochlear microphonic does not. Adaptation expresses itself as a decrease in amplitude of the compound action potential at constant stimulus intensity (Fig. 30). It has to be distinguished from fatigue. Whereas the intensity-difference threshold decreases during adaptation it increases during fatigue.[620] After termination of the stimulus, recovery from adaptation takes place within a few seconds.[259] Regarding fatigue, a longer recovery time is necessary, depending on the degree of fatigue. During adaptation, the cochlear microphonic remains unchanged. During fatigue, however, the amplitude of the cochlear microphonic decreases.† Adaptation is a certain kind of neuronal adjustment involving an improvement of performance (e.g. with respect to intensity-difference threshold) whereas fatigue implies a decrease in performance.‡

Ranke and Keidel made a significant contribution to the elucidation of the term adaptation. They demonstrated, first for the eye (Ranke's students Kern[629] and Commichau[200]) and later the vibratory sense§ and the ear,[620] how adaptation is equivalent to the adjustment of the sensitivity range of sensory organs in order to afford optimal intensity discrimination.

Ranke made a sharp distinction between the adaptation of sensory cells and central adaptation. He succeeded[557] in devising an adaptation theory that describes in a system of equations the time course of change in threshold intensity as well as the corresponding change in the difference threshold of a sensory cell. Ranke made three assumptions: (1) the excitation of a single sensory cell is primarily proportional to the velocity of a chemical reaction, but not to the concentration of an excitatory substance; (2) the velocity of reaction leading to the excitation determines the dynamic equilibrium between the velocities of dissimilation and assimilation (e.g. of a photosensible substance of the eye); and (3) dissimilation and assimilation of this substance takes place as at least a bimolecular, and probably as a polymolecular, reaction with a degree of polymerization (between 2 and 4 within the eye) comparable to that of hemoglobin.

The adaptation of sensory cells can be changed selectively by the effect of streptomycin that damages the hair cells.‖ The procedure of determining the time course of adaptation introduced by Keidel et al.[618] allows one to understand thoroughly the effect of streptomycin on the adaptation of sensory cells.

---

* There is no latency between the mechanical deflection of the basilar membrane and the onset of the cochlear microphonic.
† References 287, 400, 1031, 1210, 1211.
‡ References 555, 556, 560, 561, 584, 617, 620, 928, 931, 933.
§ References 552–554, 558, 560, 561, 618, 619.
‖ References 251, 462, 463, 465–470, 1169.

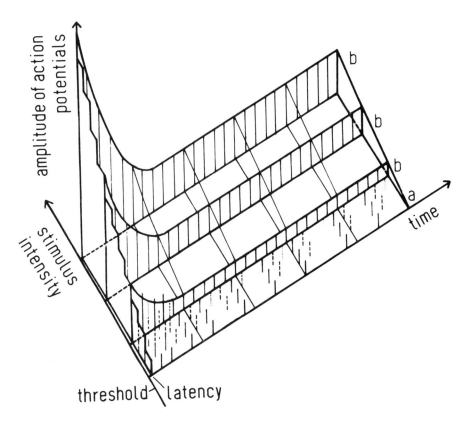

FIGURE 30. Scheme for the peripheral coding of sound. The lower most line shows the adaptation of a single element. By the addition of several elements the compound action potential is generated that, following the stimulus, adapts from the over-shoot to the steady-state value. The left front side shows that "dynamic" amplitude-intensity function while the right front side shows the "static" amplitude-intensity function. (According to Keidel et al. [620].)

If the compound action potential of the auditory nerve in the cat is recorded following presentation of a series of clicks of varying repetition rates, the first (nonadapted) as well as the last (adapted) potentials can easily be measured for different repetition frequencies as a function of stimulus intensity. Of course, peripheral adaptation increases with a higher repetition rate of clicks.

Figure 31 gives records of compound action potentials during peripheral adaptation. The hatched area shows the curves for the first response as being equal for all repetition frequencies. The curves for the steady-state portion of the responses are dependent on the repetition frequency.

If adaptation was purely electrical, being equivalent to the accommodation of the nerve, damaging the process of chemical transformation with streptomycin would change the threshold but not the time course of

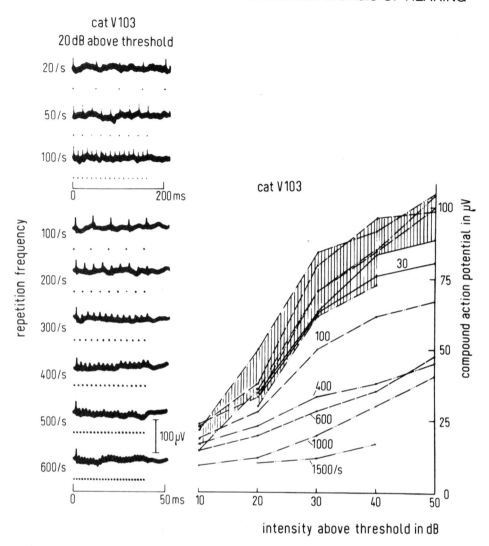

FIGURE 31. A, Time course of short-time adaptation upon stimulation with clicks as measured from the summed action potential in the cat. B, Evaluation of the dependency of the first stimulus response (dynamic curve; hatched area) and of the steady-state values on the stimulus intensity for different stimulus repetition frequencies; "adaptation fan." (According to Keidel [569].)

adaptation or the amount of adaptation. However, experiments in the cat showed that with antibiotic dosages increasing from 10 x 150 mg streptomycin per kg body weight to 10 x 200 mg and 10 x 250 mg the amount of adaptation in fact first decreases and, at the highest dosages (30 x 250 mg), increases again (Fig. 32). This holds true for the most important sound pressure levels of 50, 60 and 70 dB of the main speech area. The threshold values hardly show any change.

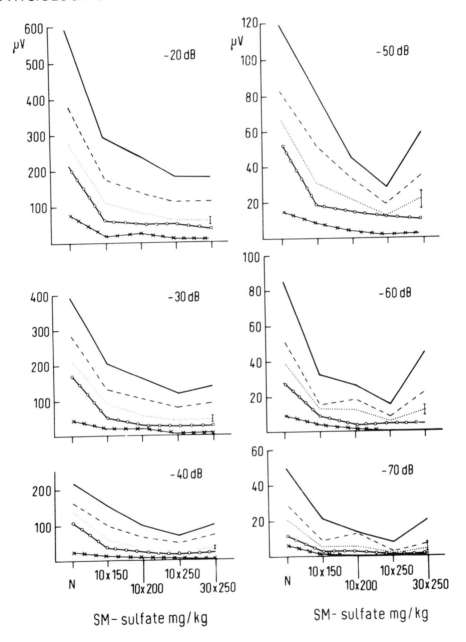

FIGURE 32. Dependency of the "adaptation fan" on different dosages of streptomycin sulfate as measured from the compound action potential in the cat. The parameter is the stimulus repetition rate. (———) rr 1/s; (— — —) rr 50/s; (....) rr 200/s; (⊖——⊖) rr 1000/s; (×××××) rr 2000/s. 0 dB = 110 dB SPL (According to Stange et al. [1096].)

These results could be interpreted as follows. First, the formation of the excitatory substance is strongly damaged, with the assimilation process still preserved. Then the amount of adaptation decreases mainly by a decrease in steepness of the curve for the first response. This applies to the dosage of 10 x 150 mg. At even higher doses the assimilation will be impaired also, the final values of the steady-state portion of the response increase, and the amount of adaptation decreases further (10 x 200 mg). At 10 x 250 mg the further damage of the assimilation process prevails, the steepness of all curves decreases further, and the amount of adaptation decreases even more. Finally, at very high doses the damage to the assimilation process proceeds with a simultaneous, apparently compensatory, recovery of formation of excitory substance; after that, the curve for the first response increases again. Consequently, the amount of adaptation expands again thereby revealing the complicated metabolism in the peripheral transformation organ. These results are in agreement with earlier measurements made by Davis et al.[251] who demonstrated a differential damage of current and action potential (among others) under streptomycin.

Adaptation has been studied also in single auditory nerve fibers.[1048, 1049]

E. Clinical Significance of the Electrical Potentials of the Inner Ear

Shortly after their first description by Wever and Bray,[1209] the cochlear microphonic (e.g. Fromm et al.[370]) and the compound action potential* were recorded in humans for diagnostic purposes. All recordings, however, could be done only during surgery.

In the last ten years techniques have been developed which allow electrocochleography to be carried out as a routine method of examination. The technique was developed independently at the same time in Japan and France.† The recording is done from the promontorium by means of needle electrodes pushed through the tympanic membrane or from the anulus tympanicus.[1254] Recordings (especially of the compound action potential) can be made without injury to the eardrum from the meatus acusticus externus,[285, 1007] the ear lobe,‡ or the tympanic membrane.§ Important

---

* References 126, 970, 989–992.
† References 46, 48–54, 908–911, 1249–1254.
‡ References 715, 1055, 1056, 1058.
§ References 194–196, 212.

technical improvements were introduced by Eggermont and Odenthal[280-283] and Odenthal and Eggermont.[863] A summarizing description of the principles and the clinical application of electrocochleography is given by Eggermont et al.[284] and Eggermont.[279] A review on the cochlear microphonic measured in humans can be found in Hoke.[491]

A procedure developed by Keidel[583, 596] deserves special notice for it allows one to record simultaneously, in the intact human, all electrical potentials recordable from the inner ear up to the auditory cortex. Different time bases were used so that the relative amplitudes of the different potentials can be compared with each other. These potentials are obtained with the electrodes located at the vertex and on both mastoids (Fig. 33).

F. Transformation of the Mechanical Stimulus into Nervous Excitation

Between the mechanical movement of the basilar membrane and the action potentials of the auditory fibers a mechanism is located transforming the stimulus into excitation.* Relatively little is known about this particularly interesting process whereas ample data are available on the preceding mechanics (page 7) as well as on the subsequent excitation pattern of the auditory nerve fibers (page 87).

The auditory receptor organ is composed of sensory cells and auxiliary structures as is the case with other sensory organs. In general, according to their architecture, sensory cells are divided into primary and secondary cells. Sensory cells are specialized nerve cells derived either from the neural canal or directly from the ektoblast. The primary sensory cells most clearly show the obligatory functional and structural tripartite composition of a neuron: a receptive area (dendrites), a conductive pathway (axon) and a presynaptic distribution area (arborization of the axon for secondary neurons—divergence principle). In this functional scheme protein synthesis is ascribed to the cell body (pericarion); it is responsible for the metabolic integrity of the neuron and its location within the sensory cell is immaterial.

The receptive area and the presynaptic distribution area represent the input and output terminals of the neuron, respectivley. The two areas are

---

* A stimulus indicates an environmental action impinging on excitable tissue. However, excitation denotes a particular change in the state of the excitable tissue that is in fact caused by the stimulus but is of an entirely different nature. Action potentials are recorded as an indication of excitation.

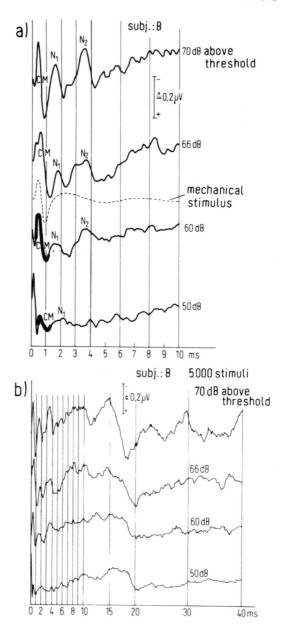

FIGURE 33. A, Averaged potential changes during the first 10 ms after stimulus onset for different stimulus intensities in dB referred to hearing threshold. CM = cochlear microphonics; N_1 and N_2 = first and second negative deflection of compound action potential. (According to Keidel [583].) B, as A, but with longer analysis time so that further potentials becomes visible especially at 30 ms following stimulus onset. (According to Keidel [583].)

always located on opposite sides of the cell. Thus, one speaks of polar arrangement as a common neuronal principle and frequently the terms receptor pole and effector pole are used. The function can be described schematically. The receptor area is in contact with the presynaptic distributive area of other neurons which, during excitation, release a chemical substance (transmitter) into the synaptic cleft (a gap, approximately 150 to 250 Å wide, between the subsynaptic membrane of a neuron and the subsynaptic membrane of the receptor area of the next neuron). This transmitter reacts with the subsynaptic membrane and eventually causes a change in the membrane polarization, named postsynaptic potential. This potential is proportional to the quantity of the transmitter substance. The receptive area of a neuron may have several thousand synapses adding either to an increase (hyperpolarization—inhibitory synapse) or to a decrease (depolarization—excitatory synapse) of the membrane polarization.* The numerous postsynaptic potentials spread electrotonically (i.e. without active membrane processes) within the cell and thereby superimpose to form a summed receptor potential. As soon as a membrane depolarization exceeds a fixed value (threshold value) at a certain location, (the initial segment), an action potential of constant form and amplitude will be triggered according to the all-or-nothing law.[276, 377] The receptor potential at the place where the action potentials are generated is called generator potential. The larger the receptor potential the more action potentials are triggered per unit of time. Thus, the magnitude of excitation is reflected by the number of action potentials per unit of time (i.e., the temporal density of the action potentials). The action potentials are conducted actively (by characteristic membrane processes) along the axon and thus arrive at the presynaptic area. Here, upon arrival of the action potentials a chemical transmitter is released through the cell membrane that diffuses† across the synaptic cleft to the postsynaptic membrane of the next neuron. Thus, generally the output of the neuron is of a secretory nature[433, 435] and acts on the input terminal of the next cell (neuron or effector, e.g. muscle or glandular cell). The presynaptic area is recognized anatomically from the numerous intracellular vessicles storing the transmitter. The secretory activity is controlled by the membrane potential and does not necessarily require true action potentials.[550] In this area action potentials of the axon can spread passively (electrotonically) so that an action potential is generated only in the proper axon upon passing the depolarization

---

* Excitatory transmitters cause an increase of permeability for the Na^+-ions in the subsynaptic membrane and thus have a depolarizing effect (References 202, 326, 1128). Inhibitory transmitters cause an increase of permeability for K^+- or Cl^--ions and thus have a hyperpolarizing effect (References 201, 325).

† In the presynaptic area the output activity can be modulated by synaptic inputs coming from other neurons (References 332, 1181).

threshold. Those areas of the membrane where this does not happen are called "electrically non-excitable." In this sense, the receptive area is "electrically non-excitable,"[433, 435] (i.e. no action potentials can be triggered here regardless of how the membrane potential is changed). Thereby it is rendered possible that the transformation into the receptor potential is approximately proportional to the stimulus[434] (Fig. 34). That is, the receptor potential is a graded response not an all-or-none response.

With regard to their general structure, the primary sensory cells are in exact agreement with the described model of a neuron. The primary difference is that the receptive area has the special ability to generate a receptor potential[376] under the action of special environmental stimuli (adequate stimulus). This receptor potential spreads electrotonically across the cell and, as a generator potential,* triggers action potentials on passing the threshold value of the axon.

Secondary sensory cells have no conductive part, they are lacking an axon; thus, no action potentials are generated. They only have the receptive and the presynaptic distributive area. Since, in general, they are synaptically contacted by several nerve fibers a divergence of excitation can occur. The sensory cells of the inner ear, as well as the sensory cells of the retina, of the vestibular system, and the taste cells, are secondary sensory cells. Upon stimulation they generate a receptor potential that, via the synapse, causes a generator potential in the innervating nerve fibers so that action potentials are triggered. Thus, the secondary sensory cells cause an excitation of the first sensory neuron. Figure 35 shows schematically the general neuronal principle of the tripartite function as well as examples of primary and secondary sensory cells.

Action potentials are triggered on the excitable membranes only when exceeding a certain value of depolarization.[490] Thus, the receptor potentials of primary sensory cells must always exert a depolarizing effect. However, the receptor potentials of secondary sensory cells can also be hyperpolarizing as was found for the retinal cones.† Regarding its amplitude, the receptor potential of secondary sensory cells does not have to meet certain threshold requirements necessary for triggering action potentials since only the secretion at the presynaptic pole of the sensory cell is determined by the receptor potential. Thus, even very small receptor potentials can lead to

---

* Frequently, the terms receptor potential and generator potential are used as synonyms. However, it is convenient to name as generator potential only the intracellular potential at the place where action potentials are triggered. In fact, in primary sensory cells receptor and generator potential can not be distinguished, but in secondary sensory cells they can be separated. Secondary sensory cells have a receptor potential but not a generator potential.

† References 64, 127, 522, 1140, 1141, 1161, 1162, 1201.

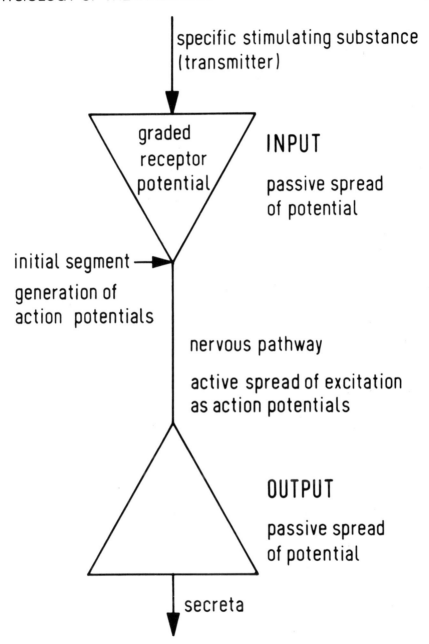

FIGURE 34. Functional scheme of neuron. The receptor potential persists as long as the stimulus is acting. Its amplitude reflects the stimulus intensity. All action potentials have the same shape and amplitude, their temporal sequence is proportional to the receptor potential. The rate of secretion corresponds with the temporal sequence of the arriving action potentials. (After Grundfest [433].)

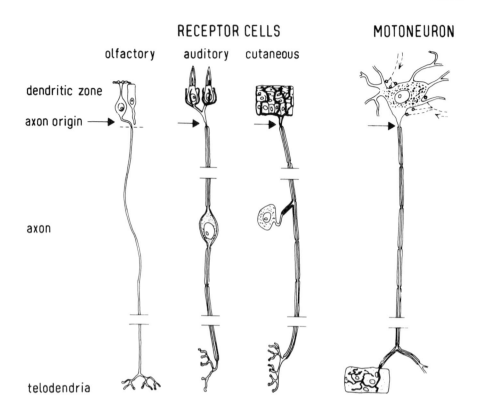

FIGURE 35. Different types of receptors and a motoneuron as an example of the functional division of a neuron into three parts. The arrow marks the place where the action potentials are generated. The cell body is not critical for the function. (According to Bodian [121].)

generator potentials of sufficient magnitude provided enough transmitter substance is released.

Only a few years ago, receptor potentials were recorded by use of microelectrodes from the inner hair cells of the mammalian inner ear. Prior to these recordings Mulroy et al.[832] and Weiss et al.[1193, 1194] recorded electrical potentials directly from the hair cells and the supporting cells of the inner ear of the alligator. They were able to show that the shape of the stimulus-related intracellular potential changes corresponded with the cochlear microphonics and the summating potential recorded extracellularly. The amplitude of the intracellular potential is larger, in agreement with the assumption that the source of these biopotentials is located in the sensory cells. Similar potentials also could be recorded from the supporting cells. The largest amplitude recorded (from these cells) was 3 mV approximately. This is in good agreement with the results obtained from the hair cells of the lateral line organ.* As a presynaptic potential it would be sufficient to modulate the transmitter release at the synapses making contact with the afferent auditory nerve fibers. The intracellular potentials found correspond well with the known discharge patterns of the afferent fibers of the cochlear nerve. Weiss et al.[108] discuss the possibility of an electrical coupling between the hair cells and the supporting cells in analogy to similar couplings already known from research with invertebrates with emphasis placed on the possibility of a lateral interaction between the hair cells. As expected, action potentials do not occur intracellularly. Figure 36 a, b shows an example of their results. Later, Russell and Sellick[997, 998] and Sellick and Russell[1027, 1028] recorded potentials from the inner hair cells of the guinea pig (Fig. 36 c, d, e). It could be shown that the receptor potential of the inner hair cells exhibits a sharp tuning comparable to the tuning curves of the auditory-nerve fibers. The maximum DC-response amplitude was 27 mV at 100 dB SPL. Also, a two-tone inhibition could be shown to exist at the level of the inner hair cells.[1028]

More recently Crawford and Fettiplace† made intracellular recordings from single hair cells of the isolated half-head of the turtle. The response of each hair cell to sound stimuli was sharply tuned with a characteristic frequency which was related to the position of the cell along the basilar membrane. The hair cells had resting potentials of about -50 mV and to low frequency tones gave periodic responses graded with the intensity and frequency of the stimulus. The voltage response to a pure tone at low sound pressure was sinusoidal for all frequencies of stimulation. At higher sound pressures a steady depolarizing component was apparent that relative to the periodic component of the response, was most prominent at high frequencies. When small current steps were injected through the intracellular electrode, the hair cell potential exhibited damped oscillations at the cell's characteristic frequency. From these results it is concluded that each hair cell contains its own electrical resonance mechanism that accounts for most of the frequency selectivity of the receptor potential (Fig. 37).

All other intracellular recordings from hair cells were obtained from sensory organs more readily accessible. However, one may assume that the hair cells of the inner ear, of the vestibular system, and of the lateral-line organ of fish and amphibians work according to the same basic principle. Many characteristic data from the hair cells of the lateral-line organ have been collected.[357] Upon stimulation with low frequency oscillations these cells exhibit a receptor potential of 1 mV maximal amplitude that reflects the temporal course of the stimulus in much the same way as the cochlear microphonic.

---

* References 362, 451, 452.
† References 207–209, 331.

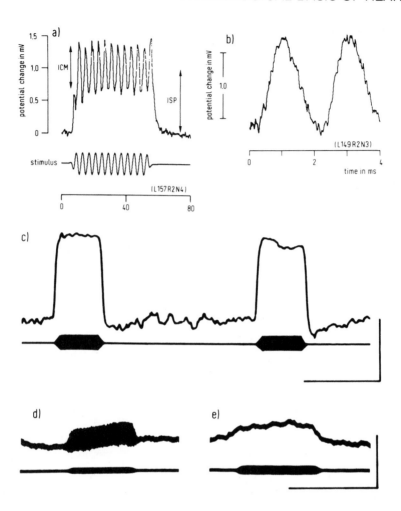

FIGURE 36. A, Averaged intracellular (supporting cell) recording upon stimulation with tone bursts. ICM = intracellular cochlear microphonics, ISP = intracellular summating potential. (Stimulus: tone bursts of 50 ms duration each, 10 stimuli per second, 250 Hz, 94 dB SPL.) (Alligator lizard.) B, Averaged intracellular recording from a hair cell upon stimulation with a continuous tone (500 Hz, 73 dB SPL). (Alligator lizard.) C, DC component of receptor potential recorded intracellularly from an identified inner hair cell in response to a tone burst at its characteristic frequency (c.f.; 17 kHz) and s.p.l. of 80 dB. Horizontal bar 100 ms, vertical bar 10 mV. (Guinea pig) D, AC component of receptor potential recorded intracellularly from an inner hair cell with a c.f. of 16 kHz in response to a 2 kHz tone burst at s.p.l. of 80 dB. Horizontal bar 100 ms, vertical bar 5 mV. (Guinea pig.) E, Depolarizing potential recorded from a supporting cell in response to a 17 kHz tone burst at 80 dB, corresponding to the c.f. of adjacent hair cells. Horizontal bar 100 ms, vertical bar 5 mV. Lower trace in all records shows the tone burst envelope. (Guinea pig.) (a and b according to Mulroy et al. [832]; c to e according to Russell and Sellick [998].)

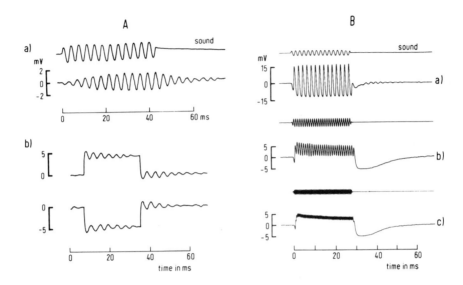

FIGURE 37. A, (a) Averaged membrane potential changes of a hair cell to tone bursts at 276 Hz, 55 dB SPL; upper trace, sound monitor. (b) Averaged responses of same cell to depolarizing and hyperpolarizing current steps. (0.024 nA) injected down recording electrode; voltage drop across electrode resistance balanced out. Hair cell resting potential -54 mV; characteristic frequency 274 Hz; maximum peak-to-peak response 34 mV. (According to Fettiplace and Crawford [331].) B, Periodic and sustained components of a hair cell's response to tones at high intensity as a function of the frequency of stimulation. Frequencies and sound pressures: (a), 500 Hz, 120 dB; (b), 1 kHz, 122,5 dB; (c), 2 kHz, 125 dB; sound pressure expressed relative to 20 μPa. The upper trace of each pair is the sound monitor. Thirty-two responses have been averaged at each frequency. Cell has characteristic frequency 425 Hz; voltages given with respect to the resting potential which was -46 mV. Temperature 25° C. (According to Crawford and Fettiplace [208].)

The chemical character of the synapses of the hair cells making contact with efferent and afferent fibers has been described. Excitatory postsynaptic potentials have been recorded from afferent acoustic-nerve fibers* and inhibitory postsynaptic potentials were recorded from the hair cells[359, 360] upon stimulation of efferent fibers. Also in electron micrographs the existence of vesicles could be demonstrated in the guinea pig and in the cat.†

The transmitters of the efferent and afferent lateral-line system apparently are acetylcholine and gamma-amino-butyric acid.[357] The transmitters in mammals are not yet known.

* References 359, 379, 513, 514.
† References 8, 292–294, 1043, 1064, 1065, 1072, 1204.

Figure 38 schematically summarizes the relationship between mechanical deformation of the cilia of the hair cells and the action potentials generated in the associated nerve fiber. If bending the hairs is the adequate stimulus leading to the receptor potentials of the hair cells, then the mechanics leading to the bending should be clarified first. This problem has by no means been settled yet. Frequently (e.g. Ranke[927]), instead of the basilar membrane proper, the whole scala media (i.e. basilar membrane, organ of Corti, tectorial membrane, Reissner's membrane, cortilymph and endolymph) is regarded as a transversely oscillating "partition." If this is correct, the twisting of the hairs can be understood according to the principle of Ter Kuile.[1137] The basilar membrane is attached on both sides and the tectorial membrane only on one side. As a result, a translatory shift between the basilar membrane and the tectorial membrane will be produced when displaced simultaneously. If the hairs are tied to the tectorial membrane and if the hair cells are firmly connected to the organ of Corti sitting on the basilar membrane, a twisting of the hairs must result (Fig. 39). Thus, either only the radial component of the deflection will be effective or the radial shearing will act on the outer and the longitudinal shearing on the inner hair cells.

Figure 40 demonstrates how radial components occur as a consequence of a bilateral attachment of the basilar membrane. Tonndorf[1145] further demonstrated that this mechanism causes a sharpening of the mechanical tuning curves (see Fig. 14) as can be seen from Figure 41.

A different hypothesis maintains that, by virtue of a different oscillating behavior of the basilar membrane with its attached structures and of the tectorial membrane, a flow of endolymph back and forth between the space underneath the tectorial membrane and the area outside the tectorial membrane takes place (Neubert's jet) thereby bending the hairs.* In connection with these hypotheses it should be kept in mind that at hearing threshold the amplitude of the oscillation of the basilar membrane amounts to only 10^{-3} to 10^{-1} Å (see page 16). The distance between the surface of the hair cells and the basilar membrane however is more than 10^5 - 10^6 Å. The hairs themselves have a length of more than 10^4 Å and a diameter of 10^3 Å.

However, one need not take the small deflections of the basilar membrane as the "motor" for subtectorial flow or for ciliary bending. We also can see the causality in the following way: the longitudinal compression waves in the canalis spiralis cochleae cause the often described transverse waves of the basilar membrane. The mechanical features of the basilar membrane determine the characteristics of the transverse wave, as to wave length and velocity. Owing to the strong coupling (analogous to coupled mechanical oscillators) the longitudinal wave mode is forced into the same

---

* References 203, 477, 478, 847, 1103, 1259–1261.

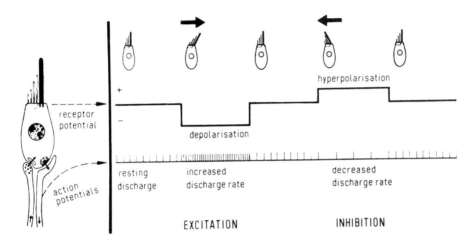

FIGURE 38. Schematic summary of stimulus, receptor potential, and sequence of action potentials. It is assumed that the deflection of the hairs in one direction causes depolarization and an increasing impulse rate, and that a deflection in the opposite direction causes hyperpolarization and a decreasing impulse rate. (According to Flock [355].)

wavelength as the transverse wave. Thus throughout the cross section of the canalis spiralis cochleae we find the same wavelength and velocity irrespective of the smallness of the amplitude of the transverse basilar membrane displacements.

The longitudinal wave—so modified by basilar membrane action—causes again transverse waves at all boundaries within the cochlear duct, also at the opposite surfaces of tectorial membrane and reticular lamina, so that shear forces may act. In this view the basilar membrane only determines the locus of minimum propagation velocity.

Still too little is known about the mechanical properties of the tectorial membrane in order to settle those processes leading to a twisting of the sensory hairs. According to the latest results it looks as if the tectorial membrane is firmly tied to the lamina reticularis as well as to Hensen's cells and to the inner border cells.*

According to the amplifier theory of Davis[227, 230] the deflection of the sensory hairs is supposed to change the electrical resistance of the cell membrane. Davis assumes that here the potential shift between EP and intracellular potential takes place (Fig. 15 a) so that the movements of the hairs, via the resistance changes, modulate a current which causes the cochlear microphonic. Thus, the stimulus merely controls an energy flow originating ultimately from the stria vascularis.

---

* References 483, 675, 986.

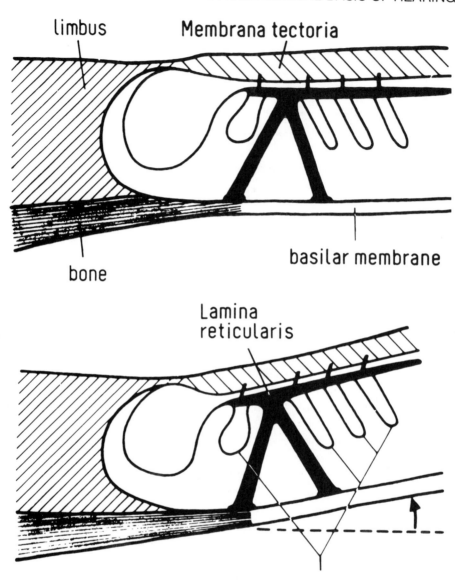

FIGURE 39. Movement of the organ of Corti and of the tectorial membrane around displaced axes causing a shearing movement of the sensory hairs. (According to Davis [228].)

However, according to Ranke[927] and Keidel[558] the movement of the hairs leads to permeability changes of the cell membrane thus causing an ionic current as the basis of the cochlear microphonics. In this theory, as in Davis' theory, the energy does not originate from the stimulus. Rather, the energy originates from the metabolism of the sensory cell.

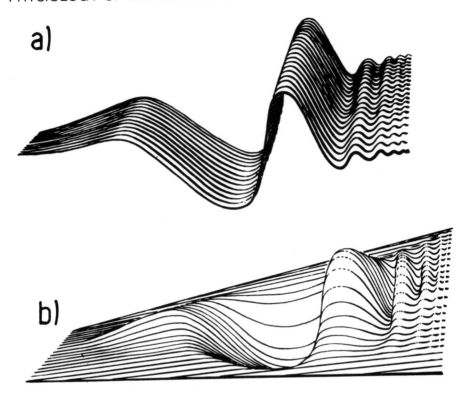

FIGURE 40. Shape of the travelling wave: A, if the membrane is not attached laterally; and B, if the membrane is attached on both sides. (According to Tonndorf [1145].)

According to Vinnikov[1176] and Vinnikov and Titowa[1177] the movement of the basilar membrane and the tectorial membrane causes a release of acetylcholine in the area of the stereocilia. It acts on an acetylcholine receptor present in the plasma membrane of the stereocilia. Here it is decomposed by acetylcholine esterase present in the stereocilia. Acetylcholine is supposed to cause the receptor potential.

In Naftalin's[835] hypothesis, however, movement of the stereocilia is not necessary. Naftalin describes the tectorial membrane as a semiconductor. He uses the EP to close the gap between the conduction band and the valence band. He then assumes that, by interaction between phonons and electrons, the energy of acoustic oscillations is transformed into electrical energy which is finally absorbed by the stereocilia. This hypothesis has two advantages: it is independent of mechanical movements of the hairs, and it describes a process of energy absorption by the hairs that is close to that found in the receptors of the eye. Nevertheless, our knowledge of the processes involved in transforming mechanical into electrical energy has not yet advanced beyond the state of working hypotheses.

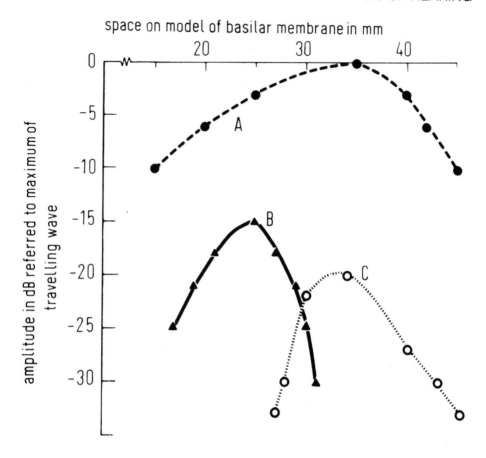

FIGURE 41. Envelopes of three modes of oscillation of a model of the basilar membrane: A, travelling wave; B, radial shearing; and C, longitudinal shearing. (According to Tonndorf [1145].)

G. Inner and Outer Hair Cells

A theory accounting for the transformations of the stimulus into excitation within the ear should explain the function of the inner and outer hair cells. The inner and outer hair cells are different in many respects. Ontogenetically, the 3400 inner hair cells develop from the margin of the huge neuroepithelial bulge. The approximately 13,400 outer hair cells, however, are derived from the small epithelial bulge (Held[476]). They can be distinguished according to their shape, number, arrangement and innervation. The inner hair cells are of ovoid shape with a fat base and a slim slightly off-center apex (Fig. 42). The outer hair cells, on the other hand, are cylinder-shaped and slim. The amount and the distribution of intracellular

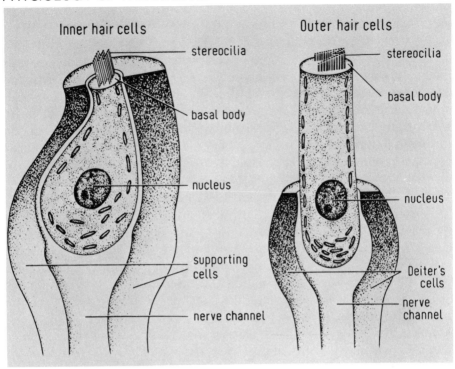

FIGURE 42. Schematic description of an inner and an outer hair cell. (According to Gulick [439].)

organelles exhibit typical differences.[8, 43] The sensory hairs of the outer hair cells (100 to 200 stereocilia) show a W-shaped arrangement, those of the inner hair cells (approximately 60 stereocilia) an almost linear arrangement (Fig. 27). The outer hair cells rest with their apex in the lamina reticularis, with their base on the supporting cells of Deiter, and are otherwise in contact with the cortilymph; the inner hair cells, however, are completely surrounded by supporting cells.[142]

The heights of the cilia show a gradient from base to apex,[726] short in the base and tall in the apex. (Inner hair cell cilia: 4.7 μm at the apex; 2.1 μm in the base. Outer hair cell cilia: 5.5 μm at the apex; 1 μm in the base.) The gradation in heights of the cilia also exists within a single bundle (Fig. 51). It is generally thought the cilia are stiff and the ciliary bundle (W-formation) may move as a unit.[295, 363]

With respect to the innervation, the differences are very distinct. The ganglion cells of the afferent acoustic nerve fibers are located in the ganglion spirale (in the canal of Rosenthal or the marginal zone of the modiolus). The dendrites of the about 30,000 bipolar neurons arrive at the organ of Corti through the habenula perforata. According to Spoendlin[1066–1072] 95% of these ganglion cells innervate the inner hair cells (inner radial fibers) and only 5% the outer hair cells (outer spiral fibers).* This means that about 28,500 dendrites make contact with the 3000 inner hair cells and only 1500 dendrites with the 13,000 outer hair cells. It is possible that those neurons innervating the outer hair cells do not have a central connection so that no afferent paths from the outer hair cells to the brain would exist.[1073] The inner radial fibers arrive at the inner hair cells via the shortest possible path and in general insert at one cell.† The dendrites to the outer hair cells first run through the inner tunnel as basilar fibers. They then pass the outer pillar cells and run in a basal direction as outer spiral fibers near Deiter's cells for about 0.6 mm before ascending to the outer hair cells. They innervate on the average 10 to 20, sometimes up to 60,[883] outer hair cells.

In addition, the hair cells are innervated efferently. According to Rasmussen[937, ‡] 75% of the efferent fibers originate from the contralateral superior olive (crossed olivo-cochlear bundle) and only 25% from the ipsilateral superior olive (uncrossed olivo-cochlear bundle).§ The efferent fibers run through the spiral ganglion and enter, together with the afferent fibers, the organ of Corti through the habenula perforata. They form the inner spiral fibers, the tunnel spiral fibers, and the tunnel radial fibers. According to Iurato,[516] in the rat all contralateral fibers innervate the outer hair cells whereas the ipsilateral fibers arrive at the inner hair cells. In addition, Spoendlin[1067] found the cat had additional contralateral innervation of the inner hair cells. Further, Perkins and Morest[883] described efferent fibers in the cat and the rat that made synaptic contact via collaterals with both inner and outer hair cells. Stopp and Comis[1109] described even fibers terminating at Deiters and Hensen cells.

At the level of the habenula perforata the number of efferent fibers is extremely small as compared with the afferent fibers. By strong arborization of these few efferent fibers, however, an extended efferent fibrous net is formed in the organ of Corti with approximately 40,000 efferent nerve endings at the outer hair cells.[1070] Whereas the inner hair cells are in contact with almost all afferent fibers (95%), the outer hair cells are innervated by a greater number of efferent fibers, although there are only relatively few original efferent fibers. The inner hair cells are innervated afferently predominantly by radial fibers (up to 20 fibers per sensory cell) and efferently by spiral fibers. On the other hand, the outer hair cells are

---

* These studies were done in the cat.
† About 0.5% of the afferent fibers innervate, possibly via collaterals of the inner spiral bundle, several inner hair cells (Fig. 45).
‡ Klinke and Galley (656) report that, according to a personal communication with W.B. Warr, in kittens 60% of the efferent fibers are of ipsilateral origin and that up to 1400 efferent fibers exist, not about 500 as assumed earlier.
§ In rats, a reticulo-cochlear bundle has also been described originating from the formatio reticularis of the pons or of the medulla oblongata (Reference 150).

innervated afferently by spiral fibers (one fiber per 10 to 60 sensory cells) and efferently by radial fibers (with a limited number of spiral fibers). Also, the kind of synaptic contact is different. Regarding the outer hair cells, the efferent fibers generally make synaptic contact with the sensory cells themselves (axo-somatic synapses). However, the synapses are mostly axo-dendritic with the inner hair cells (Fig. 43). Figures 44 and 45 schematically summarize the pattern of innervation of the organ of Corti.

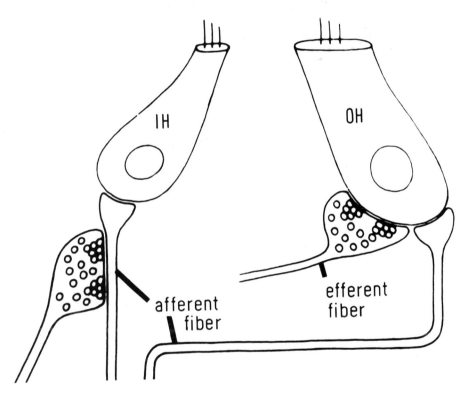

FIGURE 43. Schematic description of types of efferent contact. The inner hair cells (IH) of the cat almost exclusively show axo-dendritic synapses. The outer hair cells (OH), however, show axo-somatic synapses. (According to Spoendlin [1072].)

Among the afferent fibers essential metabolic differences must exist. After cutting the auditory nerve in the meatus acusticus internus almost all inner radial fibers degenerate. The outer spiral fibers, however, remain unchanged, even after a survival time of more than a year.[1071] During hypoxia the afferent dendrites of the inner hair cells swell rapidly; in contrast, those of the outer hair cells stay unchanged. In the degeneration experiments just mentioned, Spoendlin[1071] was able to show that at least

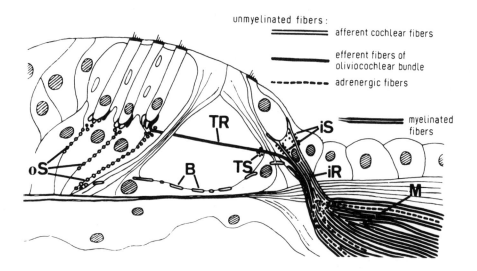

FIGURE 44. Schematic description of the different nerve fibers within the organ of Corti. Black filled lines represent efferent fibers, contoured lines represent the afferent, broken lines the sympathetic fibers. All myelinated fibers (M) lose their sheath as they exit the habenula with all nerve fibers within the organ of Corti being unmyelinated. Inner radial fibers (iR), inner spiral fibers (iS), tunnel radial fibers (TR), tunnel spiral fibers (TS), basilar fibers (B) and outer spiral fibers (oS). (According to Spoendlin [1070].)

two, perhaps even three, different types of nerve cells exist in the ganglion spirale.

Differences in function between the inner and outer hair cells can only be hypothesized. Ranke[927] and Keidel[558] assume that these systems have to be regarded as being analogous to the two receptor populations in the eye (rods and cones). The rods are more sensitive (by convergence of many receptors to one afferent fiber) but have a poorer resolving power. The cones are less sensitive but have the better resolving power (besides color selectivity). Likewise, the outer hair cells could account for the high sensitivity (energy threshold at 10^{-11} erg) of the ear by convergence of many receptors to one nerve fiber. The inner hair cells could be responsible for the excellent ability of time resolution. Stevens, Davis and Lurie[1107] had the good fortune to find a hearing loss of 30 to 40 dB at all frequencies in a cat having a degeneration of the outer hair cells with the inner hair cells preserved.* This would be in agreement with the fact (Fig. 3) that the frequency-difference threshold has its lowest value at 40 dB above

---

* However, Bredberg and Hunter-Duvar (141) reported more recently on cat "Goldie" in which the inner hair cells were selectively destroyed over a range of 2 mm leading to a hearing loss of 45 dB in the corresponding frequency range.

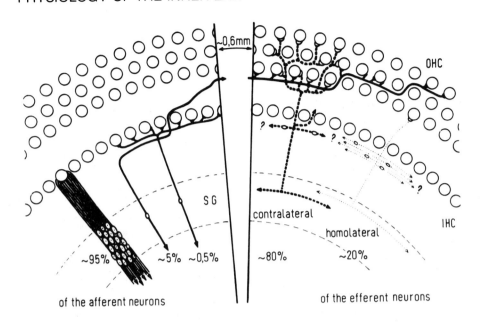

FIGURE 45. Scheme of the pattern of distribution of the different neurons in the organ of Corti. The left side shows the three types of afferent, the right side the two types of efferent neurons. About 95% of all afferent neurons run to the inner hair cells exclusively and end there without branching. OHC = outer hair cells, IHC = inner hair cells, SG = spiral ganglion. (According to Spoendlin [1070].)

threshold. In the meantime, Carlier and Pujol[172] were able to show that the break observed in the intensity function of the compound action potential that, according to this hypothesis, is accounted for by the two receptor populations, occurs in kittens together with the maturation of the outer hair cells. Likewise, adult-like tuning curves are observed in kittens and young rats following the maturation of the outer hair cells.[173] These results were obtained in continuation of the developmental studies of Pujol,[914] Pujol and Hilding[915] and Pujol and Abonnec.[916] More recently the Pujol-group* described the postnatal development of neuro-epithelial junctions and the maturation stages of receptor morphology. Two main stages of development are described. During the first postnatal days, outer hair cells look very immature with only a few afferent endings adjoining them. The inner hair cells, however, are surrounded by numerous endings with mature afferent and efferent synapses. Thus, when the efferent olivo-cochlear system begins to function during the first postnatal days, it is able to modify only inner hair cell responses. The second postnatal week is characterized by maturation of the large efferent endings below the outer hair cells. At the same time, direct

---

* References 710, 917, 918, 1032, 1033.

efferent connections become sparce at the level of inner hair cells. The maturation of hearing, at the receptor level, seems to proceed in two steps, one related to inner hair cells and corresponding to a gross and primitive hearing, the other related to outer hair cells and corresponding to more precise and discriminative hearing abilities (Fig. 46).

Although the hypothesis of Ranke and Keidel appears to be very plausible, it cannot be supported by the results of single fiber studies obtained thus far. One would expect the tuning curves of nerve fibers innervating the outer hair cells to have a lower absolute threshold but to be less sharply tuned than the tuning curves of the inner hair cells. At a ratio of 5:95 such fibers indeed would be encountered with a correspondingly smaller probability. According to the results available at present* the sharply tuned fibers reach the behavioral hearing threshold and the less sharply tuned fibers always had a significantly higher threshold than the sharply tuned fibers (see Fig. 59). However, the possibility exists that those nerve cells innervating the outer hair cells do not have a connection with higher nervous centers[1073, 1074] because after sectioning the cochlear nerve in the internal meatus those cells of the spiral ganglion that presumably belong to the outer hair cells do not degenerate (Fig. 48).†

Also, the contributions of the two systems (inner and outer hair cells) to the summed action potential of the auditory nerve (Fig. 47) appears to support the hypothesis of the outer-hair-cell system being 40 to 60 dB more sensitive.[1096] This view, however, is not in agreement with the anatomical finding according to which only 5% of the afferent fibers of the auditory nerve belong to the outer hair cells.‡

Evans§ and Evans and Klinke[314] offer a solution for this problem in connection with their "Second-Filter"-hypothesis. These authors were able to show that the additional segment of the tuning curves of the auditory nerve fibers described on page 18 Figure 14 leading to a significant increase in the low-frequency slope as well as a threshold drop of 40 to 60 dB, disappears reversibly within a few minutes under hypoxia and after administration of Cyanide and Frusemide (Fig. 49).‖

---

* References 303, 308, 317, 631, 638.

† But there are also experimental results indicating fibers which possibly belong to outer hair cells (References 672, 890).

‡ The break in the intensity function of the compound action potential can be explained in a qualitative fashion according to Özdamar and Dallos (878) also with only one fiber population. They assumed the slowly growing low-level segments to be identified with the sharp tip region of the tuning curves of the responding units, while the high-level, rapidly growing, segment is associated with the recruitment of higher frequency units that respond on the tail segment of their tuning curves.

§ References 304, 305, 307, 309.

‖ Wigand and Heidland (1231) have observed a reversible hearing loss in patients treated with Frusemide. This was described more extensively by Wigand (1230).

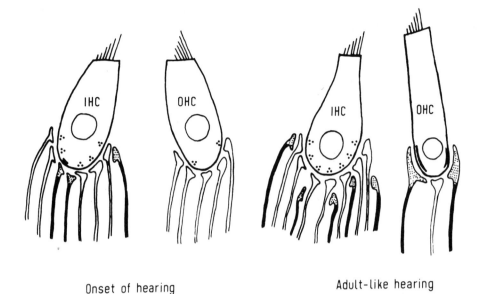

Onset of hearing   Adult-like hearing

FIGURE 46. Diagram of hair cell synaptogenesis. Afferent dendrites are unshaded. Efferent fibers are shaded and their endings contain microvesicles. Within hair cells dots represent presynaptic specializations, and dark bars indicate postsynaptic cisterns. (According to Pujol et al. [918].)

From these results they infer the existence of an extremely vulnerable "second filter 'private' to each cochlear fibre." From the good stability of the cochlear microphonic it is concluded that the mechanics of the inner ear have not changed in these experiments. From the fact that intoxication with tetrodotoxin reduces afferent activity but leaves the shape of the tuning curve unaltered it is concluded that the damage occurs prior to the auditory nerve fibers.[655] Since 95% of all fibers belong to the inner hair cells, the authors assume that the fibers studied were fibers of the inner hair cells. Since the outer hair cells are more sensitive* to ototoxic drugs[1202] than the inner hair cells, Evans assumes that the Second-Filter function possibly arises from an interaction between the systems of the inner and outer hair cells. In this connection Evans refers to the results of Kiang et al.[640] who were unable to record, in cats treated with ototoxic drugs, any activity from nerve fibers probably belonging to the inner hair cells for low intensity levels. Upon histological examination the outer hair cells of the area in question were destroyed while the inner hair cells appeared normal (under the light microscope).

---

* In fact the afferent synapses of the inner hair cells are more sensitive to hypoxia than those of the outer hair cells.

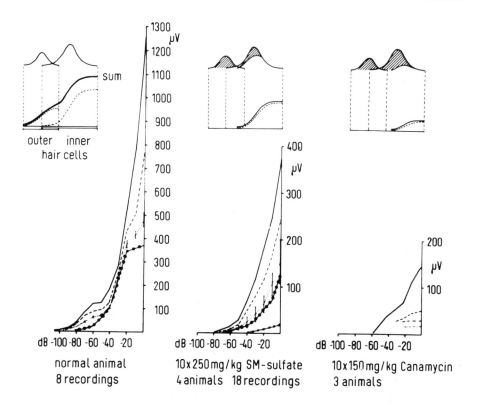

FIGURE 47. Amount of adaptation for the compound action potentials recorded from the round window in the cat following different stimulus repetition frequencies. The left panel shows the normal relations with a characteristic curve having two peaks. The middle panel shows, after administration of streptomycin, a monotonic curve with a corresponding threshold shift of 30 dB as sign of a loss of the more sensitive outer hair cells. The right panel also shows a heavy damage of the inner hair cells after administration of kanamycin. The distributions of the two populations of sensory cells are represented above. (According to Stange et al. [1096].)

Figure 50 shows tuning curves of single fibers (guinea pig) after being treated with Kanamycin for 10 days and subsequently degenerating for 14 days. Changes of the tuning curves can be seen for auditory nerve fibers arising from those areas of the cochlea in which the outer hair cells were degenerated. Similar results were described by Dallos and Harris[217] who found that (in the chinchilla) the behavioral hearing threshold, the tuning curves of single auditory-nerve fibers, and the condition of the hair cells were abnormal following treatment with Kanamycin.

As Evans notes himself, this model would of course require that the outer hair cells or their innervation be sharply tuned, whereas the inner hair cells would only reflect the mechanics of the basilar membrane. This is in contrast to the sharp tuning curves of the receptor potentials recorded from

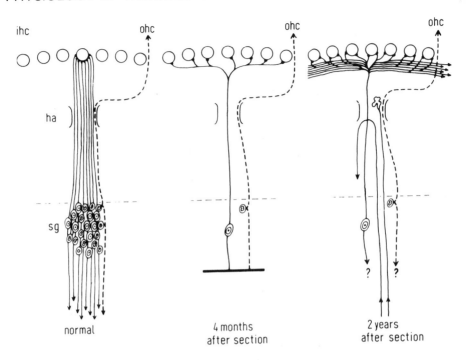

FIGURE 48. Schematic representation of the degeneration and regeneration or proliferation behavior of the afferent cochlear neurons. Whereas the area of the inner hair cells contains only very few giant nerve fibers four months after section of the VIIIth nerve, the same area is filled with proliferating branches after longer survival times. Some other fibers ending in the habenula or turning back before the habenula can be found after long survival times. They may correspond to some type of regenerating fibers. The afferent fibers for the outer hair cells are not affected by these degenerative processes. (According to Spoendlin [1073].)

the inner hair cells (page 49). Since, in general, the cochlear microphonics are regarded as generated essentially by the outer hair cells there seems to be a conflict. The small changes of the cochlear microphonic described in the experiments above (Fig. 49) do not agree with this view either. After all, the anatomical basis for an interaction is still lacking. Synaptic contacts between the system of the inner and outer hair cells have not yet been found in either the organ of Corti or the spirale ganglion. Evans assumes interaction takes place in the area of the habenula perforata where the unmyelinated radial and spiral fibers run close together. This idea has been brought up repeatedly, however, without experimental evidence proving it.

Recently, Finkenzeller[337] advanced a hypothesis. He suggests that the system of the inner hair cells is responsible for frequency analysis and that of the outer hair cells for the coding of phase information. He presupposes that the action potentials of the afferent fibers of the inner hair cells are generated in an area (e.g. the initial segment could be located close to the habenula

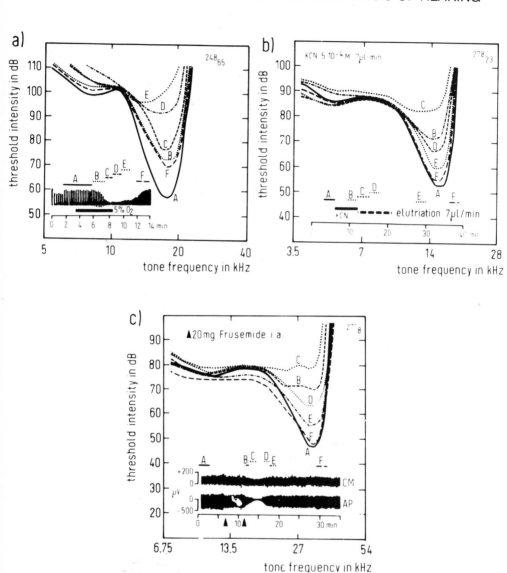

FIGURE 49. Reversible alterations of the tuning curves of single auditory nerve fibers caused by: (a), hypoxia (b), cyanide (c), frusemide. To produce hypoxia the oxygen pressure of the inspiratory air was reduced to 5% by adding N₂O. Cyanide was instilled directly through the round window. Frusemide was injected into the subclavian artery. The time span necessary for the hypoxia and the cyanide to become effective and the time of the injection of frusemide are marked on the time axis. Above the time scale, the periods of analysis for the different tuning curves are denoted by letters and symbols. Above the time scale in (a) and (c) the effect on the summed action potential (AP) is shown. The cochlear microphonics (CM) stay nearly unchanged. (According to Evans [304].)

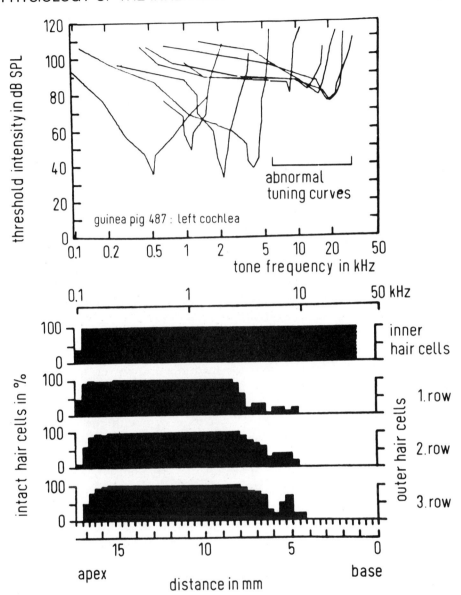

FIGURE 50. Correlation between normal and abnormal frequency response curves of single auditory nerve fibers (above) with the corresponding cochleogram (below). (According to Evans and Harrison [315].)

perforata) influenced by the cochlear microphonic that in turn is initiated predominantly by the outer hair cells. Since the generator potential represents the difference between the intra- and extra-cellular potential, and the generator potential of the afferent fibers belonging to the system of the inner hair cells necessarily has to be modulated by the cochlear microphonics.* This is supposed to be the reason for the known phase-related discharge pattern of the auditory nerve fibers.[972] In the lateral-line organ[1111] and in the cochlea of the guinea pig[497] a corresponding sensitivity to electrical potentials (threshold at 100 μV) has been shown to exist. In connection with this hypothesis, the efferent fibers could change the emphasis put on either system. On the one hand, the efferent fibers could increase the sensitivity thereby possibly decreasing the phase control (listening) while, on the other hand, they could improve the phase control thereby possibly decreasing the sensitivity (selective hearing, party-effect). Stimulation of the crossed olivo-cochlear bundle indeed causes a decrease of the compound action potential while the cochlear microphonics increased at the same time.† In order to subject Finkenzeller's hypothesis to an experimental test one would have to examine whether stimulation of the olivo-cochlear bundle would improve the phase lock of the action potentials. Of course, this would certainly not describe the significance of the outer hair cells because in order to make Finkenzeller's hypothesis work the afferent fibers of the outer hair cells would not be necessary and their existence would remain unexplained.‡

Lynn and Sayers[738] advanced a hypothesis taking into account the fibers of the outer hair cells and leading to a control of the inner afferent fibers by the outer fibers. As already mentioned, however, the necessary anatomical contact is missing.

In recent times, Lehnhardt[709] supported an idea introduced by Meyer zum Gottesberge[765] and Ranke[929] in connection with the recruitment phenomenon. According to their view the outer hair cells have a low stimulus threshold but a high intensity-difference threshold; the inner hair cells, however, have a stimulus threshold 60 dB higher but a very low intensity-difference threshold (1 dB). This is in agreement with the view of Stange et al.[1097] as well as with the electro-cochleographic recordings by Aran[47] and Portmann[907] but it does not agree with the results obtained from single-fiber recordings of the auditory nerve (see page 79). Kiang et al.[640] indicate that: "According to our data, recruitment would be based not on the selective loss of low-threshold units in the auditory nerve but on the conversion of normal units into units having abnormally high thresholds at CF but normal low-frequency sensitivity." Also, the results of Bredberg[137] and Elliott and McGee[286] disagree with this interpretation of the recruitment

---

* Unfortunately, the term cochlear microphonic is used for the intra-cellular potentials (see Fig. 36, page 50) as well as for the extracellular potentials recordable inside and outside the cochlea. Here, it is referred to the extracellular potentials.
† References 260, 261, 333, 334, 384, 656, 1053, 1054, 1226–1228.
‡ Indeed Spoendlin (1073, 1074) assumed the outer hair cells even to have no afferent connection with higher nervous centers (page 62).

phenomenon. Nienhuys and Clark[852] were able to show that in cats the frequency discrimination was not impaired after drug-induced destruction of the outer hair cells.

Finally, it should be mentioned that in the modern literature* the inner hair cells are sometimes regarded as receptors of the velocity of deflection, the outer hair cells as receptors of the deflection. This hypothesis started out from the anatomical description of the hairs of the outer hair cells as being tied to the tectorial membrane† and the cilia of the inner hair cells as standing free.[644, 724]‡

Thus, it is assumed that the hairs of the inner hair cells are deflected by the flow of the cortilymph, but the outer ones by the shear forces between the tectorial membrane and the sensory cells. Along these lines, Dallos[214] was able to show that the cochlear microphonic recorded from the inner hair cells (recorded selectively after damaging the outer hair cells with Kanamycin) exhibits a corresponding phase shift relative to recordings made from normal ears (velocity as first derivative against time) or, upon triangular stimulation, directly reflected the time differential. Zwislocki[1268] and Sokolich et al.[1059] extended this idea to a hypothesis explaining the sharpening of the neuronal versus the mechanical tuning curves by interaction of the inner and outer hair cells.

The interaction between the mechanical travelling wave and the velocity of electrotonic spread in the spiral fibers as considered by Ranke[927] was reported by Keidel on August 6, 1976 at a symposium held in honour of Prof. H.L. Wullstein on his 70th birthday in Würzburg. This interaction could explain the simultaneous increase in slope of the tuning curves and the low threshold in the area of the characteristic frequency. It will be published in the book of collected papers belonging to the symposium. Even after the destruction of all inner and outer hair cells following treatment with Amikacin, click-evoked summed action potentials could be recorded from the round window of the guinea pig. It was assumed that these potentials originated from vestibular receptors or from remaining nerve fibers.[188]

In summary, it can be concluded that in recent years the important structures of the inner ear could further be elucidated microscopically as well as electronmicrographically.§ However, the functions of the different

---

* References 214, 1267–1269.

† References 499, 644, 725.

‡ However this remains controversial because some investigators observed that the inner hair cell cilia are attached to the tectorial membrane (References 43, 499, 500, 501, 517, 986). But even if they are attached, it must be a weak attachment and the attachments are limited to only the basal turn where the inner hair cell cilia are twice as tall as the outer hair cell cilia (Reference 726). It should be noted, that in the alligator lizard the high-frequency receptor zone is covered by the tectorial membrane, but it is absent in the lower frequency zone.

§ References 42, 137–140, 142, 275, 290, 296, 515, 516, 644, 645, 728, 729, 1044.

structures are still largely unknown. The different structure of the inner and outer hair cells up to the level of the intracellular substructures is well established. However, the functional substructures of these two cell populations has yet to be resolved. The innervation pattern of the afferent and efferent fibers has been elucidated almost completely. Once again, however, no functional differences can be ascribed to the striking differences in innervation. At the time being, not even an obligatory idea exists about the significance of the tectorial membrane. Figures 51 and 52 schematically summarize the anatomical results as far as they can be shown on a transverse section of the ductus cochlearis. The reason for the gap in our knowledge about the function of the inner ear is that the structures in question are hardly accessible for suitable measuring devices.

H. Bone Conduction

Bone conduction* results when the stimulus sound waves are conducted to the inner ear via the bony skull. Vibrations are caused whenever the head is in a sound field (in air or fluid) of sufficient strength or is in direct contact with a vibrating body. Bone conduction with the skull in direct contact with a vibrating body (e.g. a tuning fork) is relatively effective because of the good coupling and is of common clinical use (Weber-Rinne-Schwabach). Bone conduction caused by sound transmitted in air is of little effect by reason of a poor coupling (the acoustic impedances of the skull and the air are different, thus a great deal of the oscillatory energy is reflected).

As von Békésy[76] demonstrated, sound transmitted by air can make the whole skull vibrate. Sufficient energy will not be absorbed to trigger an excitation of the inner ear, however, until 60 dB above hearing threshold for sound transmitted by air. Thus, there is a limited ability to block sound transmission to the inner ear by experimentally occluding the outer auditory canal. This is of significance in noise protection.

With respect to the pathway of bone conduction transmitting sound energy to the inner ear, two components can be distinguished, osteotympanic and the compression component. Regarding the osteotympanic sound transmission, the sound energy is first transmitted from the bone to the middle ear causing a vibration of the auditory ossicles either via the inertia of the ossicles[60] or via the compliance of the ear drum (compression of the air in the middle ear causes a corresponding deflection of the ear drum).[92, 430] Once

---

* Testing via bone conduction is of audiometric significance for the differential diagnosis of hearing losses and, according to Tonndorf (1157), was used even in the 16th century by Hieronymus Capivacci.

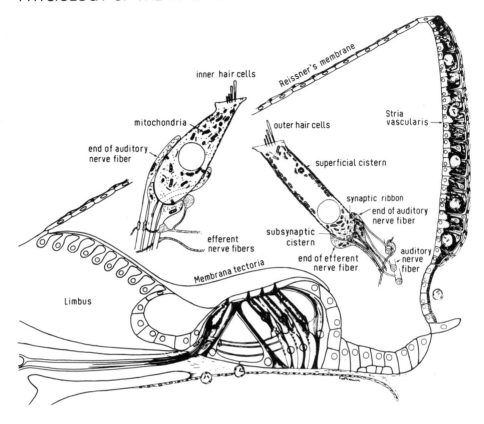

FIGURE 51. Diagram of a cross section through the ductus cochlearis (second turn) in the guinea pig. Recent findings are emphasized. (From Smith [1042]; the original was drawn by Fred M. Harwin.)

movement of the ossicles occurs the transmission to the inner ear is equivalent to that found for sound transmission in air. In the same sense, of course an osseo-meatal component can be described.[1155] The compression component results from the direct transmission of sound from the bony skull to the inner ear.*,† Concerning qualitative and quantitative descriptions of the contributions of the different components, experiments were carried out in recent times mainly by Tonndorf,‡ Tonndorf and Tabor[1158] and Tonndorf et al.[1159, 1160]

In this context it is of interest to ask why the inner ear functions irrespective of how the sound energy is conveyed to the inner ear. However, this is in exact agreement with the results obtained from the model (Fig. 12)

---

* In this connection it is referred to Ranke's (927) coupling of mass moment of inertia.
† References 481, 690, 947.
‡ References 1148, 1150, 1151.

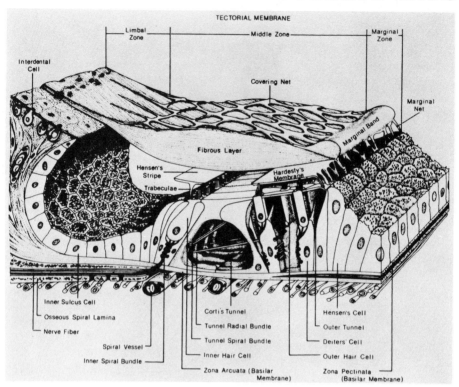

FIGURE 52. Artist's conception of organ of Corti (drawing by Nancy Sally). (According to Lim [726].)

and can be expected from the oscillatory properties of the basilar membrane as described previously. As shown previously in Figure 6, the velocity of the wave has a minimum at the place of resonance. Thus, regardless of where the wave originated from, it has its minimal velocity at the site of resonance. Asymmetric deflections of the basilar membrane occuring via bone conduction have to be space-balanced by the oval and the round window as in the case for waves conveyed by air. If the mechanics of the inner ear are described in terms of low-pass filters connected in series with the characteristic frequency decreasing systematically with the distance from the stapes, an oscillation will lead to a substantial deflection only in the suitable filter[1148, 1265] no matter where the energy input occurs.

Obviously, by superposition of oscillations conveyed to the inner ear in different ways, different effects of addition and subtraction can result depending on the phase relation between the different components. Thus, von Békésy[72] and Lowy[735] by adjusting suitable phase and intensity differences were able to compensate a tone offered via air transmission by a simultaneous tone offered via bone conduction.

II. PHYSIOLOGY OF THE AFFERENT AUDITORY PATHWAY

A. Anatomical Principles

The human auditory nerve is composed of approximately 30,000 fibers* (29,000 according to Guild,[436] 31,000 according to Rasmussen,[935] 25,000 according to Hall[443]) with fiber diameters between 3 to 10 μm.[380] Upon arrival at the cochlear nucleus every fiber splits into two branches; one branch runs to the dorsal portion and the other to the ventral part of the cochlear nucleus.† Those branches arriving at the dorsal part innervate the posterior part of the ventral cochlear nucleus also. The ventral cochlear nucleus has a complex structure so that, histologically, Lorente de Nó distinguished 13 different areas.‡

In general, the ventral cochlear nucleus is divided into a nucleus cochlearis posteroventralis (PVCN), a nucleus cochlearis anteroventralis (AVCN) and a nucleus cochlearis interstitialis (INCN). Frequently, one also speaks of an anterior part of the PVCN and of a posterior part of the PVCN and of the AVCN.

All fibers of the auditory nerve end in the cochlear nucleus. Recent studies based on tritiated-amino-acid-transport indicate the possibility of a projection of auditory nerve fibers beyond the cochlear nucleus.[178] However, a transneural transport could not be excluded.§ Each fiber makes contact with 75 to 100 cells of the cochlear nuclei. On the other hand, every cell of the cochlear nuclei has synaptic contact with many fibers of the

---

* Cat: 51,000 fibers; guinea pig: 27,000 fibers (Reference 381).

† References 475, 731, 732.

‡ For recent studies of the cochlear nucleus see references 57, 136, 440, 455, 456, 459, 539, 540, 677–679, 803, 804, 819, 822, 874, 875, 900, 1113, 1189.

§ References 178, 528, 628.

auditory nerve. Thus, the total amount of cells in the cochlear nuclei is only about two to three times larger than the number of nerve fibers in the cochlear nerve (88,000 in the monkey according to Chow[190]). This divergence-convergence principle of neuronal connection is typical for the central nervous system. With respect to the transmitter substances of the auditory nerve in the cochlear nucleus, some amino acids as well as acetylcholine could be excluded histochemically.[405, 406]

Three different fiber groups originate from the cochlear nuclei:

1. The stria acustica dorsalis (Monakow) originates primarily from the dorsal cochlear nucleus and runs to the midline (macroscopically visible next to the striae medullares in the fossa rhomboidea) across the lower cerebellar peduncle (pedunculus cerebellaris inferior or corpus restiforme), then turns ventrally and crosses the midline ventrally to the fasciculus longitudinalis medialis in order to join the medial part* of the contralateral lateral lemniscus[859, 876] and to branch off a few fibers to the contralateral superior olive.[330] Those fibers entering the lateral lemniscus end in the dorsal nucleus of the lateral lemniscus and in the inferior colliculus.[380]

2. The stria acustica intermedia (Held) is composed of neurites of a cell group of the PVCN† and ends in the periolivary nuclei of both sides.

3. The largest fiber group consists of neurites that stem primarily from the INCN and the AVCN to form the trapezoid body. The fibers of the AVCN predominantly run to the ipsilateral lateral superior olive and to the medial superior olive of both sides whereas the fibers of the INCN primarily end in the medial nucleus of the contralateral trapezoid body. Those fibers of the trapezoid body not ending in the superior olivary nuclei join the lateral part of the contralateral lateral lemniscus and end in the dorsal and ventral nuclei of the lateral lemniscus and in the inferior colliculus.

Many fibers of these three groups end in the area of the formatio reticularis ("unspecific auditory pathway," Galambos,[385] Magoun[739]). However, most fibers of the cochlear nucleus end in cell groups of the metencephalon summarized as the superior olivary complex. The nuclei of

---

* The medial and lateral part of the lateral lemniscus are separated by the nuclei of the lateral lemniscus.
† References 456, 859, 874, 1186.

the lateral lemniscus can be regarded as the rostral part of this complex and, strictly speaking, the nuclei of the trapezoid body belong to it also. One can distinguish the lateral olivary nucleus* (the S-shaped segment, nucl. oliv. sup. lat.), the medial nucleus accessorius (the nucl. oliv. sup. med.), and the ventral periolivary nuclei (the pre- and retro-olivary cell groups according to Ramón y Cajal[921]) of which the lateral preolivary nucleus passes over to the ventral nucleus of the lateral lemniscus. The ventral nucleus stretches over the whole length of the lateral lemniscus.

Those fibers originating from the lateral olivary nucleus run bilaterally in the lateral lemniscus to the lemniscal nuclei and to the inferior colliculus whereas the afferent fibers of the medial olivary nucleus run homolaterally to the lemniscal nuclei and to the inferior colliculus.[460, †] No fibers originating from the olive ascend beyond the level of the inferior colliculus. Further connections between the other parts of the olivary nucleus are not certain. The superior olivary complex certainly is of significance for reflexes triggered by acoustic stimuli. Direct fiber connections are known to exist to motor nuclei (e.g., to the abducens nucleus and to the motor nuclei of the trigeminal and facial nerve).

From the nuclei of the lateral lemniscus, fibers ascend to the inferior colliculus. There are connections also from the dorsal nuclei of the lateral lemniscus to the opposite side. In the monkey the superior olivary complex has 34,000 cells while the nuclei of the lateral lemniscus have 38,000 cells.[190]

All afferent fibers of the specific auditory pathway arrive at the inferior colliculus.[‡, 412, 859] The inferior colliculus was divided into three parts by Ramón y Cajal[921]: the central nucleus, the marginal area, and the external area. In recent times, Morest§ has examined this nucleus closer and divided it further. He distinguished a central nucleus, a dorsal and caudal marginal area, a lateral zone, an intercollicular commissural zone, and a dorsomedial nucleus.

---

* The lateral nucleus is especially well developed in the bat and in the dolphin. In the cat and in the dog it is also well developed, but it is very small in primates. On the other hand, the medial nucleus is strongly developed in primates, well developed in the dog and in the cat, but missing completely in the bat and in the dolphin; see references 327, 459, 512.

† According to Gacek (380), the fibers of the lateral olivary nucleus ascend homolaterally, those of the medial olivary nucleus ascend bilaterally.

‡ Following injections of horseradish peroxidase into the central nucleus of the inferior colliculus of the rat (Reference 113), cells within the cochlear nuclei (ipsi- and contralateral), superior olivary complex (ipsi- and contralateral) and auditory cortex (layer V) were stained. With the same technique (Reference 5) could be shown projections from the contralateral cortex, medial geniculate, hypothalamus, substantia nigra, superior colliculus and the central gray.

§ References 809, 814, 815, 817.

The central nucleus has cells with disc-shaped telodendria arranged in lamellae. The fibers entering from the lateral lemniscus run parallel to these lamellae; this is, according to Morest, of significance in connection with the tonotopic organization. Stellate cells make interlaminar connections.

The marginal zone has four layers of different cells. Collaterals and ascending fibers arrive in this region. There are also connections between the cortex and the central nucleus. The afferent fibers coming from the central nucleus end in the ventral part of the medial geniculate body.* In the monkey the inferior colliculus has 392,000 cells.[190] At the level of the inferior colliculus many connections exist to the contralateral side. The ascending projections of the inferior colliculus are highly differentially organized according to its subnuclei.[696]

The medial geniculate body is the thalamic nucleus of the central auditory pathway. All fibers originating from the inferior colliculus switch neurons in the medial geniculate. Even the afferent fibers of the unspecific auditory pathway (formatio reticularis) arrive here. Thus, the only access to the auditory cortex is via the medial geniculate. According to Chow[190] the principal part alone contains 364,000 cells (in the monkey).

In the medial geniculate, Monakow[800] distinguished two subnuclei, the pars principalis and the pars magnocellularis. The pars principalis consists of smaller, densely packed cells, whereas for the pars magnocellularis the larger, less densely packed cells are typical. This distinction has been adopted widely in later times.†

Dorsomedially, the principal part borders on the posterior nuclei of the thalamus whereas ventromedially it passes over to the magnocellular part. In the frontal and in the horizontal section the principal part has the shape of a half moon with the convex border forming the free surface of the medial geniculate and with the concave border surrounding the magnocellular part. In the principal part Ramón y Cajal[921] further distinguished a dorsal and a ventral part. Detailed descriptions of the medial geniculate have been based on Golgi preparations (besides the Nissl- and electron micrographic examinations) that have been published in recent years primarily by Morest.‡ These studies confirmed that, based on the dendrite pattern of the Golgi-type I-cells (principal cells), the principal part can be subdivided into a ventral and a dorsal part. In the ventral part§ only fascicular dendrites are encountered, in the dorsal part only radial dendrites, but in the magnocellular part both patterns occur. The architecture of the fibers is different

---

* References 40, 171, 185, 695, 806, 859, 912, 938, 1130.
† References 806, 866, 959, 975, 977.
‡ References 810, 812, 813.
§ According to Morest the ventral part is divided further into subnuclei, namely: pars lateralis nuclei ventralis, pars ovoidea nuclei ventralis, nucleus ventrolateralis and zona marginalis.

too. The ventral part has large axons (1 to 2.5 μm) and the cell bodies are surrounded by a fibrous condensation. This fiber plexus originates from the brachium colliculi inferioris. The dorsal part contains a dense plexus of thin (0.5 μm) diffusely arranged fibers. The ventral portion (pars lateralis and pars ovoidea) shows a laminar structure. Every axon entering from the brachium colliculi inferioris runs along those laminae branching off collaterals which insert with large synapses on the proximal dendrites of the principal cells. Thus, each cell of a lamina is in contact with the same axon. Thin descending corticothalamic axons insert on the distal dendrites of those cells. Further synapses were observed electron-microscopically. These are synapses between the dendrites of Golgi-type II-cells and the principal cells. Morest was able to follow the axons of the principal cells of the ventral part up to the primary auditory cortex.

The innervation of the dorsal part[*] is more complex which follows from the stellate dendrite pattern of the principal cells. Also, axons of cells located medial to the brachium colliculi inferioris and axons of cells of the pars magnocellularis have synaptic contacts to the stellate dendrites. Apparently, the dorsal part receives afferent input not only from the acoustic pathway but also from other sensory systems. This holds true primarily for the nucleus suprageniculatus and for the pars magnocellularis that receives afferent inputs from the medial lemniscus and the colliculus superior along with input from the inferior colliculus. All these subnuclei belong to the auditory system as has been proven by studies tracing the path of degeneration following sectioning,[†] even though additional connections to other sensory channels[‡] exist[§].

The axons of the principal cells of the medial geniculate ascend as radiatio acustica (in the sublenticular part of the inner capsule) to the auditory cortex. The auditory areas of the cerebral cortex are located in the Sylvian part of the gyrus temporalis superior (Gyri temporales transversi, Heschl's convolution), in the neighboring insular cortex, and in the parietal operculum.

The innervation of the auditory cortex by other sensory channels is even more pronounced than in the medial geniculate. Thus, the demarcation

---

[*] Andersen et al. (39) report that the primary region of the inferior colliculus does not project to the dorsal part.

[†] References 59, 171, 268, 530, 805, 806, 912, 939, 977, 1235.

[‡] Electrophysiologically, additional inputs of other sensory modalities have been demonstrated mainly for the pars magnocellularis. Upon stimulation of peripheral nerves, evoked potentials could be recorded here (References, 902, 1222–1224), as well as following vestibular stimulations (References 395, 766). Even multimodal sensory activation of single cells has been observed in the pars magnocellularis (References 117, 530, 733, 740–742, 1200).

[§] References 31, 134, 135, 175–177, 755.

of those areas belonging to the auditory system is extremely difficult. Demarking criteria are the cytoarchitecture,[382] retrograde degeneration and electrophysiological results. One interesting feature of the auditory conio-cortex is its extreme variability of structure. Thus, von Economo and Horn[278] were able to distinguish 11 subtypes of cortical structures in the area of the gyri temporales transversi alone. The demarcations of the auditory cortex obtained using different criteria are not identical. Figure 53 shows the auditory areas in the cat based on the cytoarchitecture. For comparison, Figure 54 shows the structure of the projection areas resulting from degeneration experiments with the auditory parts of the thalamus.

Originally it was assumed that the "primary auditory cortex" marked as AI in Figure 53 is superimposed on the "secondary auditory cortex" since Ades[7] was able to record auditory evoked electrical potentials from the secondary auditory cortex,* if he treated AI with strychnine. Based on latency measurements, Bremer[146] extended this secondary auditory cortex to AII (of Fig. 53). Kiang[630] and Dowman et al.,[272] however, demonstrated that the "secondary auditory cortex" is not exclusively activated via the "primary auditory cortex." They showed that after removal of AI, Ep and AII can still be activated by sound stimuli. Nevertheless, the existence of corticocortical connections between AI and the secondary areas AII and Ep has been proven† and it can be assumed that these areas do not work independently of each other.

There are also connections between the auditory pathway and the cerebellum. Already in 1944 Snider and Stowell[1052] discovered that, upon stimulation with clicks, bio-potentials ("evoked potentials") could be recorded from the cerebellar cortex of the cat. Similar results were reported later by several investigators.‡ Single-unit recordings from the cerebellar cortex have been described also.§ The patterns of discharge indicate a relation with the localization of the sound source. Likewise, light stimuli are apt to activate the cerebellar cortex. With auditory stimuli the latencies are short. Therefore, a short connection between the ear and the cerebellum must exist. Pathways connecting the dorsal part of the cochlear nucleus with the vermis of the cerebellum were found by Niemer and Cheng.[851] In any case, after destruction of the vermis, a retrograde chromatolysis occurs in the cochlear nucleus. The tecto-pontine pathway described by Rasmussen[936] is another possible connection with the cerebellum. On the other hand, stimulation of the "audio-visual" cerebellar cortex evokes responses in the cerebrocortical auditory cortex and vice versa. In 1932, Mettler[762] described in the cat a projection pathway from the auditory cortex to the pons. The

---

* According to Ades (7), the area marked Ep in Figure 53.
† References 266, 267, 272, 364, 529, 762, 880, 881.
‡ References 111, 323, 482, 1241.
§ References 19, 33, 366, 736, 747, 821, 1034.

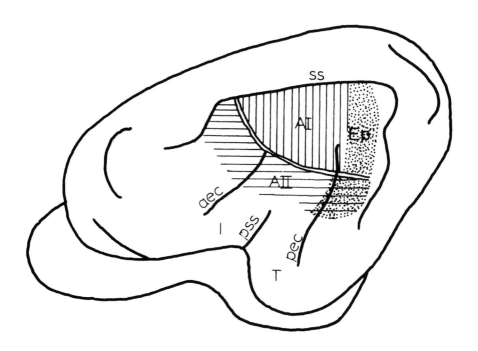

FIGURE 53. The three auditory areas defined according to the cyto-architecture. ss = gyrus suprasylvicus; Ep = ectosylvian posterior auditory area; AI = primary auditory cortex; AII = secondary auditory cortex; I = insular cortex; T = temporal auditory cortex; aec = sulcus ectosylvicus anterior; pss = sulcus cerebri lateralis; pec = sulcus ectosylvicus posterior. (According to Rose and Woolsey [975].)

proof of an anatomical (not functional) pontocerebellar auditory connection is still missing. Here, the tecto-pontine pathway described by Rasmussen[936] has to be considered.

The connection of the reticular activating system with the auditory pathway occurs according to our present knowledge at the level of the brain stem. Arousal reactions (i.e., central activations) can be triggered easily by auditory stimuli.[182, 183] They even occur in animals with a bilateral transection of the specific auditory pathways. Thus, an "unspecific" auditory system with more of a general activating function than a special function must exist. The interconnection between the specific and the unspecific pathways apparently plays an important role within the framework of the "sensory optimalization function of the CNS."[561] Figure 55 schematically summarizes the course of the auditory pathway just described.

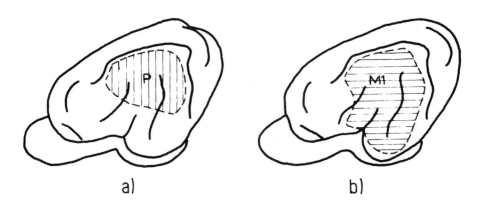

a)   b)

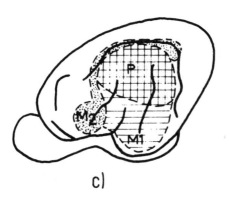

c)

FIGURE 54. A, P = cortex auditivus principalis, defined as projection area of the pars principalis of the medial geniculate. B, M_1 = multisensory auditory cortex, defined as the projection area of the multisensory parts of the geniculate. C, Combined representation showing the overlap of P and M_1, and of the multisensory area M_2 resulting as projection area of the nucleus suprageniculatus. (According to Harrison and Howe [460].)

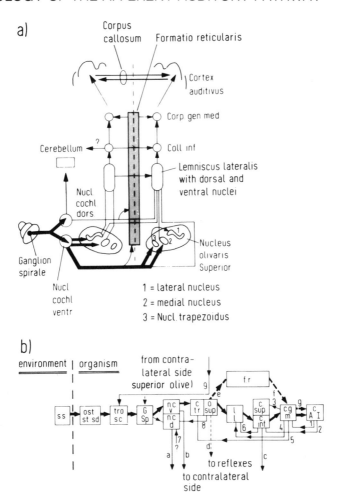

FIGURE 55. A, Simplified schematic representation of the afferent auditory pathway. For the sake of clarity the pathways of only one cochlea are shown. The commissures at the level of the lateral lemniscus and the inferior colliculus are shown in one direction only since it is generally assumed that fibers after having crossed once to the opposite side do not cross back again. However, this does not preclude the existence of connections "back" to the original side after synaptic transmission has taken place to neurons being innervated ipsilaterally on the opposite side. In this sense, the arrows could point in either direction. (According to Kallert [535].) B, Block diagram of the auditory pathway. ss = sound source; ost = organ for stimulus transmission; st = stimulus transmission; sd = stimulus distribution; tro = transformation organ; sc = sensory cells; GSp = Ganglion spirale; n.c.v. = nucleus cochlearis ventralis; n.c.d. = nucleus cochlearis dorsalis; c.tr. = corpus trapezoidum; o.sup. = oliva superior; f.r. = Formatio reticularis; l.l. = lemniscus lateralis; c.sup. = colliculus superior; c.inf. = colliculus inferior; c.g.m. = corpus geniculatum mediale; c.A.I. = cortex auditivus principalis. (According to Keidel [558].)

B. The Cochlear Nerve

The cochlear nerve has a tonotopic structure.[56, 901] That is, certain sound frequencies are associated with certain fibers, just as in the inner ear a tonotopic representation exists (place theory, see page 4). This was described by Lorente de Nó[731] and Lewy and Kobrak[716] based on degeneration experiments. This tonotopic relation has also been confirmed electrophysiologically. If one describes the single fibers by their characteristic frequency one can find that, upon advancing a microelectrode through the cochlear nerve of the cat posterodorsally to anteroventrally, fibers with a high characteristic frequency are encountered first, then fibers with a successively lower characteristic frequency and, finally, fibers having increasingly higher characteristic frequencies. Thus, fibers with a high characteristic frequency are located around the perimeter while those with a lower characteristic frequency are located more centrally.[636]

For studying the functional efficiency of the cochlear nerve, recordings of action potentials from single fibers by means of micro-electrodes are of special value. The first examinations of this kind were carried out by Galambos and Davis[386, *] later supplemented by Katsuki et al.[†] and advanced strongly by Kiang and colleagues[636-639] and by Rose and colleagues.[‡]

As a rule, the evaluation is done using statistical methods. For that purpose the same stimulus is presented several times in succession at suitable intervals and the recorded action potentials are added in a temporally correct manner with the aid of electronic computers. As a result, histograms are obtained. Since the information content of recorded action potentials is not the voltage but the temporal sequence of the spikes, time histograms are used for studying the function of single neurons. The most important time histograms are:

1. the post-stimulus-time histogram (PST-histogram);
2. the interval histogram;
3. the joint-interval histogram; and
4. the period histogram.

The post-stimulus-time histogram represents the temporal frequency distribution of action potentials. The abscissa gives the time following stimulus onset (as zero-time any other defined time before stimulus onset

---

* However, later it became likely that in these studies recordings might have been obtained from scattered neurons of the cochlear nucleus. Thus, as a rule, Tasaki[1131] is now mentioned first.
† References 545, 548, 549.
‡ References 981, 982, 984.

can be used) while the ordinate gives the number of recorded action spikes per bin* for a predetermined number of stimuli.

The interval histogram represents the frequency distribution of the time intervals between two successive action potentials. Thus, the abscissa gives the intervals in temporal units and the ordinate gives the number of such recorded time intervals per total time of analysis and per bin.

The joint-interval histogram represents the frequency distribution of interval combinations determined by successive intervals. These histograms are three-dimensional. The two axes in the drawing plane give the lengths of intervals as does the abscissa in the interval histogram and the axis vertical to this plane gives the frequency.

The period histogram is analogous to the PST-histogram, however, instead of the time the abscissa gives the phase value of the stimulus period. Most often, however, the corresponding time value is given and the stimulus period is represented as a wave line in the histogram (e.g. Fig. 64). Thus, the timing on the abscissa starts with the beginning of each stimulus period.

Interval histograms, joint-interval histograms, and period histograms can be obtained from a sequence of action spikes elicited also by a continuous tone or from a sequence of spontaneous discharges. However, for obtaining post-stimulus-time histograms, several equal stimuli are always necessary (Fig. 56).

All reports on single-fiber studies agree that most fibers show spontaneous activity. This means that action potentials can be recorded without any auditory stimulus. This spontaneous activity[†] ranges from a few spikes per minute to about 100 spikes per second.[‡] With respect to the time pattern, the spontaneous activity of the cochlear fibers is irregular[1182] as opposed to the vestibular fibers and follows the statistical laws of a Poisson-distribution[§] regarding the frequency of the time intervals between the action spikes.

---

* The term bin describes the time resolution of the abscissa determined by the computer program. These programs can be different for different histograms. If, for instance, 1 bin = 1 ms, the ordinate of a post-stimulus-time histogram would be given by the number of action spikes between 0 and 1 ms, between 1 ms and 2 ms and so forth. In an interval histogram the ordinate would be given by the number of all intervals between 0 and 1 ms, between 1 ms and 2 ms, between 2 ms and 3 ms and so forth.

† In 1979 Kim et al. (642) described a bimodal distribution of cochlear nerve fibers with respect to spontaneous rate (SR). The low-SR population with SR < 15 spikes/s comprises 24% and the high-SR population with SR ≥ 15 spikes/s comprises 76% of the total sample. The mode of the high-SR population in the pooled sample is 50 to 60 spikes/s.

‡ References 303, 636, 858, 984.

§ The Poisson-distribution obeys a mathematically defined relation following from general considerations of the theory of probability under the assumption that the

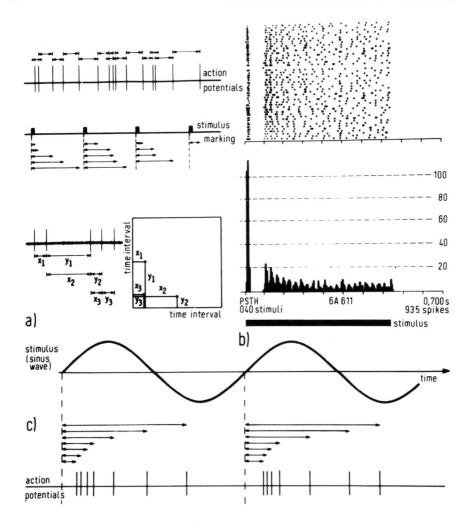

FIGURE 56. A, The upper row shows the lengths of intervals as double arrows; they represent the values on the abscissa for the interval-histograms. The middle row shows the temporal distances (arrows) of the action potentials from the stimulus onset; they are the values on the abscissa for the post-stimulus-time histograms. Below is shown how a joint-interval histogram is formed. B, Formation of a histogram. Above: the dots in each line show the sequence of action potentials triggered by one stimulus presentation. The abscissa represents the time following stimulus onset. Thus, each line gives the recording of the action potentials for one stimulus; the ordinate gives the numbers of stimuli. Below: by addition of the columns a post-stimulus time histogram results from the dotted diagram above. Only here the periodicity of the sequence of the action potential is clearly visible. C, Pure tone as stimulus and, underneath, the corresponding sequence of action potentials. With each beginning of a period (vertical lines) the timing for the abscissa of the histogram starts. The double arrows represent the value on the abscissa for the period-histogram. (According to Keidel [573].)

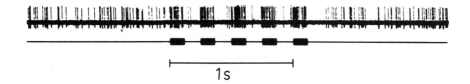

FIGURE 57. Spontaneous and stimulus-related activity of a single fiber of the cat's cochlear nerve. Upper line: record of action potentials that, for the time scale chosen, appear as spikes (needle impulses). Lower line: record of the stimuli (tone bursts of 9.5 kHz, 15 dB above threshold). (According to Evans [308].)

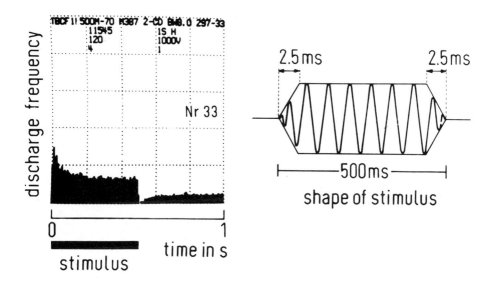

FIGURE 58. Response pattern of an auditory nerve fiber represented as a histogram. Tone bursts served as stimuli. They are 500 ms tones having a 2.5 ms rise/fall time. The envelope of the signal, therefore, is not rectangular but has the shape of a double trapezoid as shown in the right part of the figure. This is the typical discharge pattern of the auditory nerve. Discharges occur for the whole duration of the stimulus. A very strong excitation occurs at the beginning of the stimulus decreasing monotonically and, after about 20 to 30 ms, reaching a value which is maintained to the end of the stimulus (adaptation). The latency (i.e., the time difference between stimulus onset and the beginning of excitation) is only 1 to 4 ms. Correspondingly, the discharge sequence stops shortly after the end of the stimulus. (Modified according to Kiang et al. [636].)

With tone stimuli of suitable frequency and of sufficient intensity a pronounced stimulus-related increase of discharge (Fig. 57) is obtained. The description of action potentials in a post-stimulus-time histogram triggered by a series of stimuli yields an identical discharge pattern* (Fig. 58) for all fibers of the cochlear nerve.

The minimal intensity of a tone stimulus necessary to trigger action spikes depends on the stimulus frequency. The threshold intensity (minimal stimulus intensity for eliciting action spikes as function of stimulus frequency) is described by the frequency-threshold curves (FTC or tuning curves) having a characteristic shape. For each fiber a certain frequency exists at which this curve has an absolute minimum. This frequency is labeled "best frequency" or "characteristic frequency" of the fiber in question† (Fig. 59). At stimulus intensities above these curves stimulus-related discharges occur in the corresponding fiber, but they do not occur at intensities below the curve. Thus, the area above the threshold curve is called the response area.

The area of stimulus frequencies for which the fiber is excitable is very narrow at low stimulus intensities, but it becomes wider with increasing intensity. At very high intensities, excitation results for practically all frequencies below the characteristic frequency. The steep slope on the high frequency side (see page 17) is particularly conspicuous. Earlier studies showed that the threshold intensity at a given characteristic frequency varied by 40 to 60 dB. In analogy to the different innervation of the inner ear (spiral fibers and radial fibers, see page 57) a distinction between two populations of auditory nerve fibers with different thresholds and different shapes of tuning curves has been taken into consideration.‡ However, Kiang showed that, after compensation for the frequency response of the stimulator and after elimination of the middle ear muscles, the differences in curve shape§ disappear and the scatter of the threshold values is reduced to

---

events occur independently of each other. The proof that a frequency distribution (here the frequency of different time intervals between successive action spikes) agrees with a Poisson-distribution thus demonstrates the independency of the events from each other. This means that the length of an interval is independent of the following interval. In the interval distribution a deviation from the general Poisson-distribution occurs in so far as the shortest possible interval is determined by the refractory period.

* However, Kohllöffel (673) was able to record different response patterns from the spiral ganglion.

† This characteristic frequency can also be obtained using frequency modulated tones (Reference 1038).

‡ References 546, 547, 549.

§ The temporal invariance of the tuning curves was observed by Simmons and Linehan (1037) in a chronic experiment over six weeks.

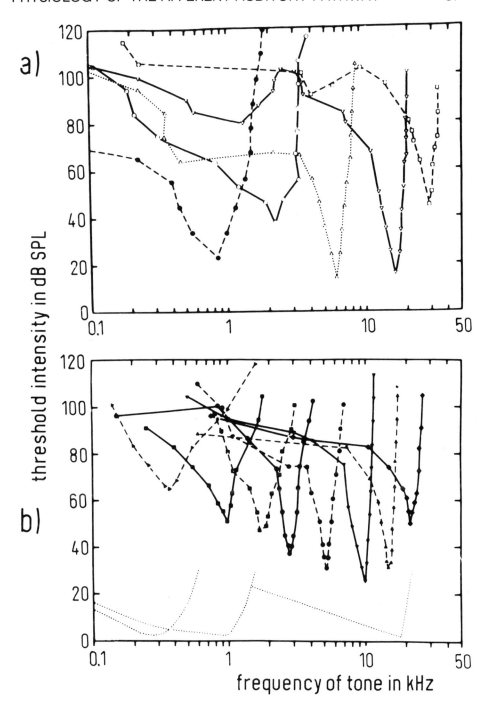

FIGURE 59. Typical examples of tuning curves of single auditory-nerve fibers: A, in the cat (according to Kiang et al. [638]); and B, in the guinea pig (according to Evans [303].)

less than 20 dB if the data are collected from one single animal (intra-individual scatter). Within this narrow range there is a tendency for fibers with low spontaneous activity to have higher thresholds and vice versa.[640] Thus, when measured appropriately there is little scatter for intra-individual threshold values. In addition, the neural thresholds approach those obtained from behavioral experiments, with the exception of these threshold values obtained from fibers with a high characteristic frequency.[308]

Whereas the tuning curves make a statement only about the excitatory behavior at threshold intensity, the reaction of single fibers to tones of any suprathreshold intensity can be described by "frequency response curves" (iso-intensity curves).[486-488] For that purpose, tones of different frequencies but of equal intensity are presented and the number of spikes per unit of time is recorded (Figs. 60 and 61). These curves also clearly show that each fiber has a characteristic frequency. Also, at higher intensities saturation can be noted affecting necessarily the range around the characteristic frequency. The frequency-response curves look less sharply tuned, this is partially due to the saturation phenomenon and partially because the scale on the abscissa is not logarithmic (as in the tuning curves) but linear. If these curves are changed into curves of equal discharge rate, they all resemble the tuning curves (Fig. 62).

The frequency-response curves clearly demonstrate how the effective frequency range is related to the intensity of the stimulus. Upon stimulation with pseudo-stochastic noise and by the use of cross-correlation techniques, Møller[792-795] also could demonstrate the frequency selectivity of single nerve fibers.

By varying the stimulus intensity the same discharge rate can be elicited in the same fiber using very different stimulus frequencies. Upon stimulation with pure tones having frequencies not higher than 4000 Hz the discharges occur phase-locked with the stimulus, irrespective of the characteristic frequency of a certain fiber, provided the stimulus intensity is high enough to elicit excitations. This behavior was thoroughly studied in modern times by Rose et al.[981-984] Anderson et al.,[41] Brugge et al.,[155] Rose[972, 973] and Pfeiffer and Molnar.[889] Interestingly, not every stimulus cycle is an effective stimulus as can be seen from the interval histogram (Fig. 63). For high frequencies with periods below 500 to 700 μs the refractory period could be a limiting factor. This may also hold for stimulus frequencies having a relatively long period. As a rule, the intervals between two consecutive action spikes are much longer than the refractory period (Table 2).

The period histogram shows that the action potentials are phase-locked to the stimulus so that most excitations occur only during one half of the period (Fig. 64). If two non-harmonic tones, either one of which triggers a phase-locked excitation, are offered simultaneously, there is of course no fixed phase relation between the stimuli themselves. The action potentials, depending on the intensity relation of the two tones, are phase-locked either

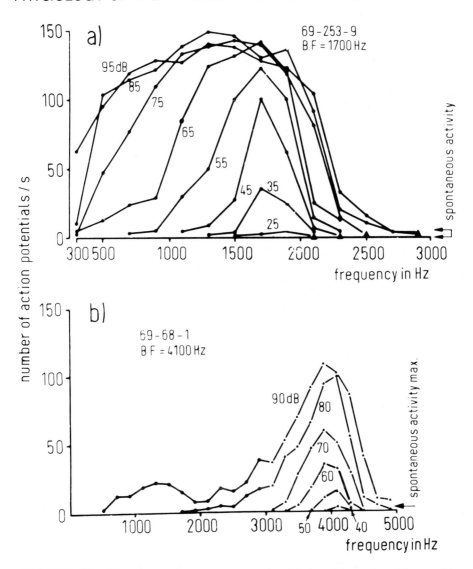

FIGURE 60. Frequency response curves obtained from two fibers of low spontaneous activity of the cochlear nerve of the squirrel monkey. (According to Rose et al. [984].)

with both tones or with one of them only (Fig. 65). The latter case may perhaps correspond with the psychological effect of masking. If however two harmonically related tones are presented simultaneously, a fixed phase relation is obtained between the two tones and a complex tone with a constant period results. If the phase angle between both tones is varied, the form of the complex tone can thus be changed. Phase shifts of this kind are of no consequence for the discharge rate. However, the period histogram shows that the time pattern of the discharges strongly depends on the

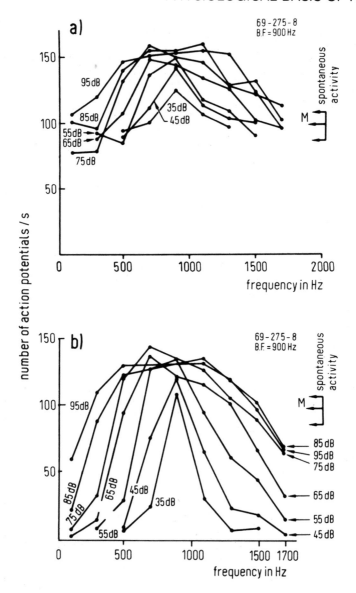

FIGURE 61. Frequency response curves obtained from a fiber of high spontaneous activity of the cochlear nerve of the squirrel monkey. A, All action potentials are taken into account. B, Only those action potentials in synchrony with the stimulus (see page 90) are considered. (According to Rose et al. [984].)

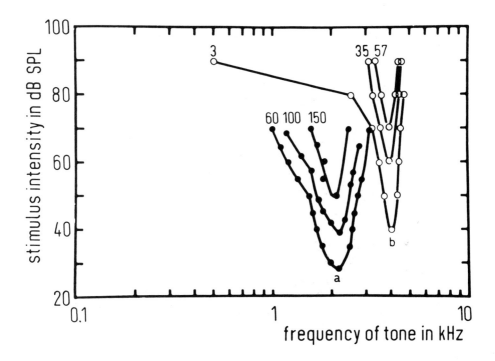

FIGURE 62. Curves of equal discharge rate (parameter: average number of action potentials per second). A, Cat; average spontaneous rate was 50 action potentials per second. B, Squirrel monkey (from the data of Fig. 60b); negligible spontaneous activity. (According to Evans [308].)

waveform of the complex stimulus (Fig. 66). Also, the intensity of such a complex tone stimulus is reflected by the period histogram (Fig. 67). Since the shape of the stimulus plotted as a continuous curve in the different period histograms corresponds with the temporal pattern of the movement of the basilar membrane (at a certain place), these results support the idea that the deflection of the membrane only in one direction causes an excitation and that the magnitude of excitation is proportional to the amplitude of basilar membrane deflection.

The phase lag occurring between stimulus onset and excitation depends on the place along the basilar membrane where excitation is triggered[891] and, thus on the characteristic frequency of the fiber. This is simply a reflection of the propagation time of the travelling wave in the inner ear (Fig. 68).

Excitations coupled with the stimulus phase support the old hypothesis of "periodicity hearing"* at least for the low frequency range (see page 4).

---

* "Periodicity hearing" as opposed to "spatial hearing" in the sense of the one-site theory and the tonotopic representation.

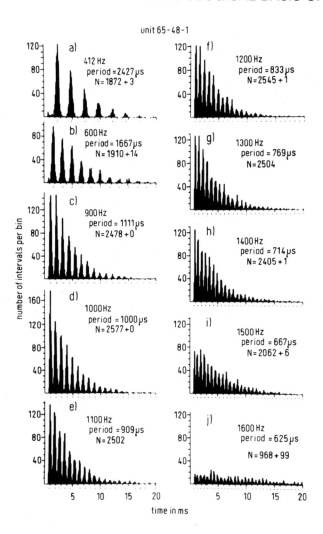

FIGURE 63. Interval histograms of a fiber upon stimulation with tones of different frequencies. Each histogram is derived for pure-tone stimuli of 1 second duration. 1 bin = 100 μs. The dots underneath the abscissa denote the integer values of the stimulus period. The two numbers for N give the number of the counted intervals (first number) and the number of intervals having exceeded the abscissa (second number). Intensity of all stimuli 80 dB SPL. (According to Rose et al. [981].)

Table 2.
Probability of occurrence of the next action potential being triggered by one of the 1st to the 10th periods of a pure tone following an action potential which had occurred at time "zero." Computed from the sequences of excitation triggered by 10 tones of 1 s duration. (According to Rose et al. [982]).

Frequency in Hz	Periods of pure-tone stimulus										Total number of action potentials triggered	Number of stimulus periods	Action potentials per period
	1	2	3	4	5	6	7	8	9	10			
408	0.16	0.16	0.19	0.20	0.17	0.19	0.18	0.18	0.25	0.25	746	4080	0.18
850	0.16	0.20	0.22	0.23	0.21	0.22	0.23	0.30	0.22	0.26	1798	8500	0.21
1000	0.14	0.16	0.18	0.20	0.20	0.19	0.18	0.24	0.18	0.18	1832	10000	0.18
1150	0.14	0.16	0.18	0.18	0.21	0.20	0.20	0.21	0.21	0.19	2077	11500	0.18
1500	0.11	0.15	0.15	0.17	0.16	0.17	0.17	0.19	0.19	0.15	2351	15000	0.16
1700	0.07	0.11	0.12	0.14	0.13	0.14	0.13	0.12	0.13	0.16	2099	17000	0.12
2000	0.04	0.06	0.08	0.08	0.10	0.09	0.10	0.09	0.10	0.09	1791	20000	0.09

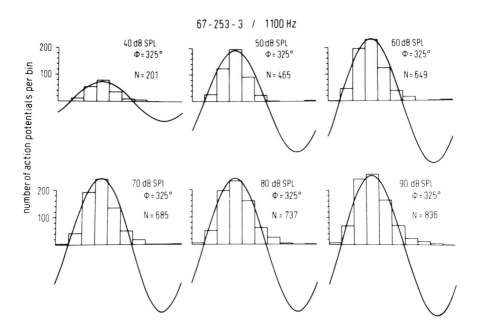

FIGURE 64. Period histogram of a fiber upon stimulation with sinus tones of the characteristic frequency (1100 Hz) and of different stimulus intensities. The smooth curve gives the respective temporal course of the pressure of the stimulus.

Length of period 912 μ s, 1 bin = 92 μ s, N = number of action potentials, Ø = phase shift of the sine wave against the origin of the coordinates, stimulus duration 5 s. (According to Rose et al. [984].)

One should consider, however, the possibility that the central nervous system is not capable of taking avantage of this temporal order. "If it can not, anything we can extract with an oscilloscope or a computer is quite irrelevant."[1213] One can assume, however, that under physiologically meaningful stimulus conditions (i.e. the stimulus intensity is substantially higher than the threshold intensity as, for instance, in the main speech area of Fig. 1), those fibers having much higher characteristic frequencies are excited by low frequency components since the stimulus intensity is above the corresponding low-frequency "tail" of the tuning curves belonging to those fibers.

In addition, tuning curves are changed, primarily in the range of the characteristic frequency, by background noise. This is especially true for low frequency background noise (Fig. 69). Thus, Kiang and Moxon[635] were able to show that the speech-elicited excitation pattern of a fiber having a high characteristic frequency stays unchanged after adding noise, whereas the pattern of a fiber having a low characteristic frequency can be suppressed completely by addition of noise (Fig. 70). From this result they infer that the loss of units having a high characteristic frequency may possibly lead, in the

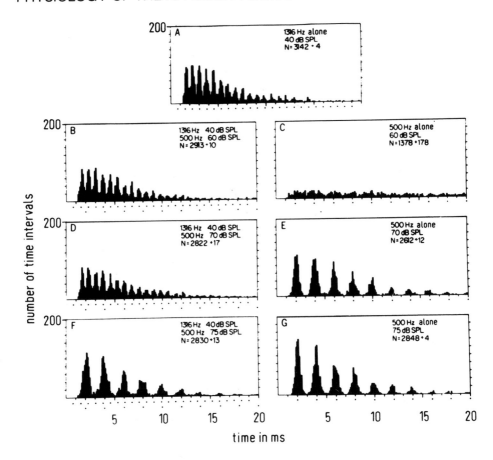

FIGURE 65. Interval histograms of the excitations of an auditory nerve fiber upon stimulation with pure tones or with combined tones of different intensities as given for each histogram. (According to Rose [973].)

old age, to a restriction of speech understanding if a low frequency background noise is present.

These results may be related to the phenomenon of two-tone inhibition. In fact, in practically all fibers the discharges triggered by one tone can be suppressed by a suitable second tone when presented simultaneously, whereas each tone presented separately is able to elicit a discharge. This is called two-tone inhibition. For each fiber, inhibition areas, like response areas, can be determined (Figs. 71 and 72).

As a rule, such inhibition areas are located on either side of the response area. With increasing intensity of the tone bursts, the discharge rate produced by the continuous tone decreases to a minimum (-10 dB in Fig. 72 b, middle line), thereafter it increases again. That is, the inhibition is not monotonically related with the intensity of the inhibitory stimulus. It is

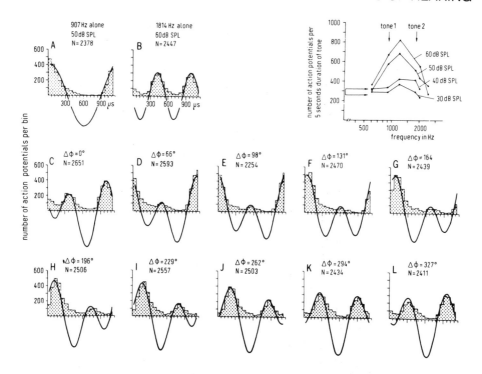

FIGURE 66. Changes of the discharge pattern of an auditory nerve fiber depending on the phase difference between the tone components of a sound stimulus composed of two pure tones acting simultaneously. Each histogram is based on 2 stimuli of 10 s duration each.

1 bin = 60 μs, period length of the complex sound stimulus = 1,102 ms, N = number of the recorded action potentials. A and B: period histograms upon stimulation with the single tone components (907 Hz and 1814 Hz) alone, C to L: period histograms upon stimulation with the sound stimulus composed of the two tones but with changing phase differences between the two pure-tone components ($\Delta\emptyset$). The smooth curve gives the respective temporal course of pressure of the stimulus. (According to Brugge et al. [155].)

further noticed (Fig. 72) that the inhibition as well as the excitation follows an "adaptation time course."

The mechanism underlying this inhibitory effect is still unknown. The most detailed descriptions are found in Sachs and Kiang,[1003] Sachs,[1002] Arthur et al.,[58] and in Abbas and Sachs.[1] Two-tone inhibition was also described by Nomoto et al.,[858] Hind et al.,[486] Liff and Goldstein[722] and by Frishkopf.[368] Schmiedt and Zwislocki[1012] found inversion of two-tone inhibition in "two-tone-summation" after cochlear lesions by exposure to impulse noise or treatment with Kanamycin which destroys initially the outer hair cells leaving the inner hair cell population apparently intact.

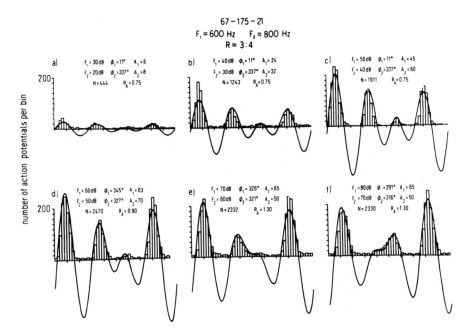

FIGURE 67. Period histograms of the discharges of an auditory-nerve fiber upon stimulation with a sound stimulus composed of two pure-tone components (600 Hz and 800 Hz) both of which were increased in steps of 10 dB. R_A = amplitude A relative to amplitude B. (According to Rose et al. [984].)

This process clearly is not mediated by efferent fibers since two-tone inhibition could be recorded from the peripheral stump of the severed auditory nerve[369, 636] and after sectioning the crossed and uncrossed olivocochlear bundles.[631] A neuronal interaction in the sense of lateral inhibition is regarded by all authors as being very unlikely. Rather, the underlying process is assumed to be located in the mechanics of the inner ear.[707]

An excitation can also be produced by tone combination. Thus, Nomoto et al.[858] were the first to demonstrate that two tones of suitable frequency, if presented simultaneously, lead to an excitation when either tone alone did not. This was examined more extensively by Kiang[631] and by Goldstein[419] with tones of the frequencies f_1 and f_2, both being outside the response area of the fiber in question, but with the frequency difference ($2f_1 - f_2$) coinciding with the characteristic frequency. The response to such tone combinations behaves as if in fact a tone of the frequency $2f_1 - f_2$ was presented.[420] The excitation caused by an additional tone of frequency $2f_1 - f_2$ and of suitable phase could abolish the response. This phenomenon has been known for a longer time from psychological experiments (e.g., Zwicker[1258]).

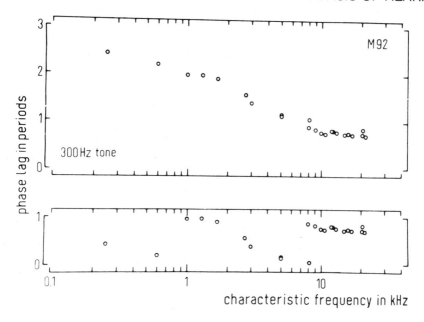

FIGURE 68. Phase delay as a function of the characteristic frequency of the fiber as recorded from 23 fibers in the cat. The stimulus was a 300 Hz tone of 83 dB SPL. The lower graph shows the phase delay between 0 and 1 period, the upper graph shows the same data with integer multiples of a period supplemented such that a monotonic curve results. (According to Kiang and Moxon [635].)

   Stimuli much more complicated than pure tones are clicks.* They are caused by short electric rectangular pulses (e.g., 100 μs duration) applied to a loudspeaker. Upon stimulation with clicks, characteristic post-stimulus-time histograms are obtained. Following click presentation several discharges occur with a regular temporal pattern showing several frequency peaks in the histogram in fibers having a characteristic frequency lower than 5 kHz. Interestingly, the latency (the time interval between stimulus onset and the first action potential triggered by the stimulus) depends on the characteristic frequency of the fiber such that latencies become shorter with increasing characteristic frequency. This is analogous to the different travelling time of the pressure wave in the inner ear and suggests that the characteristic frequency of a fiber is determined by the place of origin along the basilar membrane.†

---

* As an aperiodic event, according to Fourier, they include practically all frequencies.
† Anderson and colleagues (41), upon stimulation with different frequencies, determined the travelling time in the inner ear from the phase shift in the period histogram. In addition they found that the average phase angle between stimulus and response depends on the stimulus intensity in a peculiar way. For stimulus

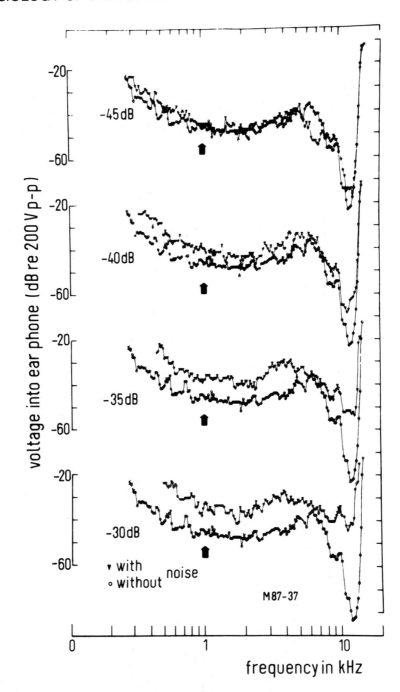

FIGURE 69. Effect of band-pass noise (center frequency = 1 kHz, band width = 500 Hz) of different intensities on the tuning properties of a fiber with a high characteristic frequency. Corresponding tuning curves without additional noise are shown for comparison. The arrow marks the center frequency of the band-pass noise. (According to Kiang and Moxon [635].)

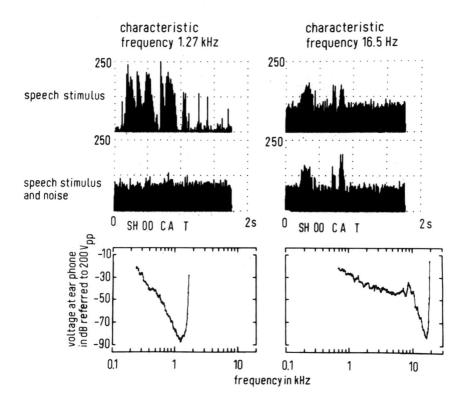

FIGURE 70. Effect of low-frequency background noise on the excitations of two auditory-nerve fibers of different characteristic frequencies (1.27 kHz and 16.5 kHz) triggered by speech stimuli. The speech stimulus was the words "Shoo-cat" shown in the correct temporal relation below the post-stimulus-time histogram. The histogram following the speech stimulus without additional noise is shown on the top, the histogram following the speech stimulus with noise is shown in the middle, and the corresponding tuning curve is shown on the bottom; on the left for the fiber with the lower characteristic frequency and on the right for the fiber with the higher characteristic frequency. According to the speech spectogram, the main frequency components of the speech stimulus ranged between 0.3 and about 3.5 kHz. (According to Kiang and Moxon [635].)

The temporal distance between the frequency peaks of a histogram is equal to the period of the characteristic frequency (Fig. 73) and, thus reflects the oscillatory behavior of the basilar membrane. If double clicks having a temporal distance of exactly half the period of the characteristic frequency

---

frequencies below the characteristic frequency, the discharge occurs later with increasing intensity; above the characteristic frequency, the discharge occurs earlier with increasing intensity; and close to the characteristic frequency, the phase angle changes little or not at all with intensity.

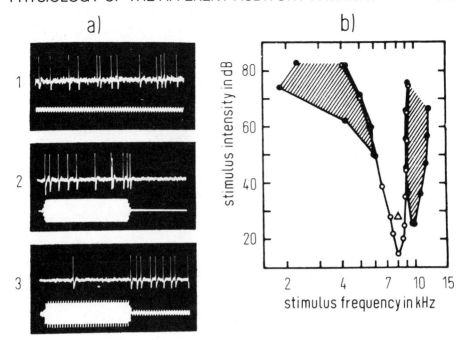

FIGURE 71. An example of two-tone inhibition (A) and excitatory and inhibitory areas (B). A, A single primary auditory neurone responds to a 40 dB continuous tone at the best frequency of 360 c/s (A1), and also to a 60 dB tone burst of 720 c/s (A2). When these two tones are simultaneously delivered, inhibition is demonstrated (A3). The duration and rise-decay time of the tone burst are 100 and 2.5 ms, respectively. B, The ordinate represents sound pressure level (dB referred to 0.0002 dyne/cm²) and the abscissa, stimulus frequency in kHz. The area above the tuning curve (open circles) is the excitatory one in which the discharge rate is more than 20% above the spontaneous rate. The hatched areas are inhibitory ones in which the response to a continuous tone at the best frequency (triangle) plus a second tone is more than 20% below the response to the continuous tone alone. (According to Arthur et al. [58].)

are used as stimuli, then the response phases following the second click coincide with the silent phases belonging to the first click and vice versa. The intensity relation can be chosen such that the silent phase of the one click abolishes the response phase of the other click. This demonstrates that the silent phases are not simply quiet periods or inactivity but that they are inhibitory phases.[402] This is in line with the idea that the deflection of the basilar membrane in one direction is excitatory, while deflection in the other direction is inhibitory.

If the post-stimulus-time histograms of a fiber obtained with clicks of opposite polarity are combined (Fig. 74), a picture is obtained which

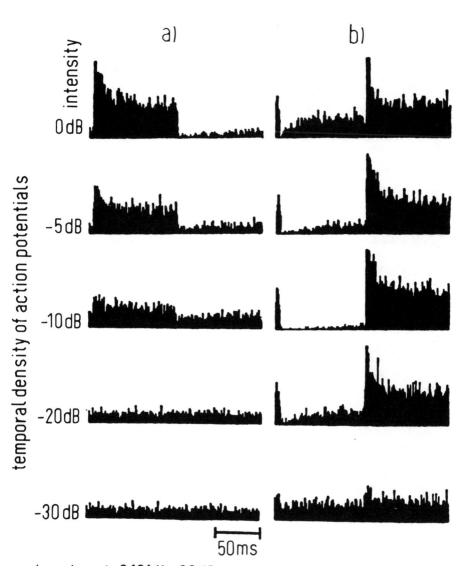

tone burst: 8161 Hz 90dB / steady tone 13190 Hz 74 dB

FIGURE 72. Post-stimulus-time histogram of a single fiber. A, Responses to 128 tone bursts per histogram of 100 ms length and of different intensities. B, Response upon combination of the tone bursts with a continuous inhibitory tone. (According to Arthur et al. [58].)

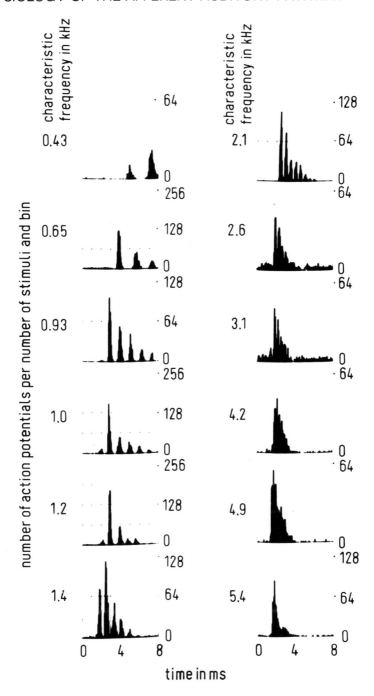

FIGURE 73. Post-stimulus-time histogram upon stimulation with clicks. It can be seen that the latency decreases with increasing characteristic frequency and that the distances between the peaks correspond with the period of the characteristic frequency. (According to Kiang et al. [636].)

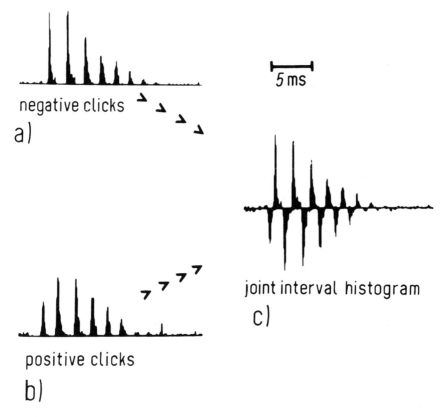

5 ms

negative clicks

a)

positive clicks

b)

joint interval histogram

c)

FIGURE 74. A, Post-stimulus-time histogram of a fiber following rarefaction clicks. B, Post-stimulus-time histogram of a fiber following condensation clicks. C, Sum of A and B being inverted. (According to Pfeiffer and Kim [890].)

corresponds with the oscillation of the basilar membrane following click stimulation as measured by Robles et al.[963, *]

With respect to the dependency of the magnitude of excitation on the stimulus intensity the discharge rate, as a rule, represents a monotonic function (Fig. 75). The dynamic range of these intensity functions typically covers only 20 to 50 dB.

Even if it is assumed that the scatter of the threshold values is about 20 dB the single fiber cannot encode the whole intensity range of about 120 dB covered by the ear. This problem has not yet been settled. Perhaps the middle ear and the efferent system must work together in order to handle the wide intensity range. In this connection, the low-frequency tails of fibers

---

* From the number of the frequency peaks Pfeiffer and Kim (890) deduced the existence of two fiber populations which were supposed to correspond with the inner and outer hair cells.

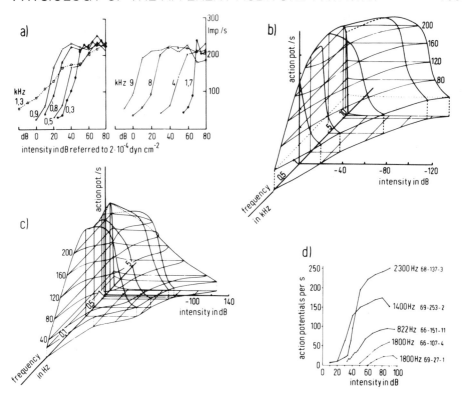

FIGURE 75. A, Intensity functions of two auditory fibers. The dashed function of the left diagram, against the rule, increases over an intensity range of more than 80 dB (at characteristic frequency), for all the other functions this range is 20 dB. B, Three-dimensional description of the intensity function of the single fiber with a small dynamic range, illustrated by the right diagram of A. C, Three-dimensional description of the intensity function of the fiber with a dynamic range of more than 80 dB, illustrated by the left diagram of A. (A to C according to Nomoto et al. [858].) D, At the characteristic frequency the discharge rate shows a large variability. It ranges between 30 and 250 action potentials per second. (According to Rose et al. [984].)

having a high characteristic frequency could conceivably play an important role. At very high intensities, the ability to discriminate pitch decreases suggesting that intensity may perhaps be encoded by the number of activated fibers. Sachs and Abbas[1004] have thoroughly investigated the relation between the discharge rate of single auditory nerve fibers and the stimulus intensity.

According to Kiang et al.[639] and Kiang and Moxon[634] at very high stimulus intensities (90 dB SPL and more) a remarkable decrease in the discharge rate of a single fiber can occur within a few dB (Fig. 76). This phenomenon too has not yet been explained satisfactorily.

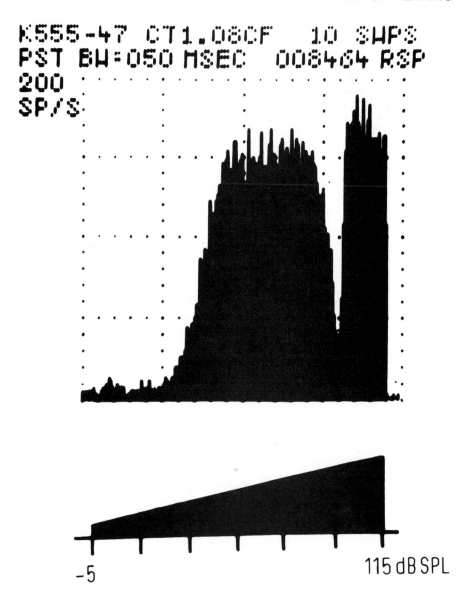

FIGURE 76. Discharge rate of an auditory nerve fiber as a function of the intensity of a tone of the fiber's characteristic frequency (1.08 kHz). For the first 10 bins (0.5 s) the stimulus was not switched on, during the next 180 bins (9 s) the intensity of the tone was changed continuously from -5 dB to 115 dB SPL, for the last 10 bins (0.5 s) the stimulus was absent. The histogram is based on 10 stimuli. (According to Kiang and Moxon [634].)

Whereas the results described so far were obtained essentially from the cat, the squirrel monkey, and the guinea pig, Gross and Anderson[431] described intracochlear microelectrode recordings from single neurons of the auditory nerve in the pigeon. The results are in good agreement with those obtained from mammals except for the following. In the pigeon, there are units responding only to frequency-modulated stimuli. A neuron was also found with a discharge rate decreasing with increasing stimulus intensity. Also, inhibition of spontaneous activity by single tone stimuli was observed. In contrast, Sachs et al.[1005] observed in the pigeon an agreement with the results obtained from mammals, except for quantitative deviations (e.g., higher spontaneous activity and higher maximal discharge rate). This agreement included phase coupling, two-tone inhibition, periodic discharge upon stimulation with clicks, and shape of tuning curves and frequency response curves. Similar results were obtained in reptiles.[654, 657]

The results obtained so far from the auditory nerve can be summarized by stating that the auditory nerve provides the input to all of the auditory afferent centers of the CNS. All performances of the auditory system ultimately are based on the processing of excitation patterns of auditory nerve fibers. However, in the auditory nerve no excitation patterns are to be expected showing signs of information processing.

In fact, all mechanical events of the inner ear are reflected by the excitation patterns of the auditory nerve. This applies even to the phase relations of the stimulus (Fig. 66, 67); that is, to stimulus properties having no sensory correlate, but perhaps being of significance for information processing (e.g., in connection with directional hearing).

Apart from the modulation by the efferent system, from two-tone inhibition (Figs. 71 and 72), and from adaptation processes, the activity of the auditory nerve provides a true copy of the stimulus. This was shown very impressively by Kiang[632] for low intensities by comparing the neural coding of speech to the acoustical speech stimulus (Fig. 77). Since every auditory nerve fiber has one and only one characteristic frequency (see page 83) such that the excitation threshold runs through an absolute minimum at this frequency (Fig. 59), the auditory nerve fibers respond to the action of a complex sound stimulus like narrow-band filters. If several fibers with sufficiently different characteristic frequencies are selected, then the neurogram is in very good agreement with the sonagram of the stimulus, provided the stimulus intensity is not too high. At higher intensities less differentiated neurograms occur as expected from the response areas of the fibers.

But if the stimulus is recognizable also at these higher intensities, it appears that there must be cues in the neural discharge patterns other than average discharge rate, which are useful. Some of these cues may be related to synchrony, some may involve the distribution of activity among different subpopulations of fibers and a short-term adaptation mechanism.*

* References 257, 633, 797, 974.

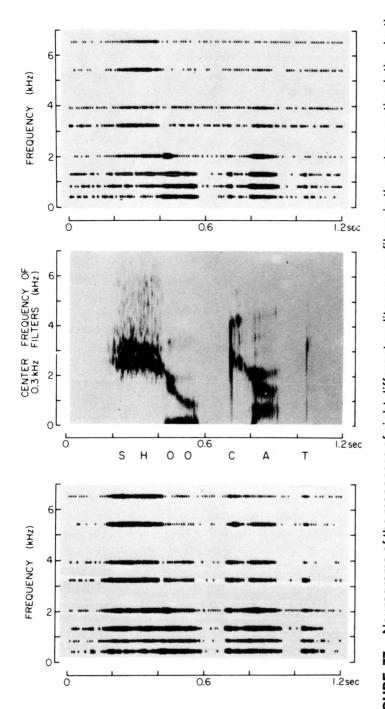

FIGURE 77. Neurograms of the responses of eight different auditory nerve fibers in the cat upon stimulation by the spoken word "SHOO CAT." The characteristic frequencies of the fibers are given on the ordinate. (Top) Neurogram for a low stimulus intensity (-57 dB referred to 200 V$_{PP}$ for the highest peaks at the 1 inch-condenser ear phone). (Middle) Spectrogram (sonagram) of the word "SHOO CAT." The center frequency of the filter is given on the ordinate. (Bottom) Neurogram of the same auditory nerve fiber at a stimulus intensity 20 dB higher. The dark areas in the neurogram are proportional to the stimulus-related discharge rate. (According to Kiang [632].)

Some of the psychophysical findings like tone masking, the residue phenomenon, and the formation of combination tones, can be explained by the results obtained from the auditory-nerve fibers. The actual processing of activities mediated by the auditory nerve, however, is of course reserved to the higher nuclei of the CNS.

C. The Cochlear Nucleus

Morphologically, the cochlear nucleus shows an extremely complicated structure regarding the shape of the cell, the fiber connections, and the synaptic contacts.[136, 271] Figure 78 represents a simplified scheme* obtained from the cat. It is not surprising that the response patterns of single units in this complex nucleus vary considerably. In the anterior part of the nucleus cochlearis anteroventralis the units tend to behave like auditory nerve fibers and in the nucleus cochlearis dorsalis they yield more complicated response patterns. Unfortunately, in some publications too little is noted about the location of the units studied so that many properties of the units of the cochlear nuclei can be described only very generally.

In contrast to the behavior of the auditory-nerve fibers, different response patterns occur in the post-stimulus-time histogram. Completely new patterns are obtained besides those already known from the auditory-nerve fibers (primary-like-patterns). These different discharge patterns were described in several early studies.[†] They are summarized systematically in Figure 79.

Only under very restricted conditions[‡] can a certain pattern be ascribed to a single unit from the cochlear nucleus, because frequently, the response pattern of a unit changes when the frequency or intensity of the stimulus is varied (Fig. 80). The octopus-cells (Fig. 81) of the pPVCN[819] are perhaps an exception. Only octopus-cells are found in the octopus-cell area, apart from a few small Golgi-type II-cells. A striking feature of the octopus-cells is that more than 50% of the surface of their somas and 70% of the surface of their proximal dendrites is covered with large synapses of afferent fibers

---

* There are also histochemical mapping experiments (References 405, 406, 407) and it is considerable evidence that aspartate and glutamate are the transmitters of the cochlear nerve (References 170, 181, 448, 1138, 1195–1199), while there are noradrenergic nerve terminals in the cochlear nucleus (References 692, 693) originating from the locus coeruleus which induce inhibition of dorsal cochlear nucleus neurons (Reference 189).

† See for example references 386, 411, 637, 772, 824, 886, 887, 978.

‡ For example, by looking only at the pattern following stimulation 10 dB above threshold at the characteristic frequency.

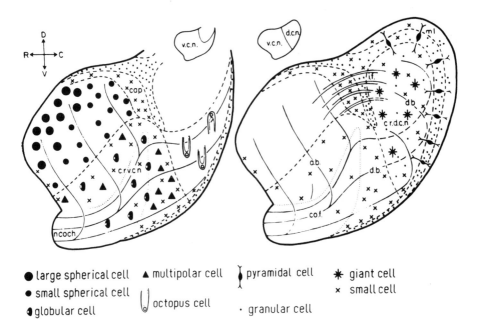

● large spherical cell   ▲ multipolar cell   pyramidal cell   ✳ giant cell
● small spherical cell   × small cell
◐ globular cell   octopus cell   · granular cell

FIGURE 78. Distribution of the nine different cell types in a schematic sagittal section of the cat's nucleus cochlearis. Left: nucleus cochlearis ventralis alone. Right: nucleus cochlearis ventralis partly covered by the nucleus cochlearis dorsalis. On the right, the pathways of the fibers are indicated: a.b. = ascending branch of the cochlear nerve; d.b. = descending branch of the cochlear nerve (see page 73); i.f. = internal fiber connections between the dorsal and the ventral nucleus; co.f. = fibers of the cochlear nerve. In the ventral area the small cells and the granular cells are indicated: D = dorsal; V = ventral; R = rostral; C = caudal; v.c.n. = nucleus cochlearis ventralis; d.c.n. = nucleus cochlearis dorsalis; c.r.d.c.n. = central region of the nucleus cochlearis dorsalis; m.l. = molecular layer; n.coch. = nervus cochlearis; c.r.v.c.n. = central region of the nucleus cochlearis ventralis. (According to Osen [875].)

belonging to the cochlear nerve. In addition, the long dendrites stretch across a large number of afferent auditory nerve fibers, a fact explaining the wide tuning curves of the octopus-cells. (In contrast, the dendrites of the star cells of the AVCN are arranged in parallel to the "isofrequency plane" of the arriving fibers.)

Apparently, these octopus-cells are the first cells of the afferent auditory pathway that have pure on-discharge patterns (i.e. they are active only at the beginning of a stimulus). If the primary-like-discharge patterns are considered, inhibitory inputs have to be assumed too in order to account for the on-patterns.

In all other parts of the cochlear nucleus, different cell types are mixed together (Fig. 78). Thus, in order to class a response pattern with a certain

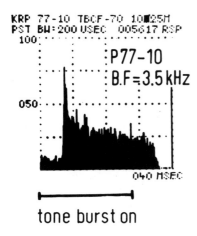

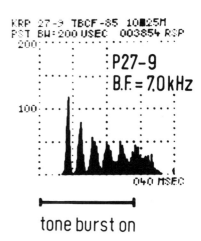

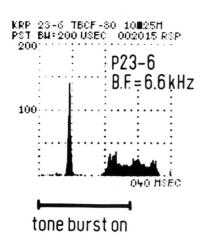

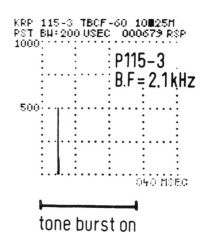

FIGURE 79. Typical post-stimulus-time histograms of different units of the cochlear nucleus upon stimulation with tone bursts. B.F. = best or characteristic frequency.

These patterns are named: Primary like (upper left), chopper (upper right), pauser (lower left), on-pattern (lower right). (According to Pfeiffer [887].)

cell type it would be necessary to mark the different cells from which the response patterns were obtained.* Such work has been initiated by Caspary.[179]

---

* Naturally, criteria other than cell morphology can be applied. As criterion for the large spherical cells in the anterodorsal part of the ventral cochlear nucleus (see Fig. 76), for example, Kiang et al.(637) and Pfeiffer (887) used characteristic potentials

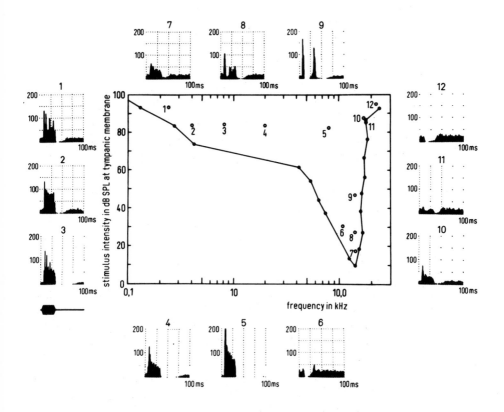

FIGURE 80. Tuning curve and response patterns (post-stimulus-time histogram) of a unit of the polymorphic layer of the dorsal cochlear nucleus. The numbers give the location of the post-stimulus-time histograms within the response area of the unit. (According to Godfrey et al. [403].)

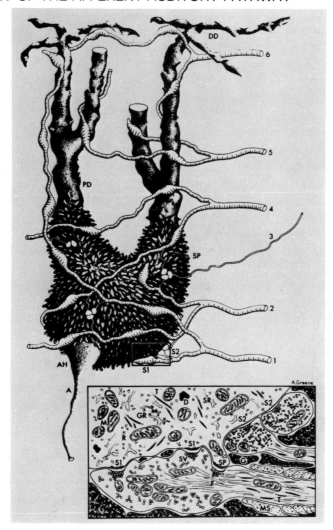

FIGURE 81.   An octopus cell. The cell body (over 35 μm in diameter) is cloaked with short stubby appendages, the somatic spicules (SP), which greatly increase the surface area involved in axosomatic synapses. S_1 is a large ending from the thick, descending branches of the auditory nerve (e.g., 1, 2, 4, 5, 6) and S_2 is a small ending. The small endings are formed secondarily by thin collaterals of the large descending branches or primarily by thin axons (e.g., 3) of undetermined origin. The large synaptic endings occur as isolated, elongated enlargements, either at the terminal or in passage. A = axon; AH = axon hillock; DD = distal dendrites; PD = proximal dendrites. The inset shows an enlargement of the area of the large (S_1) and small S_2) synaptic endings. F = neurofilaments; T = microtubules; SV = synaptic vesicle; G = glial process; GR = granular endoplasmic reticulum; M = mitochondria; D = dense body (lysosome); R = ribosomes; SP = somatic spicule; MS = myelin sheath; SR = smooth endoplasmic reticulum. (According to Morest et al. [819].)

In each of the large subnuclei the cells are arranged tonotopically.* That is, high frequencies project to dorsal, caudal, and medial parts, whereas progressively lower frequencies project to ventral, rostral, and lateral parts of these nuclei (Fig. 82).

Mainly patterns other than primary-like occur in the dorsal part of the cochlear nucleus; namely "chopper-," "pauser-," and "build-up" patterns.† All possible mixtures of excitatory and inhibitory processes as well as pure inhibitory responses ‡ (Fig. 83) can be encountered.§

According to the studies of Evans and Nelson[311, 313] the inhibitory inputs of the dorsal cochlear nucleus come from intranuclear fibers running between the ventral cochlear nucleus and the dorsal cochlear nucleus. The latency of 4 to 6 ms is too short for efferent inputs and the inhibition persists after the descending fibers have been cut.

In general, the tuning curves resemble those of the cochlear nerve fibers (Fig. 84). On the other hand, some very wide tuning curves do occur, especially in the posterior part of the nucleus cochlearis posteroventralis (the area of the octopus cells[641]). In addition, tuning curves having two distinctive characteristic frequencies with different inhibitory areas (e.g. Fig. 83) also appear in the dorsal nucleus.[780, 824]

The magnitude of spontaneous activity in the cochlear nucleus is comparable to that of the auditory-nerve fibers.[307, 312] However, the spontaneous activity of the ventral cochlear nucleus subsides after sectioning the auditory nerve, whereas the activity of the dorsal nucleus remains unchanged.[664] Further, periodic spontaneous activity also occurs in the dorsal nucleus,[888] whereas the activity of the ventral nucleus and of the auditory nerve shows a Poisson-distribution (see page 83).

---

occurring before the extracellularly recorded action potential which is missing in other cells. It is assumed that these pre-potentials have to do with the notably large synapses of the auditory nerve fibers making contact with these cells (Held's bulbi). Only a few of these synapses occur on the large spherical cells. The pre-potentials might be an expression of the excitatory events of the end of the fiber. The response patterns of these cells are "primary-like" and cannot be discerned from those of the auditory nerve fibers (Reference 641).

* References 133, 312, 680, 743, 749, 888, 971, 978, 1050.

† These patterns can be found (Reference 641) also in units of the INCN (= nucleus cochlearis interstitialis), of the pAVCN (= posterior nucleus cochlearis antero-ventralis) and of the aPVCN (= anterior nucleus cochlearis posteroventralis).

‡ This inhibition is not to be mistaken for the two-tone inhibition occurring already in the auditory nerve.

§ References 312, 403, 404, 508, 773, 779, 978, 1178, 1255.

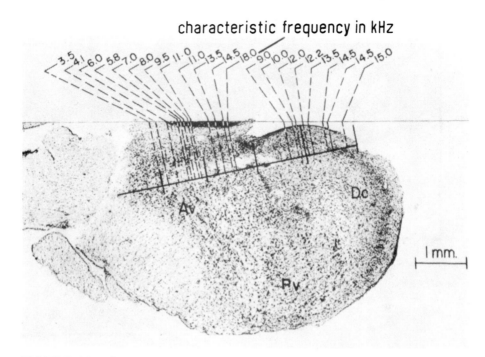

characteristic frequency in kHz

FIGURE 82. Sagittal section of the left cochlear nucleus. The path of the micro-electrode and the positions of the different characteristic frequencies are shown. In the dorsal cochlear nucleus, the characteristic frequencies decrease from the caudal to the rostral side from 15.0 to 9.0 kHz. Upon crossing the border to the nucleus cochlearis anteroventralis, a new sequence begins from 18.0 to 3.5 kHz. Dc = nucleus cochlearis dorsalis; Av = nucleus cochlearis anteroventralis; Pv = nucleus cochlearis posteroventralis. (According to Rose et al. [978].)

Regarding the intensity function, monotonic intensity curves occur primarily in the ventral nucleus* and nonmonotonic ones appear especially in the dorsal nucleus† (Fig. 85). The dynamic behavior has been studied thoroughly by Møller‡ using amplitude-modulated stimuli.

Another striking feature of the units of the cochlear nucleus is that the maximum discharge rate obtained for stimulus frequencies above the characteristic frequency is lower than that obtained for stimulus frequencies below the characteristic frequency.[772, 780]

Not all units of the cochlear nucleus respond to click stimuli. Units in the ventral cochlear nucleus responding to tone stimulation with "primary-like" patterns respond to clicks in the same way as the auditory nerve fibers. They show periodic responses[775, 776] if their characteristic frequency is below

---

* References 411, 415, 772, 778, 823, 978.
† References 411, 426, 1255.
‡ References 781, 783, 784, 787–791.

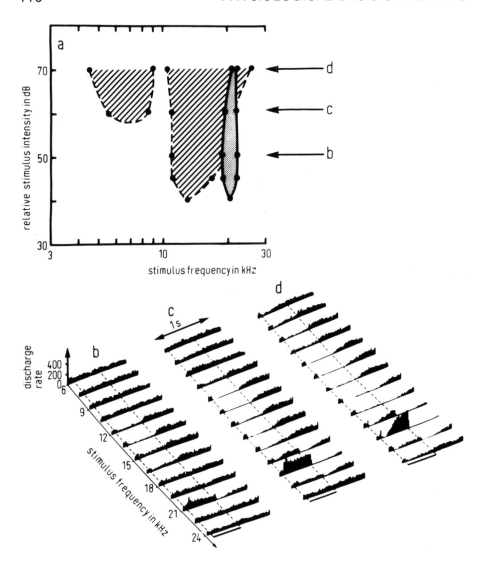

FIGURE 83. A, Tuning curve of a unit of the dorsal cochlear nucleus of the cat. Dotted area = excitatory response area, hatched area = inhibitory response area. B to D, Three-dimensional plot of post-stimulus-time histograms. Analysis time, stimulus frequency, and discharge rate are given by the three axes. The histograms of row B were obtained with a stimulus intensity of 10 dB above threshold, those of C with 20 dB above threshold and those of D with 30 dB above threshold as indicated by the arrows in A. The tone bursts were of 0.4 s duration. Stimulus presentation is marked by a line below the abscissa and by the dashed line. Especially in D an extensive inhibitory area and a narrow excitatory area with clearly delayed "build-up" pattern was noticed at 21 kHz. (According to Evans and Nelson [312].)

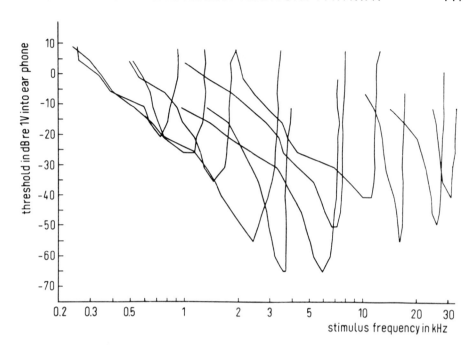

FIGURE 84. Examples of tuning curves of 11 units of the cochlear nucleus of the rat. (According to Møller [772].)

4 kHz. Units with "chopper"- and "pauser"-histogram patterns, on the other hand, respond to click stimuli with only one peak in the post-stimulus-time histogram.

Some units show a very precise 1:1 relation between action potential and click stimulus up to a critical click frequency. This critical repetition frequency ranges between 200 and 800 clicks per second.[774, 777] If the click rate increases beyond the critical repetition frequency, the cell responds only at the beginning of the click series with an on-effect, as it does at the beginning of a tone. Using tone bursts instead of clicks, Møller was able to demonstrate that the pause between two successive stimuli is the critical parameter. Another feature* is that amplitude modulation of the stimulus can determine the discharge rate, with 1 dB stimulus modulation causing up to 50% discharge modulation. Interestingly, independent of the characteristic frequency, a modulation frequency of 200 to 300 Hz causes a clear maximum of the modulation of excitation (Fig. 86).

The response patterns phase-locked with the stimulus (see page 90) and observed in the cochlear nerve can be seen again in the cochlear nucleus, especially in the anteroventral part.† They might be the basis of the

* References 781, 782, 784, 786, 788, 796.
† References 399, 418, 701, 823, 984, 985.

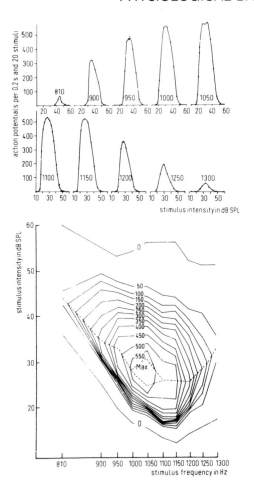

FIGURE 85. Below: contours of equal discharge rate (iso-rate curves) of a unit of the dorsal cochlear nucleus. Above: non-monotonic intensity function of the same unit corresponding to vertical sections through the iso-rate curves below. Parameter is stimulus frequency. (According to Greenwood and Maruyama [426].)

"Frequency Following Response" in the compound potential of the cochlear nucleus as described by Marsh and Worden[746] and by Starr and Hellerstein.[1100]

For the most part, intracellular recordings from the cochlear nucleus* show the theoretically expected relationship (Fig. 87) but there is also dissociation between discharge rate and membrane potential (Fig. 88). The dissociation between the recorded membrane potential and the discharge rate led to the idea of a specially branched receptive area of these neurons at

---

* References 300, 397, 968, 969, 1098, 1099.

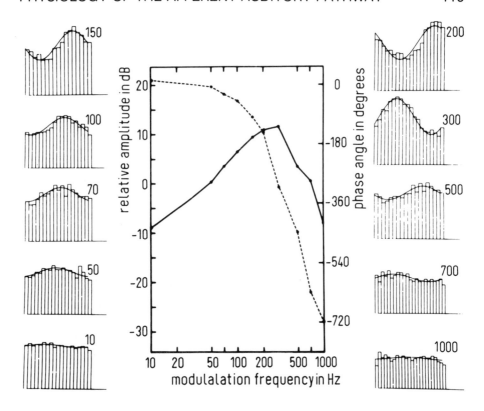

FIGURE 86. Period histograms for sinusoidal amplitude modulation of a tone stimulus. The parameter is the modulation frequency. The relative amplitude of the sine wave fit to the period histogram (the maximal change of the discharge rate) divided by the relative amplitude of the stimulus modulation is shown in the middle as a function of the modulation frequency (continuous line). The phase difference between the stimulus modulation and the sine wave of the period histograms is also shown (dashed curve). (According to Møller [782].)

some distance from the area where action potentials are generated. With suitable models, Fernald and Gerstein[328] could imitate the obtained response patterns to frequency-modulated stimuli.

Particularly notable are the binaural effects described by Mast[748, 750] for the cochlear nucleus since no afferent connections are known to exist from the spiral ganglion to the opposite side or from one cochlear nucleus to the other (Fig. 55). Thus, it has to be assumed that these binaural effects in the cochlear nucleus are accomplished via the descending system. In any case, in the pyramidal and the polymorphic cell layers of the dorsal cochlear nucleus, Mast found cells that could be activated by ipsilateral stimuli and inhibited by contralateral stimuli (Fig. 89), as well as some cells that could be activated by both ipsilateral and contralateral stimuli.

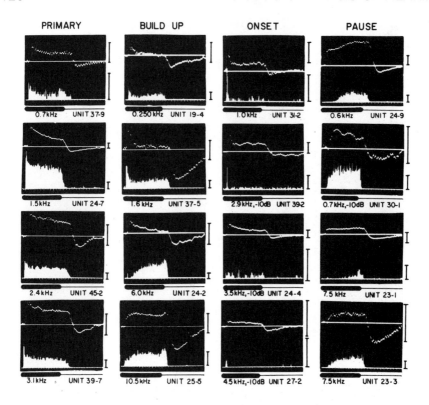

FIGURE 87. Comparison between the averaged membrane potential (intracellular recording) and the temporal discharge rate (post-stimulus-time histogram) for the four different types of discharge patterns. For each recording the membrane potential is shown above. The corresponding histogram is shown below. The stimulus and the number of the cell are shown below the abscissa. The stimulus duration is 250 ms. Calibration of the membrane potential 1 mV, calibration of the histogram 10 spikes. (According to Britt [149].)

The characteristic frequencies were of about equal value for ipsilateral excitation and contralateral inhibition (Fig. 89). Also, the latencies of both are of comparable length (contralaterally between 8 and 25 ms, ipsilaterally between 5 and 20 ms). Upon binaural stimulation, these neurons are sensitive to interaural intensity differences (Fig. 90). The eventual significance of these binaural effects with respect to directional hearing, however, is still uncertain.

As a rule, frequency-modulated stimuli elicit response patterns predictable from their response to pure tones, as in the auditory nerve. Thus, frequency-modulated tones can provide an image of the frequency response curve. Møller* could also demonstrate a dependence on the velocity of

---

* References 773, 779–781, 785, 796.

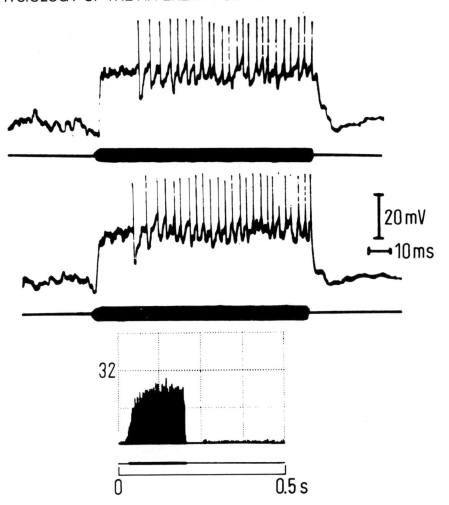

FIGURE 88. Intracellular recording from a unit of the dorsal cochlear nucleus upon stimulation with pure tone (18.5 kHz). The corresponding post-stimulus-time histogram representing a "build-up" pattern (see Fig. 79) is shown below. As can be seen, no discharges occur at first although the membrane potential is depolarized to the same degree as it is during the period of maximum discharge rate occurring at a later time. Since, even upon clear inhibition of the discharge, hyper-polarization was observed only rarely it is conceivable that the electrode was localized too far away from the inhibitory synapses. (According to Gerstein et al. [397].)

modulation, such that a certain optimal velocity causes a maximum discharge rate (Fig. 91).

Also, asymmetric response patterns were found for frequency-modulated stimuli.* That is, the response depends on whether the stimulus

---

* References 166, 300, 308, 329, 779–781, 785, 845.

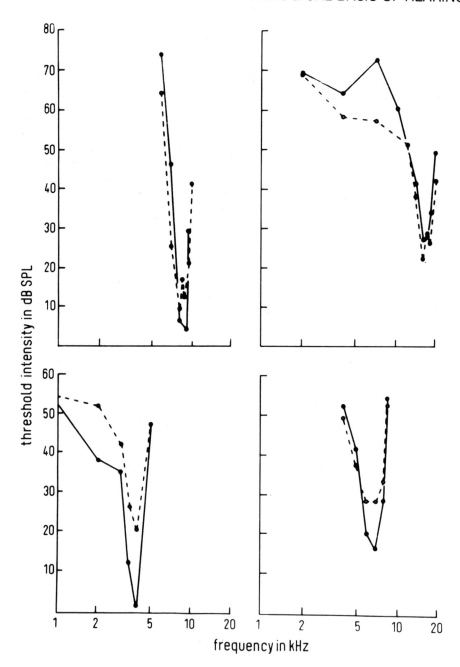

FIGURE 89. Typical tuning curves of neurons of the dorsal cochlear nucleus with contralateral inhibition. Continuous curves: ipsilateral excitatory threshold; dashed curves: contralateral inhibitory threshold. (According to Mast [748].)

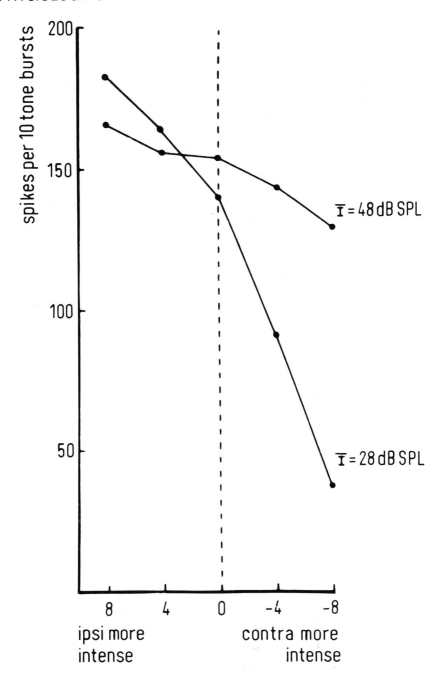

FIGURE 90. Discharge rate as a function of interaural intensity difference. The average intensity ($\overline{I}$) is constant for each curve. (According to Mast [748].)

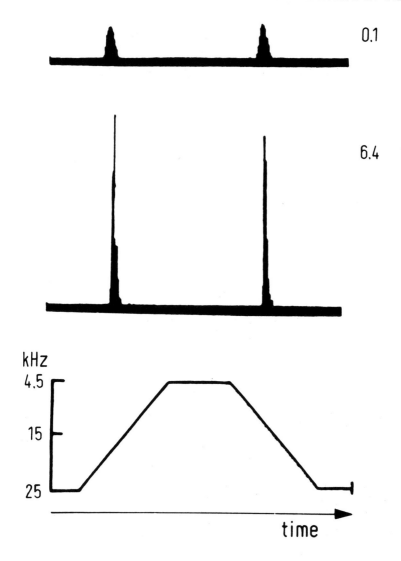

FIGURE 91. Post-stimulus-time histograms of a unit of the cochlear nucleus upon stimulation using trapezoid frequency modulation (lower panel) with different velocities of modulation (modulation rate above: 0.1 kHz per second, below: 6.4 kHz per second). (According to Møller [779].)

frequency is modulated towards higher or towards lower values. However, these patterns can also be predicted from the response to steady pure tones and can be represented by a model.[328]

In summary the anatomical structure and the electrophysiological findings yield a mixed picture pointing out the variety of mechanisms processing the information arriving via the auditory nerve. The available results do not yet allow one to draw any firm conclusions regarding the functional significance of this complex nucleus. Despite the limitations associated with the findings described, it can (perhaps somewhat simplistically) be said that the units of the cochlear nucleus show narrow tuning curves so that a tonotopic structure can be defined. An apparent exception is the octopus-cell area having wide tuning curves. In contrast to the auditory nerve, however, the tuning curves of the cochlear nucleus are surrounded on either side by inhibitory areas, an effect presumably based on lateral inhibition. Also, the latency values are widely scattered partly resulting from inhibitory processes (according to Møller,[787] latencies up to 50 ms are encountered; Mast[748] gives values between 5 and 25 ms, see Fig. 88). However, an average latency of 2 to 5 ms for the ventral cochlear nucleus and of 4 to 12 ms for the dorsal cochlear nucleus can be quoted (Fig. 92). Of course, the latency time depends also on the intensity and the frequency of the stimulus (sinus tones), (Fig. 93).

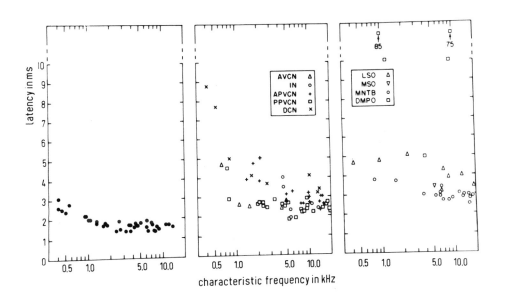

FIGURE 92. Comparison of typical latencies in the auditory nerve (left panel), in the cochlear nucleus (middle panel), and in the superior olive (right panel) following stimulation with clicks. AVCN = nucleus cochlearis anteroventralis; IN = nucleus cochlearis interstitialis; APVCN = anterior part of the nucleus cochlearis posteroventralis; PPVCN = posterior part of the nucleus cochlearis posteroventralis; DCN = nucleus cochlearis dorsalis; LSO = lateral nucleus of the superior olive; MSO = medial nucleus of the superior olive; MNTB = medial nucleus of the trapezoid body; DMPO = periolivary complex nucleus. (According to Kiang et al. [641].)

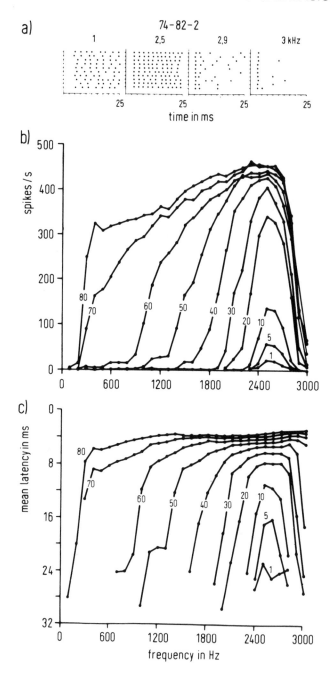

FIGURE 93. Data for neuron 74-82-2. A, Dot-response patterns for indicated frequencies at 70 dB SPL; 10 consecutive trials. Each dot represents a spike. B, Rate-response area. C, Latency-response area. Numbers indicate sound pressure levels rel. 0.0002 dyne/cm². Stimulus: tone burst 50 ms in duration. Each data point based on 50 presentations. Rate: 4/s. Cell located in AVCN (According to Kitzes et al. [648].)

If one wants to speculate about functional significance, one may well assume that the large spherical cells of the anteroventral nucleus (see Fig. 78) act as relay cells for the binaural processing of temporal information since they have a bilateral tonotopic connection with the middle nuclei of the superior olive.[460, 874] They are the input stage for the binaural processing of temporal information taking place in the superior olive (see page 133).* The small spherical cells, however, project tonotopically into the lateral nucleus of the ipsilateral superior olive.[460, 874] Thus, they could be relay cells serving frequency analysis, especially since they are innervated by all parts of the cochlea.[460] The "primary-like" response pattern observed for both cell populations is in favor of the relay function.

The globular cells project into the centrolateral nucleus medialis of the trapezoid body where every cell is innervated by only one of the large calyces of Held.† From there, fibers run to the lateral nucleus (S-segment) of the superior olive[939] so that the lateral nucleus also is innervated bilaterally.

It is known that the axons of the octopus-cells (stria acustica intermedia) end in the periolivary nuclei.[859, 1186] Thus, they may be of importance for the descending olivocochlear bundle originating here. They cannot be regarded as relay cells because their response pattern (mostly the on-effect) indicates real information processing. The more complex response patterns of the dorsal nucleus exhibit a further processing of the excitation patterns of the auditory nerve, but their significance is still completely unknown. The axons of the pyramidal cells of the dorsal nucleus form the stria acustica dorsalis (see page 33) and end in the dorsal nucleus of the lateral lemniscus and in the inferior colliculus. Here, they join again the ascending fibers that arrive in the lateral lemniscus and the inferior colliculus via the ventral nucleus and the superior olive.

Figure 94 shows how the generation of the different response patterns can be explained by means of a model. The existence of the postulated interneurons, however, has not yet been proven.

Figure 95 gives a survey of the different response patterns occurring in the auditory nerve, the cochlear nucleus, and the superior olive. Upon stimulation with short (25 ms) tones at the characteristic frequency and low intensity, these patterns typically are encountered in the specified areas and form the basis of the speculations outlined above.

If the distribution of the different cell types of the cochlear nucleus as shown in Figure 78 is considered, the correspondence between discharge pattern and cell type as carried out in Figure 96 can be assumed. Figure 97 shows the connection between those different cell types and the nuclei of the superior olive.

---

* The large spherical cells receive their inputs only from the apical and middle parts of the cochlea.[1189] Correspondingly, the response area of the middle nucleus and the superior olive is reduced.[413]

†References 454, 457, 461, 859, 1110.

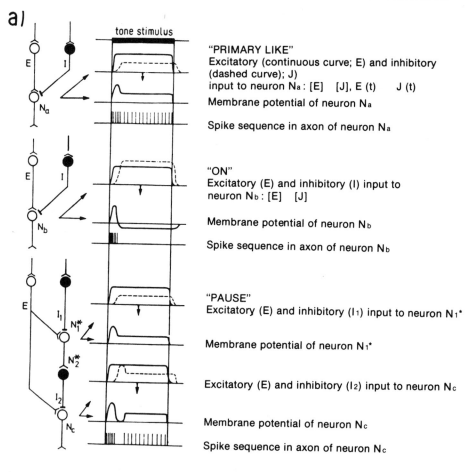

FIGURE 94. A, Models of functional neuronal connections for the generation of "Primary like," "On" and "Pause" response patterns under the
assumption of linear inhibition. B, (see page 129) Model of a functional
neuronal connection for the generation of a "Chopper" pattern in neuron
Na—see spike sequence in the axon—under the assumption of an additive
linear inhibition. (According to Dunker and Krämer [273].)

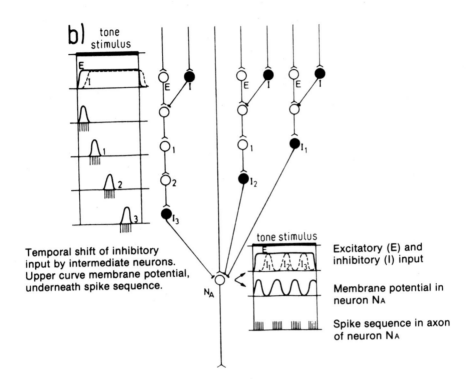

Temporal shift of inhibitory input by intermediate neurons. Upper curve membrane potential, underneath spike sequence.

Excitatory (E) and inhibitory (I) input

Membrane potential in neuron N_A

Spike sequence in axon of neuron N_A

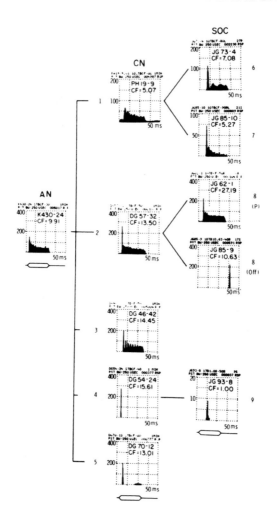

FIGURE 95. Typical response patterns (post-stimulus-time histograms) upon stimulation with short tone bursts (25 ms) using the characteristic frequencies of units of the following parts of the auditory pathway: AN = auditory nerve; CN = cochlear nucleus; SOC = superior olive. AVCN = nucleus cochlearis anteroventralis; IN = nucleus cochlearis interstitialis; APVCN = anterior part of the nucleus cochlearis posteroventralis; PPVCN = posterior part of the nucleus cochlearis posteroventralis; DCN = nucleus cochlearis dorsalis; LSO = lateral nucleus of the superior olive; MSO = medial nucleus of the superior olive; MNTB = medial nucleus of the trapezoid body; DMPO = periolivary complex nucleus. The analysis time was 50 ms. The symbol below each column is the envelope of the stimulus. The null point of the histograms was 2.5 ms before the beginning of the stimulus. (According to Kiang et al. [641].)

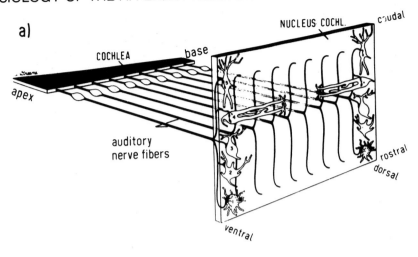

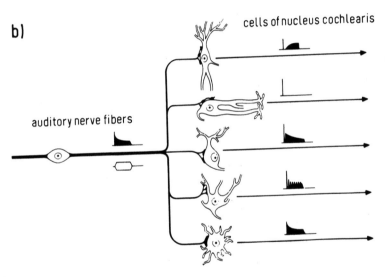

FIGURE 96. A, Schematic description of the anatomical relationship between the auditory nerve fibers and the different cell types of the cochlear nucleus. Note that the cochlear nucleus is not disk shaped and that the indications of direction give only a rough orientation. 1 = spherical cells; 2 = multipolar cells; 3 = globular cells; 4 = octopus cells; 5 = pyramidal cells. B, Correspondence between cell types and the characteristic response patterns. The stimuli are short tones (25 to 50 ms) of low intensity at the characteristic frequency. Characteristic frequency is assumed to be high since at low frequencies periodic discharge patterns occur. The post-stimulus-time histogram above the auditory nerve fiber shows the typical pattern belonging to those fibers, the stimulus marking is shown underneath. The patterns of the units of the cochlear nucleus are "Primary like" for the spherical cells, "Chopper" for the multipolar cells, "Primary-like with incision" for the globular cells, and "On" for the octopus cells. (According to Kiang [632].)

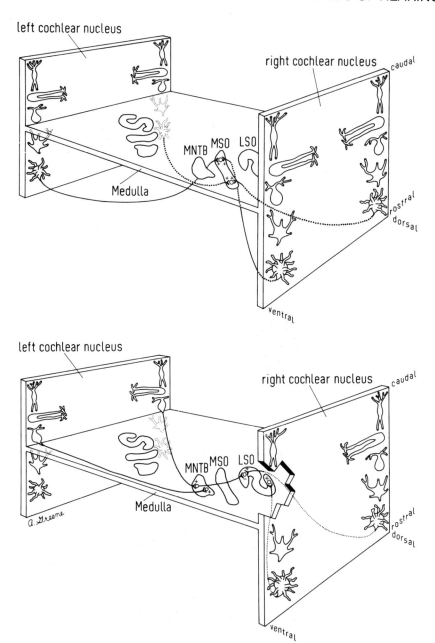

FIGURE 97. Schematic description of the connections between the different cell types of the cochlear nucleus and the nuclei of the superior olive. + and - signs indicate excitatory and inhibitory synapses respectively. MNTB = nucleus medialis corporis trapezoidi; MSO = nucleus medialis olivaris superior; LSO = nucleus lateralis olivaris superior. (According to Kiang [632].)

D. The Nuclei of the Superior Olive and the Lateral Lemniscus

The superior olive is also composed of several subnuclei (Fig. 98). The largest three are the lateral olivary nucleus (S-segment), the medial olivary nucleus (nucleus accessorius), and the trapezoid body (see Fig. 55). In the lateral lemniscus, there are two different cell groups, the dorsal and the ventral nucleus of the lateral lemniscus.

1. The S-segment

As illustrated in Figure 55, the S-segment is innervated directly from the ipsilateral side as well as via the trapezoid body from the contralateral side.[859, 939] As a rule, the cells are activated upon ipsilateral stimulation* and they are inhibited (about 90% of the cells) upon contralateral stimulation† (Fig. 99). The contralateral inhibition includes an inhibitory interneuron most probably located in the ipsilateral trapezoid body. This inhibitory pathway also must be organized very precisely because the characteristic frequency for ipsilateral excitation and for contralateral inhibition are identical.‡

The monaural tuning curves of single units of the S-segment are similar to those of the cochlear nerve and the cochlear nucleus.[132, 1167] Frequently, they are flanked by inhibitory areas[408] as was described already for the cochlear nucleus. For the S-segment, Tsuchitani and Boudreau[1167] proved the existence of a precise tonotopic structure representing the whole audible frequency range.

The tuning curves for contralateral inhibition and for ipsilateral excitation are in good agreement, the only difference being a tendency toward somewhat wider inhibitory tuning curves. However, there are also excitatory units which can be activated by either ipsilateral or contralateral stimulation. The latter are termed EE- (excitation—excitation) while the others are called EI- (excitation—inhibition) cells. Thus if the tuning curves for ipsilateral and contralateral stimulation are of different width, then a tone deviating from the characteristic frequency may be located in the response area on one side, and in the inhibitory area on the other side: the feature EE or EI becomes frequency dependent.

Upon ipsilateral stimulation with tone bursts, the first action potentials of all cells of the S-segment have a very stable latency.[132] This amounts to

---

* References 388, 416, 1167.
† References 131, 132, 1168.
‡ References 131, 132, 1168.

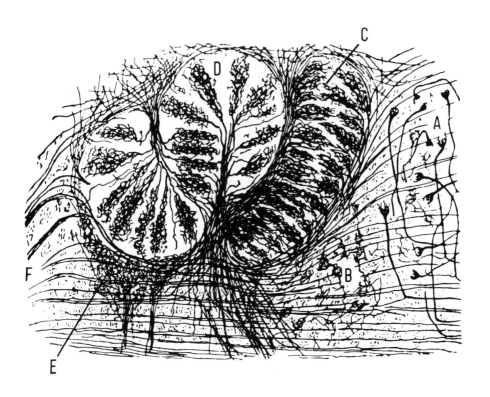

FIGURE 98. Fiber pattern of the olivary nucleus (Golgi-staining) in a cat of a few days of age. A = nucleus trapezoidus; B = preolivary nuclei (internal); C = nucleus accessorius; D = S-segment; E = preolivary nuclei (external); F = fibers of the trapezoid nucleus. (According to Ramón y Cajal [921].)

about 8 ms for tone stimuli 10 dB above threshold at the characteristic frequency.

The monaural intensity functions are S-shaped with a proportionality range of 20 and 40 dB followed by a plateau. This is true regardless of stimulus frequency. With frequencies other than the characteristic frequency, however, the threshold naturally changes in agreement with the tuning curve. This causes, for frequencies below the characteristic frequency, a parallel shift of the intensity function. For frequencies above the characteristic frequency, the maximal discharge rate is diminished drastically. This was observed also in the cochlear nucleus. For binaural stimulation, the intensity function depends on the intensity relation between the stimuli offered to both ears (Fig. 100).

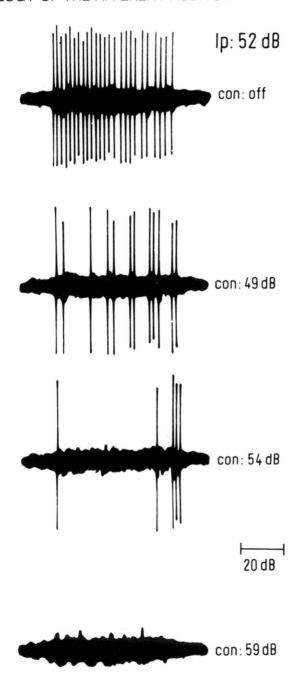

FIGURE 99. Discharges of a cell of the S-segment upon monaural and binaural stimulation with a tone at the characteristic frequency (35 kHz, 60 ms). The intensity is given in dB SPL. (According to Boudreau and Tsuchitani [132].)

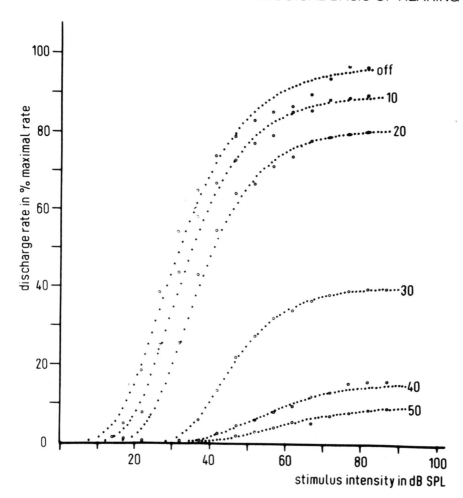

FIGURE 100. Binaural intensity functions of an EI-cell of the S-segment upon stimulation with tones at the characteristic frequency and of 200 ms duration. Abscissa: ipsilateral stimulus intensity. The parameter is the intensity of the contralateral stimulus in dB above threshold. (According to Boudreau and Tsuchitani [132].)

2. The Nucleus Accessorius

It has been demonstrated by Goldberg and Brown[413] and by Guinan et al.[438] that the nucleus accessorius has a tonotopic structure. This nucleus is innervated bilaterally to a large extent (Fig. 55).

As early as 1959, Galambos et al.[388] observed that, upon binaural stimulation with clicks, the magnitude of excitation of single units clearly depended on the time difference between the clicks presented to both ears (Fig. 101). Apart from the commonly encountered relation between latency

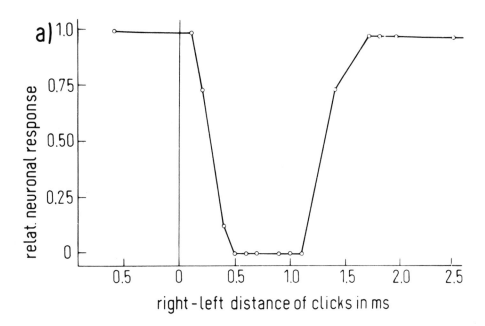

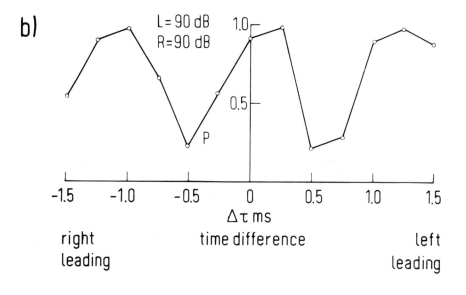

FIGURE 101. Relative number of action potentials of a neuron of the nucleus accessorius upon binaural stimulation with clicks as a function of the right-left time difference with which the clicks were delivered to both ears. A, According to Galambos et al. [388]; B, According to Hall, from Whitfield [1212].)

and stimulus intensity (the latency shortens with increasing intensity), they found cells in which the latency of the action potentials elicited by the clicks did not depend on the intensity and cells in which paradoxically the latency increased with increasing intensity.

In many cells, the action spikes triggered by clicks still occur in the periodic sequence observed in the cochlear nerve. Since this sequence corresponds exactly with the period of the cell's characteristic frequency, it has been related to the oscillation of the basilar membrane.*

Hall[444] described units responding with excitation to both ipsilateral and contralateral stimulation. Under binaural stimulation, summation of excitation occurs which is largest when the click stimuli are offered to both ears at exactly the same time. If, however, the clicks are temporally shifted against each other, then, with increasing interaural time difference, the discharge rate runs through maxima and minima (Fig. 101b). Some cells were excitable only contralaterally and reacted almost according to the "all-or-nothing" law. (Only within about 8 dB they showed a connection between discharge probability and intensity.) Although ipsilateral clicks alone had no effect on these cells, they modified the response to contralateral stimuli. Whereas Moushegian et al.[827] described cells that could be excited with contralateral clicks but inhibited with ipsilateral clicks, Hall[444] studied a population of cells reacting in just the opposite way. In general, time-sensitive EI-cells are also sensitive to interaural intensity differences.[444, 995] Thus, these cells exhibit a time-intensity-compensation effect resembling, at least formally, the psychophysical "trading effect" in directional hearing. From the beginning, these results were viewed in connection with directional hearing.

The direction from which the sound is coming can be recognized in two ways: either by the sound stimulus arriving at one ear earlier than at the other or by the sound being meaningful louder at one ear than the other. Under physiologically stimulus conditions, the two effects are combined such that the ear receiving the sound with some delay is stimulated less intensively than the other, since the sound shadow of the head is interposed between the two ears. However, there is no doubt that either one of the effects alone is able to evoke a clear impression of directionality. If in electrophysiology both mechanisms take effect, two kinds of cells must exist. Namely, cells measuring time differences with an extraordinary accuracy and processing them by bilateral comparison and other cells that are able to transduce intensity differences into time differences. That at least the first group of cells must be located in the relative periphery of the auditory pathway follows from the high accuracy of the time measurement being on the order of some 10 μs. This would be impossible if the signal had

---

* Reference 437, 825, 829.

to pass a large number of synapses, since every synapse decreases the accuracy of timing at least for the single event.

The response of cells in the nucleus accessorius to tone stimuli was studied by Moushegian et al.* and by Goldberg and Brown.[413, 414] They found phase-locked response patterns (as in the cochlear nerve, see page 90) as well as cells firing with a fixed cell-dependent periodicity after stimulation with different frequencies (Fig. 102).

For click stimuli, the excitation depends on the time separation between the clicks presented to both ears. Similarly, it depends strongly on the phase difference between ipsilateral and contralateral pure tones (Fig. 103 above). Also, the locking of the phase of excitation with the stimulus phase depends on the interaural phase difference (Fig. 103 below). As index for the degree of phase-lock the so called "vector-strength" is used that ranges between 0 and 1, where a value of 1 means perfect synchronization.[†] However, the behavior of the vector strength does not have to parallel the discharge rate, as is the case in Figure 103.[829]

For tone stimuli, the cells can also be classed as EE- and EI-cells. Goldberg and Brown[414] found that, out of 105 cells studied, 65% were EE- and 24% were EI-type cells, about 11% could be affected monaurally only. EE-cells with low characteristic frequency show a phase-locked discharge and, upon binaural stimulation, are sensitive to time differences as well as intensity differences. On the other hand, the discharge rate of the EE-cells having a high characteristic frequency is insensitive to intensity differences but depends on the average stimulus intensity. All EI-cells were sensitive to both time and intensity differences.

This means that two cell populations can be distinguished of which only one population allows an intensity-time compensation (trading effect). This might perhaps be the physiological correlate of the psychophysical "double image"-phenomenon.[441, 519] According to it, a complete compensation of the time factor by interaural intensity variation is impossible.

The electrophysiological results are in good agreement with the capabilities of directional hearing since the magnitude of excitation is sufficiently affected by both interaural time differences and interaural intensity differences. For instance, if it is assumed that the higher nervous centers are able to discriminate a difference in excitation of 10%,[572] then from Figure 101a right-left time difference threshold of 10 to 50 μs may result which is in good agreement with the psychophysical findings (Fig. 104).

Although the latencies of the neurons in the nucleus accessorius are 5 to 10 ms,[388, 413] both click and pure-tone stimuli having right-left time differences of 10 to 20 μs result in clear alterations of excitation. This may

---

* References 826, 827, 829.

† References 414, 701, 829.

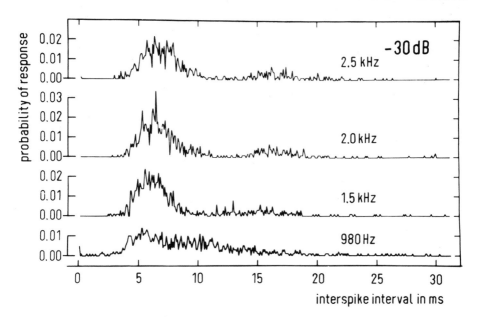

FIGURE 102. Interval histogram of a cell of the nucleus accessorius upon stimulation with tones of different frequencies (980 Hz to 2.5 kHz). (According to Moushegian et al. [827].)

result in the need for the independence of latency on intensity, as well as for the "paradoxical" latency-intensity behavior, mentioned above.

Binaural excitation showing sensitivity to time and intensity difference has been described for all higher nuclei (e.g. for the dorsal nucleus of the lateral lemniscus,[22, 157] for the inferior colliculus,[392, 485] for the medial geniculate body,[12] for the cortex,[156, 446]). These electrophysiological results are a typical example of how the function can be recognized from the neural response pattern. After all, one has to assume that for directional hearing a processing of time and intensity differences is necessary. Certainly not all excitation patterns appearing to be suitable at first sight are in fact qualified for this purpose. Moushegian et al.[828] point out, for instance, that in the kangaroo rat the characteristic delay times* range between 100 and 400 μs.

---

* By characteristic delay time (Reference 980) is meant the following: Binaurally excitable neurons show cyclic discharge rates as a function of interaural time differences (see Fig. 103). The period of this cyclic rate is equal to the period of the stimulus frequency (for phase-locked excitation). If different stimulus frequencies are used separately within the response area of the cell, either maximal or minimal discharge rates are encountered which coincide. The interaural time difference at which this coincidence occurs is called the characteristic delay time of that particular neuron. It is invariable with intensity and frequency. Thus, preferably the characteristic delay time is viewed in connection with the ability of directional hearing.

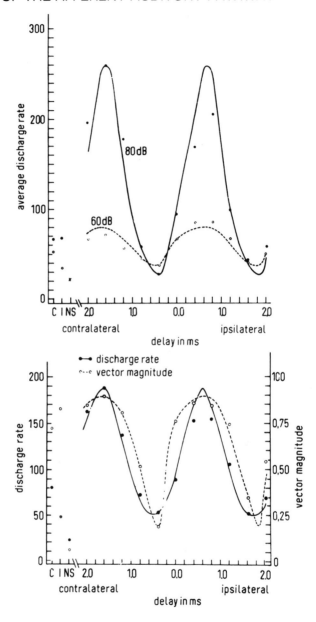

FIGURE 103. (Top) Dependence of the discharge rate of a unit of the nucleus accessorius on the phase delay between ispilateral and contralateral stimulus (pure tone at the characteristic frequency of 444.5 Hz, 1 s duration, ipsi- and contralateral at the same level). The data points on the very left give the discharge rate upon monaural stimulation. C = contralateral stimulation, I = ipsilateral stimulation, NS = spontaneous activity. (Bottom) As above. Here, however,the magnitude of the vector is also shown as a measure of the phase lock between stimulus and excitation. Stimulus intensity 70 dB SPL. (According to Goldberg and Brown [414].)

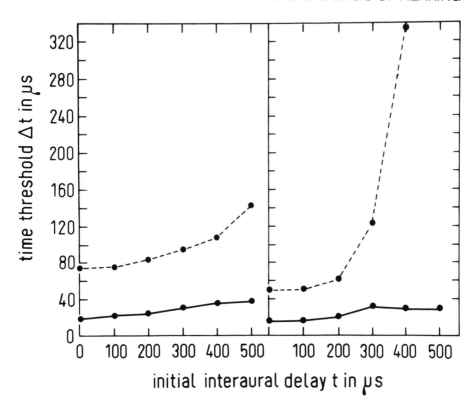

FIGURE 104. Just noticeable interaural time differences (Δt) of two subjects as a function of the initial time difference (t). The lower curves were obtained with clicks of low frequency composition (0.1 to 2 kHz), the upper curves were obtained with clicks of a higher frequency composition (3 to 4 kHz). The stimulus intensity was 48 dB SPL. (According to Hafter and DeMaio [442].)

For a distance between the two ears of 3.5 cm for the kangaroo rat, however, a maximum interaural time difference of 105 μs can occur.

Another experiment demonstrates that in this connection important questions still remain to be answered. Strominger and Oesterreich,[1112] after sectioning the cat's brachium colliculi inferioris on one side, observed that the animal had a defective ability to localize the sound source if it was located in the sound field contralateral to the brain section. As a rule, the discharge rate of bilaterally excitable neurons are effective for a temporal leading of either the ipsilateral or contralateral stimulus. The asymmetry of defects cannot be understood from the excitatory behavior of single neurons. Even if one postulates a further right-left comparison of binaural excitation patterns at a higher level, for instance, then a unilateral lesion would have to lead to symmetrical defects also.

In connection with binaural effects, the experiments reviewed by Green and Yost[425] should be mentioned. Noise and a signal were offered simultaneously to both ears of a subject. The intensity of the signal was adjusted by the subject to an intensity that was just detectable. If the intensity of the signal was diminished by 5 dB, the signal was lost in the noise. If, however, the attenuated signal is offered to one ear only with the noise still acting on both ears, the subject again recognizes the signal. The difference in signal intensity at threshold between a special stimulus condition and the normal case where signal and masking noise are presented identically to both ears, is called "masking level difference" (MLD). If, for example, the same noise is offered to both ears, but the signal is presented to the two ears with an interaural phase difference of 180°, the MLD amounts to 15 dB.

3. The Nucleus Trapezoidus

The trapezoid nucleus receives afferent input primarily from the contralateral side (see Fig. 55). Thus, most cells respond to contralateral stimuli only.* The trapezoid nucleus also has a tonotopic structure. High frequencies are represented in the ventromedial part, low frequencies in the dorsolateral part.[437]

The principal cells[816] are innervated by the thickest fibers of the trapezoid body via the large calyces of Held (Fig. 105). Both facts contribute to the fast conduction of neural impulses via the trapezoid nucleus. The latency values are about 1 ms shorter than in other nuclei of the superior olive. The principal cells are innervated by a peridendritic plexus formed by collaterals arriving at the nucleus accessorius.[816] The functional significance of those synapses, however, is unknown. Many axons of the neurons belonging to the trapezoid nucleus run through the nucleus accessorius on their way to the S-segment and may also make synaptic contacts in the nucleus accessorius. Possibly, they have synapses with all nuclei of the superior olive. Apart from the principal cells, Morest[816] described two more cell types, the star cells and the elongated cells. Those may be the cells that are also excitable from the ipsilateral side, having longer latencies and a somewhat more regular discharge pattern (Fig. 106, right) or responding only to the end of the stimulus.[437]

In any case, these two types of responses belong to cells that can be activated by both ipsilateral and contralateral stimuli. They are encountered considerably less often than the typical discharge patterns of the units of the trapezoid nucleus (Fig. 106, left) that can be elicited only by contralateral stimuli.

As described in the footnote on page 113, typical triphasic potentials were used as criterion in order to class the recordings with the principal cells.

---

* References 388, 413, 416, 437.

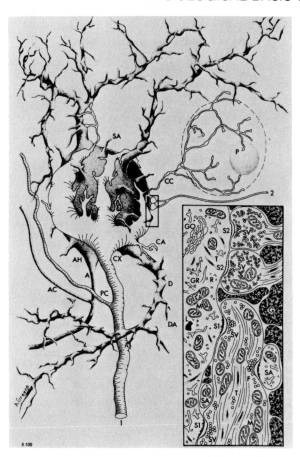

FIGURE 105. A principal neuron of the nucleus trapezoidus. Each cell receives one, and only one, calyx (CX) projecting from the contralateral ventral cochlear nucleus. Only principal cells receive the calyces. Thin collaterals of the calyx (CC) form a network of small terminal boutons, typically associated with the bodies of several nearby principal cells (P). A number of thin axons (2) form smaller synaptic endings on the cell body and dendrites. These fine axonal endings are especially numerous among the distal dendrites, where a conspicuous peridendritic plexus occurs (not shown here). The origins of most of these small endings are undetermined, except for a small contingent, supplied by collaterals of the axons projecting to the medial superior olive from the contralateral anteroventral cochlear nucleus. The axon (A) of the principal cell has a collateral (AC) that projects to the dorsomedial periolivary nucleus along with the precalcyne collateral (PC) of the calciferous axon. The other projection sites of the principal cell axon are uncertain but probably include the lateral superior olive. CA = calcyne appendage, SA = somatic appendages, AH = axon hillock, AC = axonal collateral, D = dendrite of peripheral cell, DA = dendrite appendage, GO = Golgi apparatus, S_2 = synapses of small endings, T = microtubuli, SV = synaptic vessicles, GR = granular endoplasmic reticulum, R = ribosomes, M = mitochondria, G = neuroglia, L = lysosome, S_1 = synapses of calyx, F = neurofilaments (According to Morest et al. [819].)

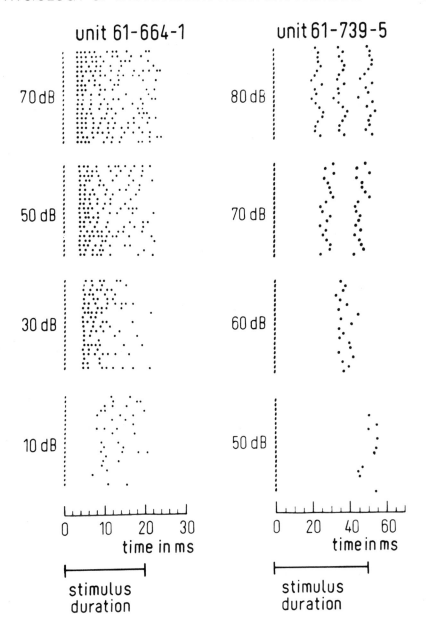

FIGURE 106. Discharge patterns of two units of the nucleus trapezoidus. On the left the most frequently encountered response pattern, probably belonging to the principal cells. On the right the less frequently encountered pattern of a LDR (low discharge rate) cell. For both recordings, 20 equal stimuli were presented. The first dot of each line marks the beginning of the stimulus. Each following dot stands for an action potential. The stimuli were tone bursts (9.0 kHz) of the characteristic frequency. Unit 61-664-1 could be activated only by contralateral stimuli. (According to Goldberg et al. [417].)

The tuning curves resemble those of the cochlear nerve and of the cochlear nucleus (Fig. 107).

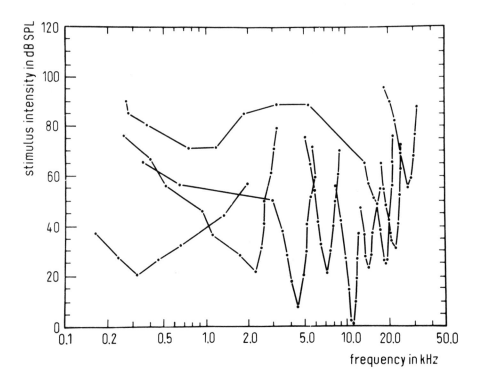

FIGURE 107. Typical tuning curves of units (probably principal cells) of the trapezoid nucleus. (According to Guinan [437], from Goldberg [408].)

Thus, the superior olive is composed of a number of subnuclei the functional significance of which is not known completely. It is, however, the first stage of the auditory pathway having afferent inputs from both ears. Therefore it is only natural to associate the excitation patterns of binaurally excitable cells with directional hearing, especially since they match in a meaningful way with the abilities of directional hearing (processing of time and intensity difference). The superior olive is also the deepest nucleus of the auditory pathway from which descending fibers project to the periphery. Thus, for this reason alone other abilities of the nucleus are to be expected.

Many details regarding the connection between the location of the cells and their response to monaural and binaural stimulation, their tuning curves, tonotopic arrangement, typical excitation pattern, and their intensity functions (magnitude of excitation as function of stimulus intensity) were published by Tsuchitani.[1166]

Noteworthy is the fixed relation between the numbers of cells in the nucleus accessorius and the number of fibers in the abducent nerve as described by Harrison and Irving[457] for various mammals. They interpret this finding as evidence for involvement with reflexive orientational movements of the eyes towards the sound source.

The different states of development of the lateral and medial olivary nucleus in various animals (page 75, footnote) were related to functional differences of the two nuclei by Masterton and Diamond.[752] In the medial nucleus the interaural time difference (Δt) is more effective while in the lateral nucleus the intensity difference (Δi) is more effective. Another possibility is that the difference of the spectral composition at the two ears (Δf) has a stronger effect on the magnitude of excitation. Naturally, for little animals the time difference is of minor significance; the same is true for the dolphin. In these animals, those structures processing Δi and Δf have to do the work.

4. The Nuclei of the Lateral Lemniscus

The normal population of neurons and their distributions within the nucleus of the lateral lemniscus were studied by Kane and Barone.[541] The dorsal nucleus receives contralateral afferent inputs from the cochlear nucleus* and binaural afferent input from the medial nucleus of the ipsilateral superior olive and from the S-segments of the superior olives of both sides. Another source of binaural convergence is Probst's commissure which links the dorsal nuclei of the lateral lemniscus of both sides together.[412, 694] The ventral nucleus receives fibers almost exclusively from the contralateral cochlear nucleus† and only a very small restricted input from the ipsilateral cochlear nucleus[1186] (the latter is not shown in Fig. 55).

The most extensive electrophysiological studies of these nuclei were carried out by Aitkin et al.[22] and by Brugge et al.[157] For both the dorsal and the ventral nucleus they found a tonotopic structure. In both nuclei, the low frequencies are represented in the dorsal part and the high frequencies in the ventral part.

The majority of neurons of the dorsal nucleus can be activated binaurally whereas those of the ventral nucleus as a rule, can be activated only contralaterally. Based on certain discharge patterns alone, the neurons cannot be classed with one or the other nucleus. The discharge patterns often change with tone frequency and intensity. Thus, pure on-discharges, discharges sustained for the whole duration of the tone, and the pause-pattern described on page 108 can be recorded from the same cell depending upon the stimulus conditions.

---

* References 61, 330, 859, 1185, 1186.
† References 61, 330, 859, 1185, 1186.

The response areas given by the tuning curves are flanked by inhibitory areas as observed in the cochlear nucleus. A phase-locked discharge can be observed up to 1 kHz. For all intensities, the latency has a relative minimum in the area of the characteristic frequency. For a fixed frequency, however, latency is generally a monotonic function of intensity (Fig. 108).

Under conditions of binaural stimulation, Brugge et al.[157] found in the dorsal nucleus a dependency of discharge rate on the interaural time difference, such that the cell's activity approaches a periodic pattern for low stimulus frequencies (Fig. 109) whereby the period of the function corresponds with the period of the stimulus. Since these same cells show a phase-locked discharge for monaural stimulation, this supports the assumption of a convergence of afferent inputs composed of periodically alternating discharge and inhibition. Neurons activated by contralateral but inhibited by ipsilateral stimuli are very sensitive to interaural intensity differences and are less dependent on the average intensity of the binaural stimulus (Fig. 110).

Given the present state of knowledge, one should not speculate about the possible functions of the lemniscal nuclei. Additional information is needed.

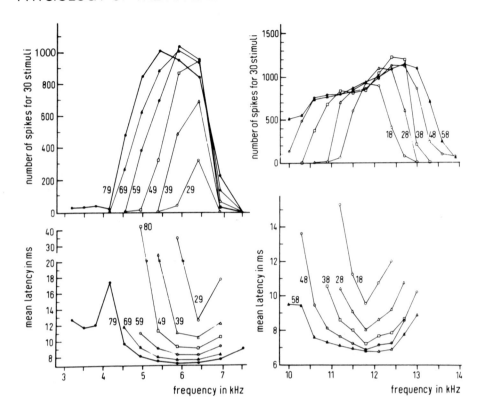

FIGURE 108. The two upper graphs show the frequency response curves of a unit for different intensities. Below are shown the corresponding curves of the latency of the first action potential triggered by the stimulus. Stimulus duration: 200 ms, stimulus repetition rate: left 2/s, right 1/s. (According to Aitkin et al. [22].)

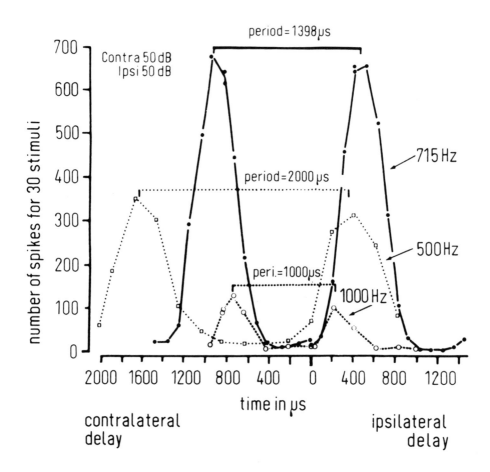

FIGURE 109. Number of action potentials of a unit of the dorsal nucleus of the lateral lemniscus triggered by 30 stimuli of 200 ms duration as a function of the interaural time delay (the parameters are the frequency and the intensity). (According to Brugge et al. [157].)

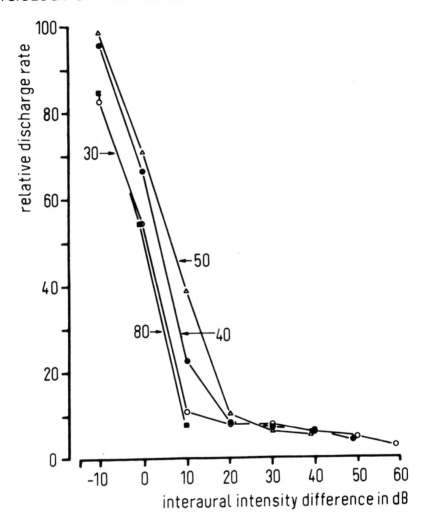

FIGURE 110. Relative discharge rate as a function of the interaural intensity difference for four different intensities (given in dB SPL) of the contralateral stimulus. (According to Brugge et al. [157].)

E. The Inferior Colliculus

In earlier times, primarily reflexive functions were assigned to the inferior colliculus, in analogy to the functions of the superior colliculus in the visual system. It was assumed that the axons of the primary auditory pathway ran from the lateral lemniscus directly to the medial geniculate and from there to the cortex. However, today there is no doubt that very few lemniscal fibers go directly to the medial geniculate. Most of the lateral lemniscal fibers end in the inferior colliculus.

The anatomical structure of the inferior colliculus is dominated by the conspicuous large central nucleus.* It contains laminellar organized cells with the dendrites arranged in discs that are contacted by the afferent fibers of the lateral lemniscus. Osen[876] topographically described the projection of the cochlear nuclei to this central nucleus and proved anatomically the tonotopic structure of the central nucleus which was found electrophysiologically by Rose et al.[979] and confirmed by Aitkin et al.,[23, 26] Semple and Aitkin,[1030] Aitkin and Moore,[20] Clopton and Winfield,[193] Adams and Teas,[6] and Merzenich and Reid[758] (Fig. 111).

The functional significance of this unusual attachment of a whole area in the central nucleus of the inferior colliculus to one point or, at the most, to one linear segment of the cochlea is unknown. From the currently popular mathematical approach to neurophysiological problems, it is a matter of transforming a two-dimensional space into a three-dimensional one. In other sensory systems (e.g. the visual and the somatosensory system), a point-to-point projection dominates the picture. Thus, it can be assumed that this structure reflects a principle specifically suited for auditory function. A theory on the functional principle of the central auditory pathway would have to explain this structure. According to van Noort[859] the inferior colliculus receives inputs from the lateral and medial nuclei of the superior olive, the dorsal and ventral nuclei of the lateral lemniscus, the dorsal and ventral nuclei of the cochlear nucleus, and the contralateral inferior colliculus. (Recent findings are described by Beyerl.[113]) Yet, it is surprising how precisely the tonotopic order is preserved.

In the central nucleus star cells also occur with their dendrites crossing as well as running parallel to the laminellar arranged telodendra of the disc-shaped cells.[393, 811] The wide tuning curves described by Erulkar,[297] Rose et al.[979] and Bock et al.[120] may perhaps belong to those star cells whereas the much more common sharp tuning curves[25, 1120] probably belong to the more numerous cells with the disc-shaped telodendra.

The central nucleus has been subdivided by Rockel[964] and Rockel and Jones[965, 966] into a dorsomedial and a ventrolateral part. The dorsomedial

---

* References 112, 393, 412, 809, 815.

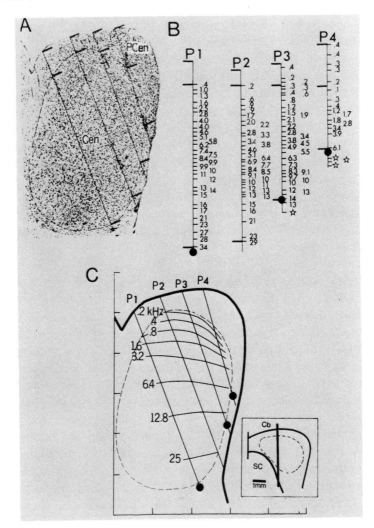

FIGURE 111. A, Sagittal section of the inferior colliculus at the location shown in the inset of C (right = caudal; left = rostral). Four microelectrode paths are shown. The cross bars at the paths mark the border between the central nucleus (Cen) and the pericentral areas (PCen). The approximate border line of the central nucleus is indicated by a dashed line. B, Reconstruction of the 4 electrode paths shown in A. Again, the heavy cross bars mark the borders of the central nucleus. The numbers give the characteristic frequencies in kHz of single units or groups of units found at those places marked by light cross bars. At those locations marked with an asterisk a response of the unit was obtained only with very high stimulus intensities. The filled circles show the locations at which the position of the electrode was marked by a lesion. C, Schematic presentation of iso-frequency contours thus obtained for characteristic frequencies. The iso-frequency contours are spaced at intervals of 1 octave and run parallel to the cellular laminae. Cb = cerebellum, SC = superior colliculus. (According to Merzenich and Reid [758].)

part receives efferent fibers from the auditory cortex, and the ventrolateral part receives afferent fibers from the lateral lemniscus.

The central nucleus is surrounded dorsally and caudally by the pericentral nucleus and laterally and rostrally by the outer nucleus (nucl. ext. coll. inf.). According to Geniec and Morest[393] the pericentral nucleus has a cortical character. Rockel and Jones,[967] however, described a laminar structure instead.

Ascending fibers of the dorsal lemniscal nucleus are believed to arrive in the pericentral and in the central nucleus. Other fibers of the lemniscus do not project to the central nucleus. The lateral sector of the outer nucleus receives both somatosensory and auditory inputs.[27] Thus, the vast majority of fibers from the lateral lemniscus end in the central nucleus.* As mentioned above, a few lemniscal fibers end in the outer nucleus also, but this nucleus presumably is innervated primarily by fibers originating from the central nucleus.[807, 1130]

Morest[814] and Geniec and Morest[393] described lemniscal fibers branching off collaterals into the 4th layer (IV) of their cortical formation (pericentral nucleus) together with collaterals of fibers originating in the central nucleus. This would allow an integration of the input and output activity of the inferior colliculus. Layers I to III presumably do not receive any lemniscal inputs. According to Geniec and Morest, layer III is qualified best for an integration of ascending and descending activities, especially via internal connections between the neurons of layers II and IV that receive the most external inputs.

Since the inferior colliculus has a quite differentiated structure its functional role probably is relatively complicated. In electrophysiological studies an accurate localization of the recording site is indispensable.

Aitkin et al.[25] compared the response behavior of cells of the central nucleus, the pericentral nucleus and the nucleus externus. The cells of the central nucleus were characterized by very sharp tuning curves† (Fig. 112 b) and by responses to binaural stimuli whereas the other cells frequently had very wide tuning curves and less pronounced characteristic frequencies (Fig. 112 a). However, in these other cells the recording of tuning curves is very difficult since they show rapid habituation and they do not respond any more after two to five repetitions of the same stimulus. If the frequency of the stimulating tone is changed, a prompt response results.[23] The function of these cells could be viewed in connection with arousal reactions.

A rule generally accepted earlier which maintained that the spontaneous activity decreases while proceeding from the periphery to the central

---

* References 393, 412, 694.

† The development of these tuning curves and of their tonotopic localization was described by Aitkin and Moore (20) in kittens between the 6th and 28th day after birth.

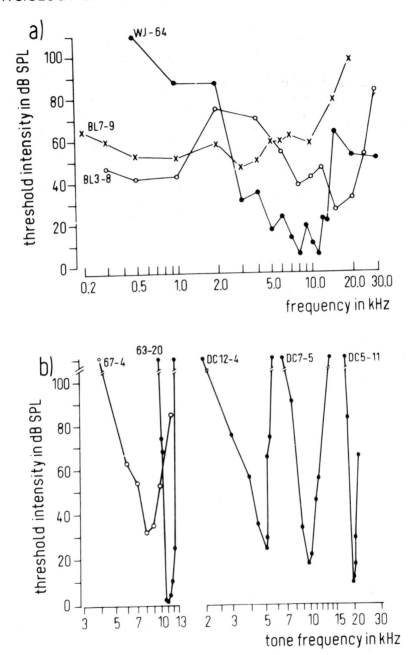

FIGURE 112. A, Typical tuning curves of units of the pericentral nucleus (WJ-64) and of the nucleus externus (BL 3-8, BL 7-9). B, Typical tuning curves of units of the central nucleus. (According to Aitkin et al. [25].)

parts of the auditory pathway seems actually to be due to anesthesia. In the awake cat, Bock et al.[120] observed spontaneous activity in all cells studied (average discharge rate 12.3 spikes per second in the awake cat* as compared to 4.7 spikes per second in the anesthetized cat). Interval histograms of the spontaneous activity show that, apart from the Poisson-distribution, fixed discharge frequencies also occur in the inferior colliculus (Fig. 113).

Both monotonic† and non-monotonic‡ intensity functions have been described. As a rule, the average discharge rate is lower than in the deeper nuclei.

In the post-stimulus-time histograms very different response patterns occur (Fig. 114), namely:

1. pure on-effects, i.e. activity is triggered only at the beginning of the stimulus;
2. sustained discharges, i.e., for the whole duration of the stimulus, discharges occur either as "primary-like" pattern with an initial overshoot then leveling off to a steady state (adaptation), or as "pause" pattern with a silent period after an initial overshoot followed by the sustained discharge, or as sustained discharge building up without an initial overshoot;
3. pure off-effect patterns, i.e. discharges occur only after termination of the stimulus; and
4. inhibition for the whole duration of the stimulus.§

Phase-locked discharges are also found in the inferior colliculus.‖ For lower frequencies the shortest discharge interval is equal to the tone period, for higher frequencies the shortest discharge interval approaches an integer multiple of the tone frequency (Fig. 115). The reduction of the higher periodicity of the stimulus to the lower periodicity of excitation, as can be seen very impressively in Fig. 115c, is called demultiplication.[575] It enables the occurrence of excitation periods of 10 to 30 ms that correspond with stimulus periods on the order of 0.1 ms.

These response patterns cannot be regarded as a characteristic property of the respective cell because, upon varying stimulus frequency and intensity, practically all response patterns can occur in the same cell. If the response patterns are to be classified, one has to keep standard conditions of

---

* In the awake Rhesus monkey the mean value is 14.7 spikes/s (Reference 1001).
† References 120, 219, 1001.
‡ References 297, 485, 979, 1001.
§ References 120, 219, 586, 599, 600, 604, 980, 1118.
‖ References 120, 211, 575, 578, 587, 588, 604, 980.

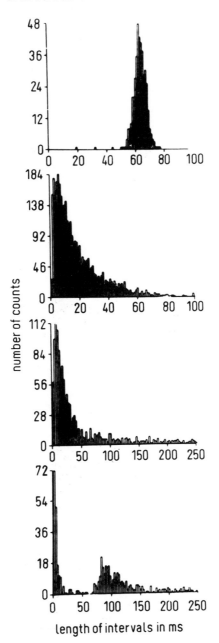

FIGURE 113. Interval histograms of the spontaneous activity of different units of the inferior colliculus. Top histogram: the discharges occur at a fixed frequency (average period length slightly above 60 ms). Second and third histogram from the top: the discharges occur approximately according to a Poisson distribution (see page 83). Bottom histogram: bimodal distribution of the lengths of intervals. (According to Bock and Webster [118].)

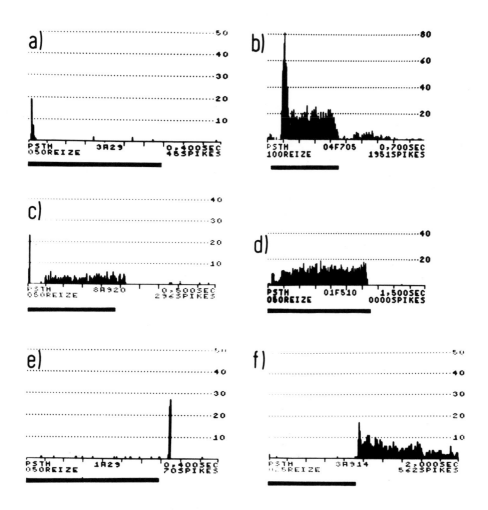

FIGURE 114. Typical response patterns obtained from the inferior colliculus shown as post-stimulus-time histograms. A, On-discharge; B, "Primary-like"-pattern; C, Pause-pattern; D, steady discharge without initial overshoot; E, off-discharge; F, steady inhibition. (According to David et al. [219] and Kallert [535].)

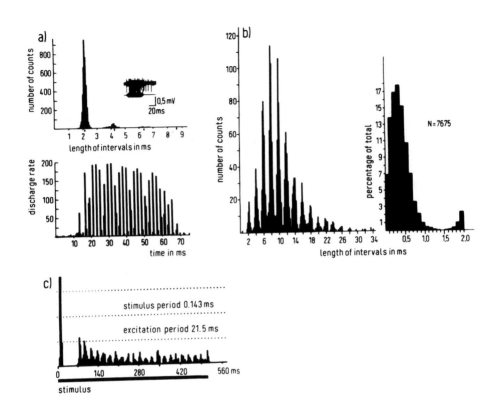

FIGURE 115. A, Above: interval histogram, below: the corresponding post-stimulus-time histogram of the response of the unit of the inferior colliculus. Stimulus: 480 Hz tone, 50 ms. The histogram is based on 200 stimuli. Stimulus repetition rate: 1/s. (According to Bock et al. [120]. B, Left: interval histogram, right: period histogram of a unit of the inferior colliculus upon binaural stimulation with a continuous tone of 500 Hz for 10 s. Whereas in A almost exclusively the length of the stimulus period occurs as discharge interval, in B the length of the stimulus period can also be observed, but an interval length of four times the period encountered is most frequent. Also, interval lengths of 10 times the period length occur. (According to Rose et al. [980].) C, Section of the post-stimulus-time histogram of a unit of the inferior colliculus (the initial discharge is not shown completely at this scale). Stimulus: pure tone of 7 kHz, 500 ms. The histogram is based on 20 stimuli. Here, the lengths of intervals are longer than 100 times the period of the stimulus. (According to David et al. [220].)

stimulation (for instance, stimulation with tones at the characteristic frequency 10 dB above threshold, as was done in the experiment of Fig. 95). If an early action potential always occurs (thus enabling a comparison), the latency of this first stimulus-related action potential depends on both intensity and (for tone) frequency of the stimulus. Typical changes of the latency with stimulus intensity are shown in Fig. 116.

In the inferior colliculus, binaural effects with EE and EI character are also encountered.* Fig. 117 shows a few typical results.

Regarding the discharge behavior upon binaural stimulation with clicks, Benevento and Coleman[106] were able to distinguish four different neuronal populations:

1. neurons sensitive to interaural intensity differences;
2. neurons sensitive to interaural time difference;
3. neurons sensitive neither to interaural time nor intensity differences; and
4. neurons sensitive to both time and intensity differences.

As in the complex nuclei of the superior olive and in the nuclei of the lateral lemniscus, these binaural effects are viewed as being related to directional hearing. Therefore, at this point a summary of the results of behavioral experiments carried out on these lines after brain stem lesions in the cat will be added.

Whereas sectioning the corpus callosum and the brachium of the inferior colliculi[801] causes no impairment of directional hearing, irreversible loss of directional hearing results[184] from sectioning the trapezoid nucleus and the commissures of Held and Monakow (see page 74). If, however, the anterodorsal part of the trapezoid nucleus is left intact, localization ability is not impaired.[843] Since according to Warr[1185] fibers in this very part run from the cochlear nucleus to the medial olivary nucleus, the significance of the nucleus accessorius for directional hearing is thus supported. Masterton et al.[753] could show that species with a marked nucleus accessorius were able to localize the source of low-frequency tones, whereas species with a poorly developed nucleus accessorius have directional hearing for high-frequency stimuli only.

Unilateral sectioning of the lateral lemniscus or of the brachium colliculi inferioris results in localization errors for the contralateral auditory field.[1112] Bilateral sectioning of the brachia colliculi inferiores or of the lateral lemnisci causes a complete loss of directional hearing. The ventral part of the inferior colliculus proved to be very important for directional hearing.[843] After destruction of one ear, an animal can learn to localize tone stimuli by skillful head movements that result in intensity fluctuations.

---

* References 24, 119, 345, 392, 485, 980, 1126.

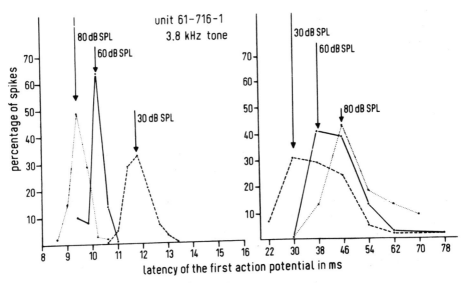

FIGURE 116. Distribution of the latency of the first potential of a unit of the inferior colliculus upon stimulation with clicks of different intensities. Left: early first action potential, right: late first action potential. As can be seen, the long latencies, as shown in the right figure, increase with increasing stimulus intensity, probably as a result of inhibition being the basis of the long latencies. (According to Hind et al. [485].)

However, after sectioning the trapezoid nucleus, there is no way to improvize directional hearing. Finally, Neff and Casseday,[841] in agreement with Whitfield,[1215] were able to demonstrate that with respect to spatial perceptions each ear was associated with the contralateral cortex. In the owl, Knudsen and Konishi[659-662] discovered cells in the midbrain that were either strictly spatially selective (localization of the sound source), or strictly frequency selective. A similar segregation of cells might exist also in the cat.[1030]

The significance of directional hearing should not be disregarded. It enables one to envisage a sound source that possibly was outside the visual field or was at first optically not perceptible.

In the inferior colliculus much more neurons than in the cochlear nucleus show a response selectivity to special features of amplitude-modulated or frequency-modulated stimuli. Stimulus properties to which such cells are particularly sensitive include the change of velocity, the change of direction, and the change of the value of the stimulus frequency and amplitude. Many patterns of excitation obtained from single cells of the inferior colliculus indicating a feature extraction of acoustical signals were described primarily in the bat.* Yet it seems as if even these responses can be

---

* There are a large number of reports concerning the inferior colliculus in bats (References 289, 427–429, 799, 904, 905, 1018–1020, 1115–1121, 1171, 1172).

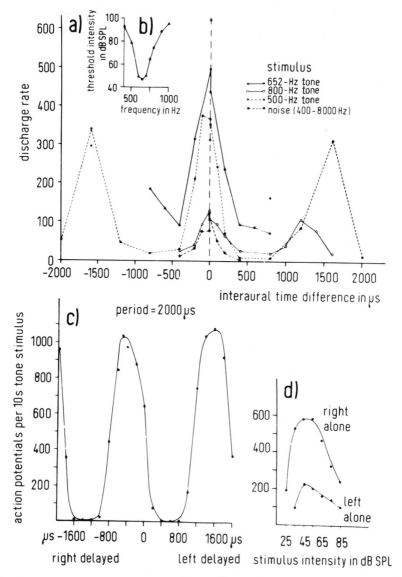

FIGURE 117. Variation of the number of action potentials triggered by binaural stimulation, if the stimulus offered to one ear has a temporal delay with respect to the stimulus offered to the other ear. A, The intensities of the different stimuli were for the 500 Hz tone: 87 dB ipsilateral, 91 dB contralateral; for the 652 Hz tone: 59 dB ipsilateral, 62 dB contralateral; for the 800 Hz tone: 84 dB ipsilateral, 87 dB contralateral; for the noise: 71 dB ipsilateral, 74 dB contralateral. B, threshold curve (= tuning curve) of the same unit as in A upon monaural contralateral stimulation (monaural ipsilateral stimulation did not result in a recordable response for any frequency range). C, Stimulation with a 500 Hz steady tone of 10 s, offered bilaterally at 45 dB SPL. D, Intensity functions of the same unit as in C. (A and B according to Geisler et al. [392]; C and D according to Rose et al. [980].)

predicted from their behavior following pure-tone stimuli, especially if the inhibitory response areas flanking the tuning curve and the latency times are taken into consideration.* Response patterns to frequency-modulated stimuli have been described, however, which did not seem to be explicable from the response to pure tones.† Such response behavior is much more characteristic for the medial geniculate and the auditory cortex. It is still assumed that the inferior colliculi, as mesencephalic nuclei, are responsible primarily for reflex activities. Thus, in animals having motor functions strongly dependent on acoustically controlled reflexes, as is the case in the bat, they might be an important stage of integration. Other results, however, indicate that the patterns of discharge are influenced by activities connected with the stimulus.[1000]

F. The Medial Geniculate Nucleus

The anatomical structure of the medial geniculate body was described more extensively on page 76. The Golgi-type-II cells mentioned above and described by Morest might play an important role. With their short axons they are regarded as being intranuclear interneurons. Figure 118 shows their typical innervation pattern while Figure 119 somewhat schematically summarizes the intercellular relations.

The distance of the synapses from the site of generation of the action potential probably indicates a predominance of the input via those synapses. Thus, if the descending fibers insert at the distal dendritic area of the principal cells but the afferent fibers insert at the middle dendritic area, then the relative effect of the afferent inputs per synapse could be larger than that of the efferent ones.

Because of the very intimate connection between the cortex and the medial geniculate, ablations of the auditory cortex always cause a marked degeneration of large parts of the medial geniculate. Thus, lesion experiments do not allow a differentiation between function of the cortex and the

---

* References 1117–1120, 1122.
† References 298, 301, 905, 946, 1170.

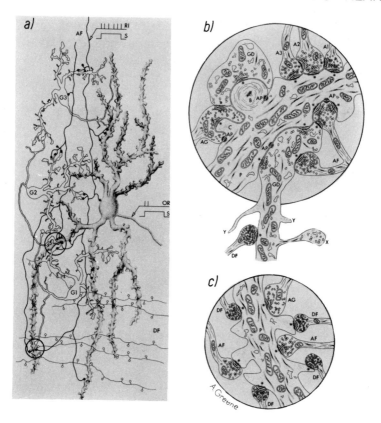

FIGURE 118. A, Synaptic organization of the ventral part of the pars principalis of the medial geniculate body. The principal cell sends its axon (OR) to the auditory cortex and receives synapses of ascending fibers (AF) from the posterior colliculus. Most ascending axons synapse in the synaptic nests on intermediate dendrites (B), fewer on distal dendrites (C), and very few on the soma. Many ascending afferents also synapse on distal dendrites of Gogi-type-II cells (e.g., G1 and G2), fewer on intermediate dendrites (G3), and relatively few on the soma (e.g., G3). Descending fibers (DF) from the cortex end predominantly on distal dendrites of principal cells and on intermediate dendrites and somata of Golgi-type-II cells (e.g., G1). Different response-patterns have been recorded from posterior colliculus (RI) and medial geniculate (OR) in response to acoustic stimuli (S).

B, Organization of a synaptic nest (from A, large circle). P = principal cell dendrite with "ball" (B) and "claw" (C) appendages. GD = Golgi-type-II cell dendrite with pre- (X) and post- (Y) synaptic filiform appendages just outside the nest. AF = ascending axonal endings; AG = axon of Golgi-type-II cell or of an undefined extrinsic source; A1, A2, A3 = sequential axo-axonic and axodendritic synapses involving small, large, and medium-sized afferent axons respectively, and the principal cell dendrite; * = postsynaptic sites; AP = attachment plaques; DF = corticogeniculate axon.

C, Distal dendrite of principal cell with typical hatchet-shaped and dentate appendages (from A, small circle).

(According to Morest [818].)

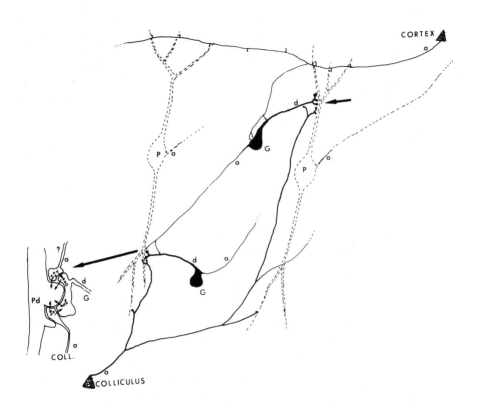

FIGURE 119. Semi-schematic diagram showing some of the principal synaptic relationships in the ventral nucleus of the medial geniculate body. Descending axons (a) from the auditory cortex end on the distal dendrites of principal cells (P) and on the proximal dendrites and somata of Golgi-type-II cells (G). Ascending axons from the posterior colliculus end on the distal and intermediate dendrites of Golgi-type-II (d) and principal neurons. The dendrites and axons of Golgi-type-II cells end on the intermediate dendrites of principal cells in the axonal nests (large arrows). The axonal nests seen in rapid Golgi preparations correspond to the synaptic nests in electron micrographs. An inset shows the sequential arrangement of the synaptic contacts (small arrows) in a typical nest at the lower left: a Golgi-type-II dendrite (G, d) synapses on a principal cell dendrite (Pd) and receives synapses from axons (a) of collicular and non-collicular (?) cells that also synapse on the principal cell's dendrite. (According to Morest [818].)

medial geniculate.* Therefore, electrophysiological studies appear to be particularly necessary for a functional diagnosis.†

The first microelectrode studies of the medial geniculate were carried out by Thurlow et al.,[1139] Galambos,[383] Galambos et al.,[387] and by Rose and Galambos.[976] They found short (8 to 24 ms) as well as long (50 to 200 ms) latencies for click stimuli and the "pause"-pattern described above for tone stimuli.

The most extensive studies carried out recently were by the Australian group of Dunlop, Aitkin and Webster. The same response patterns as described for the inferior colliculus occur in the medial geniculate. The stimulus-phase-locked discharge, however, has been found only in a few cells of the pars magnocellularis and of the ventral part for stimulus frequencies up to 1000 Hz.[956, 988] In addition, discharge patterns occur that have not been observed in responses from deeper nuclei. Specific features of single units are:

1. Periodic spontaneous activity with periods on the order of 10 to 100 ms;‡
2. Very long excitation, inhibition and latency times§ (Fig. 120).
3. Periodic discharges during and especially after the stimulus with periods of 100 to 200 ms‖ (Fig. 121).

---

* Nevertheless, excellent results are available showing that decorticated cats are able to discriminate between different frequencies and intensities almost as well as normal cats (References 165, 204, 206, 262, 409, 410, 763). However, they lose the ability to discriminate between temporal features of the stimulus such that the direction of frequency modulation (References 165, 623, 625) can be discriminated only very poorly. In addition, tone patterns of different temporal sequence cannot be discriminated at all (References 264, 265). Likewise, the ability to localize a sound source in space can be affected (References 206, 751, 840, 842, 943). Whitfield (Reference 1217) could show that normal cats hear harmonic triads as having a pitch equivalent to the missing fundamental (Reference 474). Bilateral removal of the auditory cortex destroys the learned discriminations both of the complex pitch and the pitch of simple tones. The latter can be rapidly recovered by retraining. It is also possible to retrain the animals to discriminate the high frequency triads but they now do this on the basis of the individual frequency components and not on the basis of the fundamental pitch. This supports Whitfield's (Reference 1216) view of sensory cortex as being concerned with the "constancies" (of size, shape, position, etc.) associated with the external world. In all these cases of cortical ablation, large parts of the medial geniculate degenerate also.
† The method of reversibly blocking the cortex by cold may perhaps lead to a solution of this problem (References 536, 537).
‡ References 21, 220, 538, 575, 579, 580, 586.
§ References 14, 169, 222, 532, 586, 590, 591.
‖ References 13–15, 21, 223, 274, 532, 586, 590, 591.

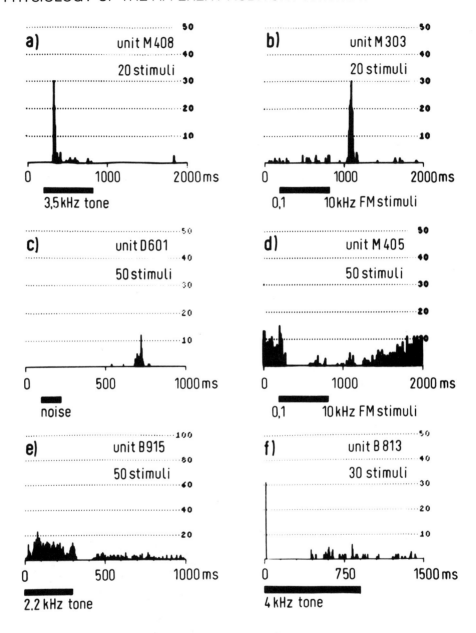

FIGURE 120. Post-stimulus-time histograms showing the long latencies or inhibitory effects or after effects. (Each histogram is based on 20 stimulus presentations. Bar below panels indicates stimulus.) Note the long latencies (100 to 1000 ms), well outside the range of typical values (5 - 60 ms) for units throughout the auditory pathway. A, on-effect with latency ca. 100 ms. B, off-effect with latency ca. 100 ms. C, latency ca. 400 ms. D, inhibitory effect nearly 1000 ms longer than stimulus. E, inhibitory off-effect ca. 100 ms. F, inhibitory on-effect ca. 300 ms (silent period). (According to Kallert [532].)

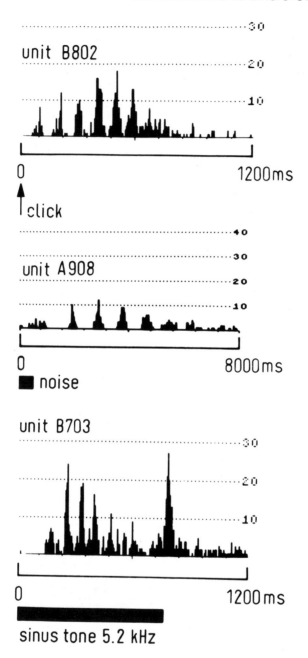

FIGURE 121. Examples of periodic unit discharges during the following stimulus presentations. Long lasting (up to 1 s) post-stimulus unit activity with a period around 10 Hz (after click unit B802, after short noise burst unit A908). Discharge periodicity during stimulus presentation unit B703. (According to Kallert [534].)

4. Although units with single-peak frequency response curves occur (as is the rule in the deeper nuclei), there is a strikingly high number of cells having frequency response curves with several peaks.* Thus, the term tonotopic organization should be used with reservation† (Fig. 122).
5. Dynamic stimuli (e.g. frequency-modulated or amplitude-modulated stimuli) are much more effective than pure tones. The response to dynamic stimuli generally is not predictable from the response to steady pure tones‡ as was the case for the deeper nuclei[808] (Fig. 123).
6. There are units that respond vigorously to complex stimuli, but do not respond at all or only very poorly to single components of these stimuli. §

Such characteristic discharge properties of course lead to speculations about their possible functional significance. The multi-peak frequency response curves and the response to complex stimuli suggest that frequency discrimination‖ takes place at a level below the medial geniculate, which is in agreement with the results obtained from behavioral experiments after cortical ablation.** However, these factors also suggest that this response behavior may be related to the recognition of complex natural stimuli,††,[1051] covering a broad frequency range (Fig. 124 top, middle) (e.g. the formants of the vowels). Pure tones as used in the laboratory do not occur naturally.‡‡

Excitations triggered primarily by frequency modulation could be related with the recognition of natural stimuli in so far as many natural stimuli include rapid frequency transitions (e.g. in some consonants, Fig. 124 bottom). For frequency-modulated stimuli, the long latencies and stimulus after-effects could be the basis for the dependence of excitation on the direction and the velocity of frequency changes. They also could be

---

* References 220, 274, 387, 532, 575, 579, 580, 586, 590, 591.
† However, tonotopic organization has been described for the medial geniculate (References 16, 17, 432). These results are still under discussion (Reference 1220).
‡ References 534, 586, 590, 591, 1187.
§ References 532, 586, 590, 591.
‖ Intensity discrimination too seems to take place at a lower level than the medial geniculate (References 840, 843) which also follows from behavioral experiments after cortical ablation or after sectioning the brachia of the inferior colliculi.
** References 206, 410, 717, 843.
†† In fact, in neurons of the medial geniculate responding poorly to pure tones vigorous discharges are frequently observed following very soft natural sounds like whisper or rustle. But there is also the opposite opinion described (Reference 1127).
‡‡ Recently, vowel-selective discharge behavior was observed also in the cochlear nucleus (References 180, 996).

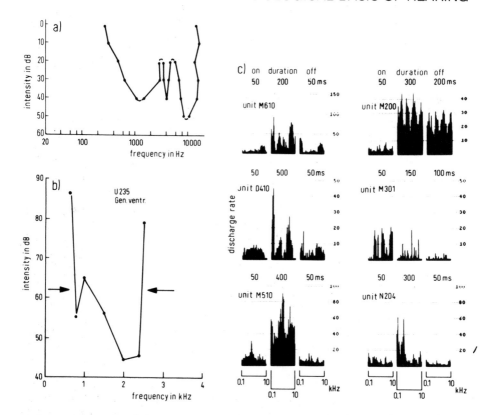

FIGURE 122. Tuning curves (A, B) and frequency response curves (isointensity curves) (C) of single units of the medial geniculate showing several characteristic frequencies. The areas under the frequency response curves are filled out black. Three frequency response curves having different intervals were recorded from each unit. "On" stands for the first 50 ms after the beginning of the stimulus, "Duration" stands for the whole remaining length of the stimulus, "Off" stands for the first time interval following the end of the stimulation. The length of the different time intervals is specified for each histogram. (A, according to Galambos [383]; B, according to Dunlop et al. [274]; C, according to Kallert [532].)

related with the ultra-short-time memory* necessary for the recognition of natural stimuli. This also would be in line with the results obtained from behavioral experiments (footnote on page 166).

---

* That is, a memory necessary for understanding a word since the whole length from the beginning to the end of the word has to be taken into consideration. In order to discriminate, e.g. between "season" and "reason" the "s" resp. "r" still must be effective during the period of "eason."

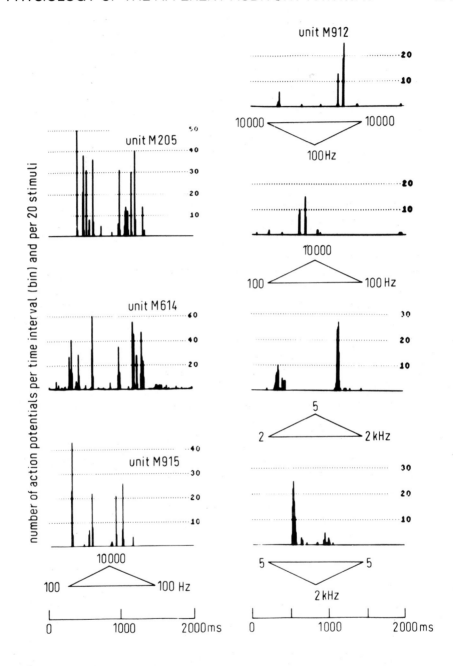

FIGURE 123. Left: response patterns of three single units of the medial geniculate to frequency-modulated stimuli. Each histogram is based on 20 stimuli. The stimulus symbol shows the direction of the change of frequency in time, namely from 100 Hz to 10000 Hz and back to 100 Hz. Right: dependence of the discharge pattern on the direction of the change of frequency. (According to Kallert [532].)

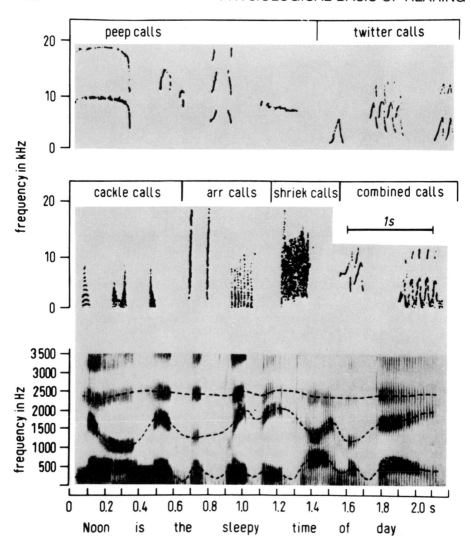

FIGURE 124. Above: sound spectrum of some calls of the squirrel monkey (according to Winter [1238]). The simultaneous combination of several frequencies and the variation of frequency in time can clearly be seen. Below: sound spectrum of the sentence "noon is the sleepy time of day" with idealized curves for the first three speech formants. (According to Flanagan [350].)

These ideas were advanced primarily by Keidel.[575–607] In general, such functions are expected to be accomplished only by the cortex. Quite similar response patterns following frequency-modulated stimuli as well as multi-peak frequency response curves and tuning curves have been obtained from cortical recordings. Stimulated by the work of Winter and Funkenstein,[1239] cortical neurons of awake animals were studied following stimulation with natural sounds. To a certain degree, stimulus-selective behavior was found.

This is not in conflict, however, with Keidel's hypothesis in which the medial geniculate begins the processing of natural vowel-like and consonant-like stimuli. It is not surprising that the response patterns developed in the geniculate appear again in the subsequent level of the auditory pathway, the primary auditory cortex. In addition, the neo-cortex developed at a relatively late state of evolution. Even lower animals, however, had to be able to recognize sounds of their own species and sounds indicating danger or food.

If the discrimination of sounds takes place already in the thalamus, storage functions of the cortex with respect to the "analysis of speech" can be expected. These functions are necessary for recognition and are much more exacting in human language using words, whole sentences, and even long lectures than in elementary sound discrimination.

Keidel connected the stimulus-independent rhythmic spontaneous activity (length of period 10 to 100 ms) with the strongly demultiplied stimulus-evoked periodicity such that by measurement of coincidence between the spontaneous activity and the periodic stimulus response a maximum of coincidence occurs at even-numbered multiples of the stimulus-related periodicity of excitation (Fig. 125). This could be the basis for the sensation of octaves.

Such frequency-response curves could of course be the result of simple convergences. This would explain multi-peak frequency response curves having characteristic frequencies that are not related to each other in an even-numbered way.

Binaural effects for both interaural intensity and time differences,[12, 13] quite similar to those in the inferior colliculus, have also been found in the medial geniculate (Fig. 126). Altman et al.[32] were able to prove a special sensitivity to movements of the source of sound.

Naturally, disturbing effects have to be expected from anesthesia at the level of the thalamus and the cortex. Thus, recordings from awake animals are desirable. Particularly striking differences between the results obtained from awake pharmacologically unaffected cats and from anesthetized cats are:[18, 534]

1. a substantially higher spontaneous activity and, thus, much more inhibitory patterns in awake animals;

2. the discharge periodicity following termination of the stimulus with a characteristic period of about 100 ms was not encountered in awake animals;

3. under anesthesia on- and off-effects dominate whereas, in the awake cat, response effects are generally present during the whole length of the stimulus; and

4. frequently, the discharge pattern of the same cell changes while the stimulus stays constant in awake animals, probably in connection with attention.

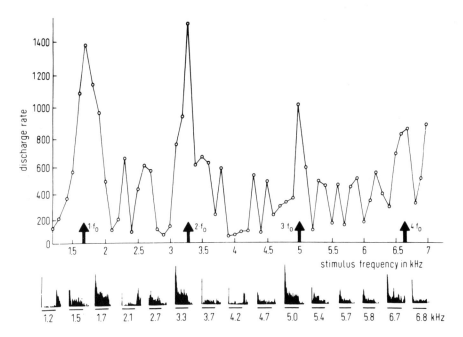

FIGURE 125. Lower line: Post-stimulus-time histograms of a unit upon stimulation with tone bursts of equal intensity but different frequency. Above: frequency response curve of the same unit with maxima of excitation at integer multiples of the fundamental frequency (arrows). (According to David et al. [220].)

Higher spontaneous activity in the awake cat has also been observed in recent times in other parts of the auditory pathway, namely the inferior colliculus[120] and the cochlear nucleus.[312, 313] Here, it causes a higher incidence of stimulus-related inhibitions in the awake cat than in the anesthetized animal. Evans could show that in the nucleus cochlearis dorsalis inhibition can be observed less frequently during anesthesia not only because of the low spontaneous activity, but that inhibition itself is probably suppressed because of barbiturate-sensitive synapses required for inhibition. A low or high incidence of inhibitory effects might be responsible for the reversal of polarity of the evoked potential associated with anesthetization (Fig. 127).

In the cat, however, the spontaneous activity of the single cell in the medial geniculate is not constant. Rather, it varies according to the general activity of the animal, as has also been reported for different cortical areas.* Together with the variability of the discharge patterns following presentation of identical stimuli this may lead to a larger variability in the statistical

---

* References 210, 318–320, 834, 856.

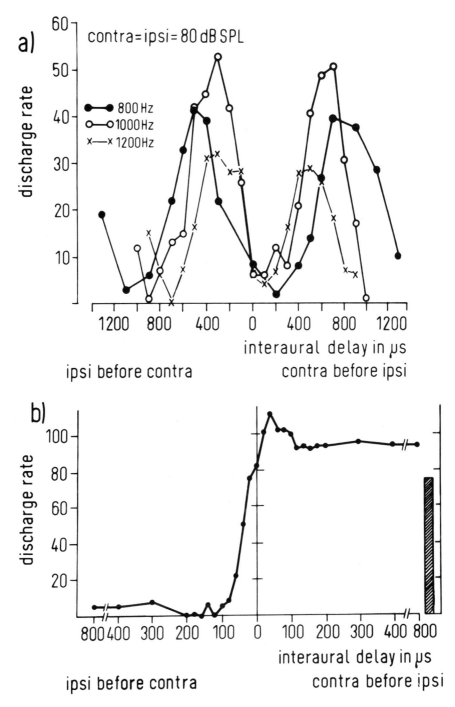

FIGURE 126. Discharge rate as a function of the interaural time delay upon binaural stimulation for a single unit from the medial geniculate. A, Tone stimuli (according to Aitkin and Webster [17].) B, Click stimuli (according to Starr and Don [1101].)

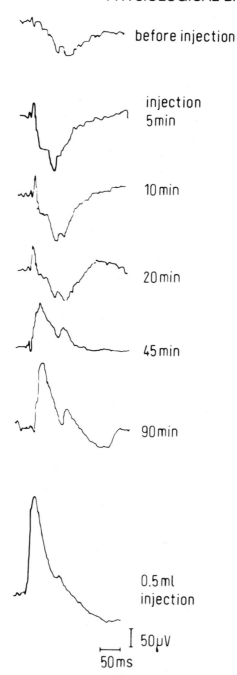

FIGURE 127. The effect of barbiturate on a click-evoked potential recorded from the medial geniculate. The time span between the injection and the recording is specified for each curve. (According to Webster and Aitkin [1190].)

evaluation of responses. Therefore it may be the reason that the frequency-response curves in the awake cat have maxima even less sharply tuned than those in the anesthetized cat.

The intra-fiber variability of the stimulus response-elicited may be related to the cat's attentiveness to the stimulus. Wickelgren,[1225] for instance, found that during habituation the responses triggered by click stimuli were clearly attenuated in the medial geniculate and in the cortex, although not in the deeper nuclei. Hall[447] has observed a similar behavior, while Kitzes and Buchwald[646] and Holstein et al.[494] have found alterations in the lower parts of the auditory pathway associated with habituation, even though the changes were more pronounced in the geniculate and the cortex. The effect of habituation could be explained by the efferent connections. Amato et al.,[34] for instance, could suppress click-evoked potentials of the geniculate and the inferior colliculus by electrically stimulating specific sites of the primary auditory cortex. By stimulation of the cortex, Katsuki[544] could obtain both facilitation and inhibition in the geniculate. Such effects, moreover, are not restricted to the cortex. By stimulating different sites of the septum, Powell et al.[913] were able to exert either excitation or inhibition in different units of the geniculate. By electrically stimulating the nucleus caudatus, La Grutta et al.[700] were able to inhibit click-evoked discharges of single units in the geniculate. Thus, in the geniculate not only may an analysis of complex sound take place in the sense described above (e.g. vowel and consonant detectors) but an essential control by the cortex and possibly the limbic system becomes effective here.

An unresolved physiological feature is the 10 Hz periodicity. This periodicity has been observed by Bremer[143] and Bremer and Bonnet[148] in the auditory cortex and in the medial geniculate, by Adrian[10, 11] in the somatosensory cortex and in the thalamic nuclei, and was also confirmed later by microelectrode studies (somatosensory thalamic nuclei,[35-38] medial geniculate,[21, 532, 533] lateral geniculate[159-161]). With the aid of intracellular recordings, corresponding hyperpolarizations were demonstrated[37] that apparently were responsible for the periodicity. Even after brain-stem sectioning at the level of the colliculi[1175] and after decortication[14, 35] the periodicity persists. Thus, it seems to be a property of the thalamus and it can be triggered by antidromic stimulation. From the invariable latency difference—between antidromically triggered excitation and hyperpolarization—of about 1.5 ms, the existence of inhibitory interneurons was inferred. These might be the Golgi-type-II cells (see page 57) described by Morest. It is assumed that, upon excitation, thalamic neurons (projection cells) activate—via collaterals of the thalamo-cortical axons—a system of thalamic interneurons* generating recurrently an inhibitory postsynaptic potential of

---

* The same process can be initiated by electrical stimulation of the brachia colliculorum inferiorum and by antidromic stimulation of the thalamo-cortical axons.

about 100 ms duration in the projection cells. By virtue of some kind of post-anodal excitation, discharges will ensue again followed by subsequent inhibition. This process is repeated over and over again. During its course, one neuron is supposed to activate several interneurons and one interneuron to inhibit several neurons in such a way that, like an avalanche, grouped discharges occur which can also be recorded as evoked potentials.[1190] A gradual desynchronization causes the periodicity to subside. It remains to be tested whether this 10 Hz periodicity is related to attention and whether it possibly blocks the conduction of auditory information to the cortex when the attention is to be shifted to another sensory channel.

G. The Auditory Cortex

The auditory cortex is even more complicated than the subcortical nuclei, in two respects. First, as described on page 78, its demarcation is much more difficult than that of the nuclei, especially with regard to the subdivision into primary, secondary and tertiary areas. Secondly, in the auditory cortex larger differences between the human and the animal are to be expected so that the results obtained from the animal can hardly be applied to the human. In the human, the most important functions of the auditory cortex should be related with the speech as a typically human achievement.

In this context, memory plays an important role. Also, those peculiarities of the auditory system expressing themselves in its characterization as "time sense"* must be evident from the cortical functions. Thus, Colavita,[198] for instance, was able to show that cats trained (avoidance reaction) to discriminate between light-stimulus sequences dark-bright-dark and bright-dark-bright lost this ability irreversibly by bilateral decortication of the insular cortex, whereas ablation of the primary and secondary visual cortex does not affect the avoidance reaction. Thus, the perception of changes of

---

* The auditory system preferably is termed "time sense" because the content of auditory information is based on the temporal change of sound. In fact, it is impossible to process information with a stationary, i.e. time-independent sound stimulus, whereas stationary visual stimuli (e.g. writing) are apt to transmit information. This is by no means in conflict with the principle of visual function that for the perception of time-independent structures, avoids a stationary image on the retina by continuous scanning movements of the eye balls. Moreover, this principle of visual function enables the eye to perceive stationary environmental structures. Thus, for describing auditory stimuli, a time axis is always necessary as shown in Figure 124.

temporal patterns of stimuli activating *different sensory modalities* in the cat seems to depend on the function of the insular cortex. With regard to temporal properties of auditory stimuli, this was described on page 166.

The auditory cortex receives its input primarily from the geniculate. These cortical projections of the medial geniculate, as well as the intracortical, the commissural and the corticothalamic connections of the auditory cortex in the cat, have also been studied again recently* (Figs. 128 and 129). According to electrophysiological results, additional cortical areas (e.g. motor cortex,[1006] frontal cortex[1243]) subserve auditory function (Fig. 130).

As mentioned earlier, many descending connections exist between the cortex and the geniculate. According to Pontes et al.,[906] efferent fibers run from the deeper layers of AI through the deeper layers of the dorsal part of the pars principalis and through the pars magnocellularis to the ventral nucleus of the geniculate. From AII, fibers run through the magnocellular part and end in the superficial and deeper layers of the dorsal nucleus. Fibers from AII also originate from the posterior ectosylvian auditory cortex and run diffusely to all subnuclei of the medial geniculate including the pars magnocellularis. Among the periauditory cortical areas, fibers also run from the suprasylvian margin to the dorsal subnucleus and from the anterior ectosylvian auditory cortex to the pars magnocellularis. The insular cortex does not project to the geniculate, although there are many connections to deeper nuclei of the auditory pathway.†

Since the time that Woolsey and Walzl carried out their early studies [1244-1248] on the tonotopy of AI and auditory cortical areas surrounding AI, a variety of investigators have confirmed their findings.‡ Several authors, however, deny cortical tonotopy in the same sense that applies to the cochlear nucleus and to the lower nuclei of the auditory pathway. § Multi-peaked frequency response curves[616] and tuning curves with several minima, ‖ wide response areas covering almost the whole audible range,[1212] and unstable response behavior**, [768] all argue against tonotopy. Also, the behavioral experiments (see page 163) described in connection with the medial geniculate indicated that in cats pitch discrimination ability was

---

* References 39, 185, 199, 263, 344, 498, 509, 627, 761, 853, 854, 867, 919, 920, 1060, 1237.

† See also references 39, 199, 627.

‡ References 141, 152, 154, 423, 658, 757, 759, 760, 895, 944, 1179, 1180.

§ References 299, 302, 316, 374, 375, 484, 547, 959, 1212, 1214.

‖ References 3, 421, 544, 691, 857, 870.

** More than 85% of cortical cells studied in the awake monkey responding to a certain stimulus with a vigorous discharge reduced this response so much after repetition of the stimulus that, following 4 to 8 repetitions, eventually no response occurred. Presentation of a different stimulus, however, immediately restored the activity. This behavior makes the recording of tuning curves difficult.

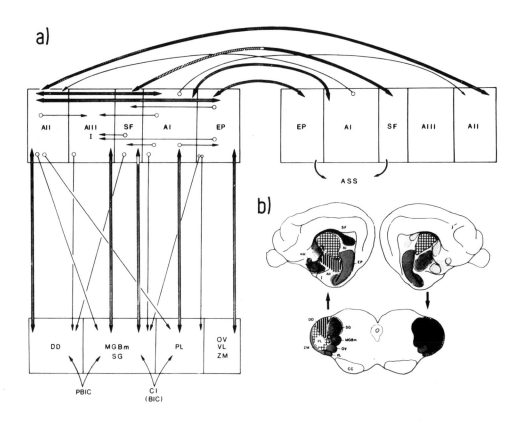

FIGURE 128. Diagram of the connections of the cat auditory cortex as revealed by silver impregnation studies of anterograde degeneration. In A all connections are shown schematically. The association and commissural interconnections of the auditory cortex are shown as demonstrated by Diamond et al. (266, 267). In B maps of the interconnected parts of the auditory cortex and of the MGB in a less diagramatic manner are shown. Connected areas are indicated by identical symbols based on the results of several authors (471, 268, 1060).

AI, II, III = primary, secondary and tertiary auditory area; SF = suprasylvian fringe; EP = posterior ectosylvian area; DD = dorsal principal part of the medial geniculate body; MGBm = magnocellular part of the medial geniculate body; PBIC = parabrachial auditory pathway; CI = colliculus inferior; SG = nucleus suprageniculatus; PL = pars lateralis of the ventral part of the pars principalis; OV = pars ovoidea of the ventral part of the pars principalis; VL = ventrolateral part of the ventral part of the pars principalis; ZM = marginal area of the ventral part of the pars principalis; I = insular cortex; ASS = association area with early component;

(According to Sousa-Pinto [1060].)

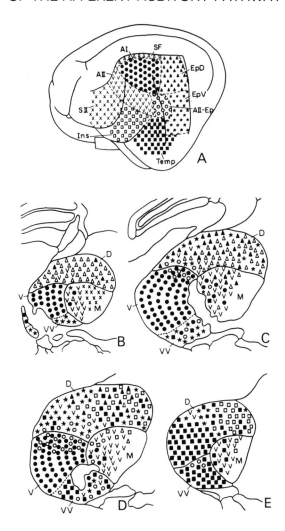

FIGURE 129. Summarizing diagram showing the organization of afferent cortical projections of MGB as it can be demonstrated by horseradish peroxidase technique. A represents the divisions of the auditory cortex. B, C, D, and E indicate the representative transverse sections of MGB from various levels: solid circles, projections to AI, V shape, to AII; open triangles, to SF; solid triangles, to dorsal Ep; stars, to ventral Ep; open squares, to insular area; solid squares, to temporal area; crosses, to SII; open circles, to AII-Ep transition area.

AI = primary auditory area; AII = secondary auditory area; AII-Ep = AII Ep transition area; D = dorsal principal part of MGB; Ep = posterior ectosylvian area; EpD = dorsal division of Ep; EpV = ventral division of Ep; Ins = insular area; M = magnocellular part of MGB; MGB = medial geniculate body; SF = suprasylvian fringe; SII = second somatic sensory area; Temp = temporal area; V = main laminated portion of ventral principal part of MGB; VV = ventromedial portion of ventral principal part of MGB;

(According to Niimi and Matsuoka [854].)

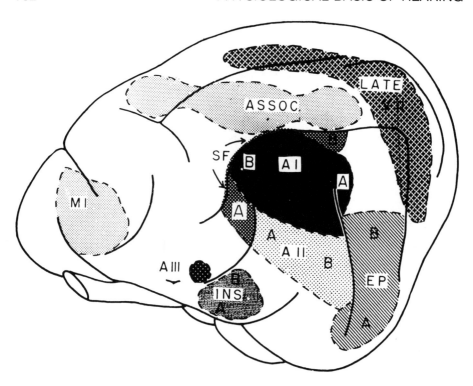

FIGURE 130. Cortical areas of the cat from which auditory evoked excitations could be recorded. AI, II, III = primary, secondary and tertiary auditory cortex; SF = suprasylvian fringe; MI = primary motor cortex; ASSOC = association cortex with early potential component; LATE = association cortex with late potential component; EP = ectosylvian auditory cortex; INS = insular cortex. With respect to a tonotopic projection, A and B refer to the apex and the base of the cochlea respectively. (According to Woolsey 1960, 1961, from Woolsey [1246].)

preserved after complete ablation of the auditory cortex. Consequently, this function cannot be assigned to the cortex. Thus, a tonotopic organization does not appear to be necessary.

In behavioral experiments (see footnote on page 163), the significance of the cortex for the recognition of time patterns and, in a certain sense for spatial localization,* was demonstrated.* Electrophysiological results also

---

* Heffner and Masterton (473), for example, found that cats deprived of primary auditory cortex bilaterally were able to indicate the direction of a moving sound with near-normal acuity but they were unable to locate its source while Cranford (205) concluded that the neocortex has no primary sensory role in sound localization. Sovijärvi and Hyvvärinen (1062) could show that some cells in AI respond only to movements of the sound source.

† References 472, 473, 624, 626, 1214, 1215, 1221.

indicate a special sensitivity to temporal frequency changes* depending on the direction and velocity of the frequency changes (Fig. 131). Also, the binaural effects as described for the lower nuclei (e.g. Figs. 101, 103, 109, 117) were observed the same way in the cortex.†

A most interesting idea about the functional meaning of the auditory cortex is shown by Whitfield.[1216] Based on impressive behavioral results he concluded that we should not seek further specific analytic functions in the classical sense ("... the classical ideas of cortical functions continue to infect our thinking"), but we should see the possibility of sensory cortex as being concerned with the constancies (of size, shape, position, etc.) associated with the external world.

Goldstein et al.[424] and de Ribaupierre et al.[955] studied the response behavior of the cat's AI-cells to click stimuli and found that four classes of cells could be distinguished. About 40% of the cells ("lockers") responded precisely to each click up to a maximum click-repetition rate ranging for the different cells between 10/s and 1000/s. About 25% did not respond at all to clicks and the rest could be divided evenly into two classes. One class ("special responders") showed different response patterns depending on the click-repetition rate while the other class ("grouper") responded only following a low click-repetition rate and in poor synchronization with the clicks.

Aside from these response patterns, response patterns like those observed in the medial geniculate also occur in the primary auditory cortex.‡ Likewise, the response pattern of the same cell changes upon variation of the stimulus parameters as was the case for cells of the medial geniculate (Fig. 132). Also, as in the geniculate, the intensity functions have a monotonic as well as a non-monotonic shape[893, 895] (Fig. 133). Many cells, however, frequently do not react (as described also for the geniculate) to tone bursts but only to more complex or natural stimuli. These findings and the idea that the meaning of the stimulus could be decisive for cortical activities led to experiments employing complex and natural stimuli.§ Thereby it became evident that in some cells the response to the complex stimulus was predictable from the response behavior to simple stimuli. For many cells, however, this was not true.

---

* References 857, 1115–1117, 1218.
† References 109, 153, 156, 446, 767, 896.
‡ References 3, 4, 152, 153, 310, 374, 396, 422, 857, 1123, 1124.
§ Müller-Preuss and Ploog (831) described inhibition of auditory cortical neurons during phonation for more than half of those cells which reacted to the play-back of tape-recorded selfproduced vocalization while the others did not differentiate between selfproduced and loudspeaker transmitted vocalizations. References 375, 745, 848, 1188, 1239, 1240, 1242.

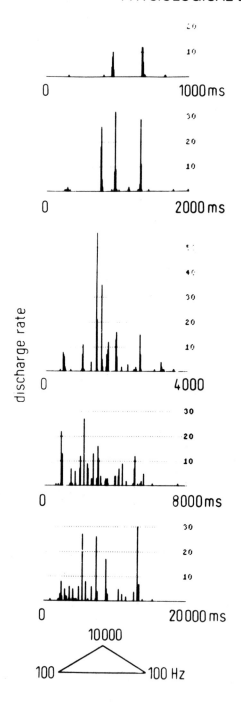

FIGURE 131. Response patterns (post-stimulus-time histograms) to frequency-modulated stimuli of varying velocities of frequency change. The velocity of change results from the time scale of the abscissa. The recording was obtained by means of telemetry in the awake free-behaving cat. (According to Keidel and Kallert [616].)

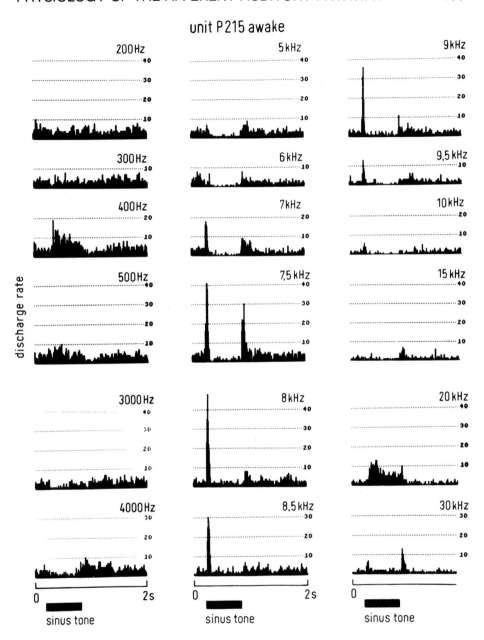

FIGURE 132. Typical example of the dependence of the response pattern of the unit of the medial geniculate in the awake cat (recorded telemetrically) on the stimulus frequency. The stimuli are shown in the correct temporal relation. The stimulus frequency is specified for each graph. The stimulus intensity was -30 dB referred to 4 V$_{PP}$ at the loud speaker. (According to Kallert [534].)

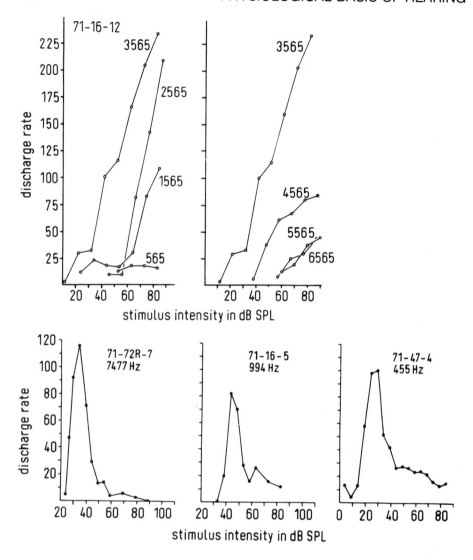

FIGURE 133. Discharge rate of cortical units as a function of the intensity of contralateral stimuli of different frequencies. Above: monotonic functions. Below: non-monotonic functions. (According to Brugge and Merzenich [153].)

Finally, single-cell recordings from AI were done by simultaneously combining them with behavioral experiments.* In trained animals, a higher response activity was found if the animal fulfilled the task it was trained to do. Response activity was reduced if the animal did not react correctly to the stimulus and was very unstable if the animal was not trained to the stimulus.

---

* References 66, 270, 110, 489, 647, 769, 770, 892, 893.

Intracellular recordings[954] showed that most cells of AI are under inhibitory influences and that responses occur after abolition of inhibition or after EPSPs prevailed. IPSPs and EPSPs could be recorded.

The architecture of the primary auditory cortex does not show a columnar functional organization as convincingly as in the visual cortex.[503] However, Abeles and Goldstein[3] observed a certain columnar tendency in the arrangement of those cells that have simple tuning curves. In addition, Brugge and Imig[154] found columns of cells formed by neurons with binaural properties while Sousa-Pinto[1061] described vertical cylinders with an outer diameter of 50 to 60 μm and having a sparsely-packed center in the fourth cortical layer.

Robertson et al.[961] and Irvine and Huebner[511] carried out microelectrode recordings from single cells of the association cortex (posterior part of the middle gyrus suprasylvii in the cat). They found many polysensory cells (about 80% of all cells). These cells reacted both in the anesthetized and in the awake animal in a comparable way. As a rule, they had a short latency (35 to 60 ms) but a refractory period of 200 ms to 30 s. Stimulus repetition rapidly caused habituation. During anesthesia, the average spontaneous activity was only 0.6 discharges per second. In the awake animal, however, it was 14.6/s. Tuning curves obtained from this cortical area are very wide.[511, 1207] The action of anesthesia and of different states of vigilance on the activity of the middle suprasylvian gyrus was also studied by Noda and Adey.[856] With progressive deepness of sleep, the discharge rate of about 85% of the cells studied decreased, whereas the activity of about 15% of the cells increased. During REM-sleep 94.8% of the units had their highest discharge rate. The activity of the cells during anesthesia cannot be compared with that occurring in a certain state of sleep. The discharge rate during anesthesia was only 30 to 50% of that occurring during the deep states of sleep (δ-wave sleep). Also, during anesthesia, long periods of absolute silence can be observed. These results are in good agreement with the comparative studies of the activity of the different parts of the auditory pathway during wakefulness and anesthesia.[493, 494]

In the squirrel monkey (Saimiri sciureus), Newman and Lindsley[850] carried out microelectrode studies in the area of the frontal association cortex.* As stimuli they used not only clicks and tone bursts but also sounds produced by that species since it is known that structures participating in vocalization were located in close anatomical relation.† Of all cells studied, 20% proved to be excitable with auditory stimuli. Out of these cells, only 39% reacted to tone bursts, whereas in AI, the figure was 70%.[374] In the

---

* The existence of connections between AI and these frontal areas has been proven anatomically (References 529, 880, 881) and auditory-evoked activities have been found (References 114–116, 844, 1009).

† References 531, 836, 837, 903.

frontal cortex, 65% responded to clicks as opposed to 23 to 52% in AI.[306, 374] Sounds of the species evoked a response in 68% of the frontal cortex units, but only 19% responded exclusively to such sounds. In contrast to the AI-cells frequently reacting to different sounds with characteristically different response patterns* the cells of the frontal lobe show little specificity in the response to different sounds. The tuning curves were found to be very wide.

Finally, acoustically excitable cells in areas 17 and 18 were also found.[343] All of these cells can also be activated by visual stimuli. Among the cells of areas 17 and 18 there are cells responding to an auditory stimulus only if the source of sound is located in the receptive field of the cell. Obviously, such cells play an important role for the spatial localization of sound sources.

Of the studies described so far in this chapter most were carried out on cats, monkeys, rats and bats. Quite analogous results have been obtained also from birds.† Thus, in the comparative physiology of the auditory system features applying universally to animals have been found. In the field of averaged evoked potentials recorded with larger electrodes extensive results have also been obtained from humans.

---

* References 848, 849, 1242.
† References 711–713, 1021, 1023, 1256.

III. SLOW* EVOKED POTENTIALS [OBJECTIVE AUDIOMETRY; ELECTRIC RESPONSE AUDIOMETRY (ERA); BRAINSTEM ELECTRIC RESPONSE AUDIOMETRY (BERA)]

Stimulus-related potentials recordable from the exposed cortex with the aid of macroelectrodes have been described by several investigators during the past century.[†] After some pioneering work in the field of evoked potentials[‡] these potentials (recordable from the intact skull of the human, just like the EEG) were subject to a closer analysis with the aid of modern electronic computers and, thus, became available for clinical application. A detailed description of ERA was given by Davis[242] and of the physiological bases of ERA and BERA by Keidel.[607] Zöllner and Stange[1257] have recently reviewed clinical experience with ERA as have Glasscock et al.[401]

---

* The term "slow" is used since the potential changes occur substantially slower than in the action potentials.
† References 67–69, 186, 187, 351.
‡ References 144, 145, 147, 688, 723.

The slow evoked potentials can be extracted from the EEG only through use of an averaging procedure. The temporal course of such an averaged potential shows several negative and positive waves generally labelled as N_1, N_2... and P_1, P_2, P_3..., respectively. With regard to the latencies, an early response (with latencies of less than 50 ms, amplitudes less than 1 μV) is distinguished from a late response (latencies between 50 and 300 ms, amplitudes between 1 to 50 μV). In order to denote an early response, subscripts are used (P_1, P_2..., N_1, N_2...), while late responses are named P1, P2..., N1, N2,...[607] Other marks of identification have also been used.

A report on the first electronically averaged recordings (by means of a self-made small electronic computer) was given by Keidel[559] at a CORLAS-meeting in Athens.[609] Even then, Keidel proposed the late response as the basis for objective audiometry. At about the same time, Davis in St. Louis worked with the late response component for use in audiometry. On this topic, Davis gave a report at the CORLAS-meeting in Würzburg in 1964. Since then, numerous contributions to this topic have been made by these two groups.* Careful studies on the influence of the location of the recording electrodes were carried out by Finkenzeller[336] (Fig. 134). Keidel and Spreng first studied the dependence of these potentials on stimulus intensity and frequency (Fig. 135).

Since the slow evoked potential represents a complex of several components, it is clear that different intensity functions can be obtained depending on the component measured. This has been a matter of frequent controversy. The data published most recently[1039] confirm the results obtained in Erlangen[167, 168] and show that, in a double logarithmic coordinate system, the intensity function exhibits a linear increase over an intensity range of at least 50 dB with an exponent of 0.2 to 0.3. Thereafter, the steepness decreases (Fig. 136). This discontinuity of the intensity function was studied in detail by Moore and Rose[802] and by Spreng.[1084, 1085] Beagley and Kellogg[65] determined the difference between intensity functions obtained under monaural and binaural stimulation.

The distribution of the evoked potentials was thoroughly investigated by Vaughan and Ritter[1173] (Fig. 137). According to them, the evoked potentials have their largest amplitude at the vertex so that the waveform obtained from this recording site was used to introduce the nomenclature. A small and variable positive component (P_1) appears first with a latency of 16 to 60 ms. P_1 is followed by two large deflections with relatively little variability; N_1, with a latency of about 100 ms, and P_2, with a latency of approximately 200 ms. Following an aperiodic stimulus pattern, a further positive deflection, P_3, occurs after about 300 ms. All these deflections

---

* References 229–242, 244–246, 252–255, 559–605, 607, 609–613, 1075–1089, 1091–1093.

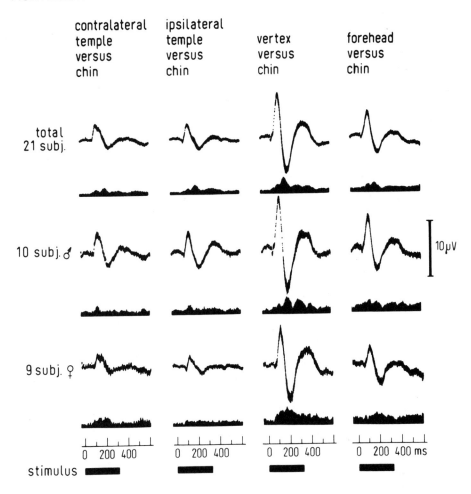

FIGURE 134. Auditory evoked potentials averaged from a total of 21 subjects. The thickness of the curves gives M± σ. The dispersion 3 σ (σ = standard deviation) is shown below. In addition, the average values of the male and female subjects are shown separately. (According to Finkenzeller [336].)

decrease in amplitude with increasing distance of the recording electrode from the vertex. Further, N_1 and P_2 show a reversal of polarity in a plane denoted 00 in Figure 137b. P_3 shows no reversal of polarity in this plane. From that the authors infer that a layer giving rise to N_1 and P_2 exists in the supratemporal plane (the primary auditory cortex). In 1975, Arezzo et al.[55] convincingly supplemented these results by intracerebral recordings in the monkey.

Naturally, the stimulus repetition rate or, better, the interstimulus interval is of high significance for the amplitude of the evoked potentials. Rau[940] could show that the amplitude increases up to an interval of 30 s.

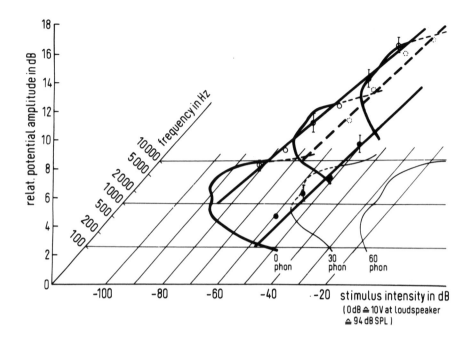

FIGURE 135. Three-dimensional diagram of the characteristic curves relating the amplitude of the potential with the stimulus intensity. The "objective" hearing threshold thus obtained is in good agreement with the "subjective" threshold. (According to Keidel [564], and Keidel and Spreng [611].)

Recent studies dealing with this topic were carried out by Scheuler and Spreng.[1010]

For clinical application it is important to select a reasonable length of the analysis time. Thus, Spreng[1084] proposed to use a single stimulus length not shorter than 300 ms and an interval length not shorter than 5 s.

The amplitudes of the potentials and their intensity functions depend on the frequency of the tone* (see also Fig. 135). However, adaptation,† habituation,‡ attention,[897] vigilance,[158, 372] deepness of sleep,§ anesthesia, the meaning of the stimulus,‖ and noise[1081, 1085] also have an effect on the amplitude and, to some extent, on the latency (transcendental meditation has an effect only on the latency[663, 1184] of the evoked potential).**

---

* References 44, 45, 163, 611.
† References 560, 561, 730.
‡ References 371, 447, 518, 898, 899, 1205, 1206.
§ References 872, 873, 877, 894.
‖ References 653, 987, 1086.
** Interhemispheric asymmetry following speech stimuli has also been described (References 367, 754, 820).

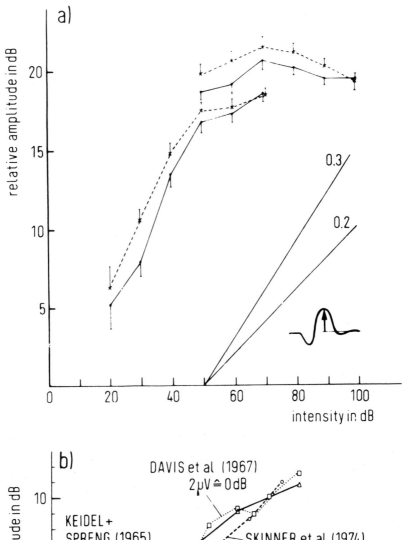

FIGURE 136. Intensity function shown in a double-logarithmic plot and compared with recent data. (A, According to Butler et al. [167, 168]). B, According to Spreng [1084].)

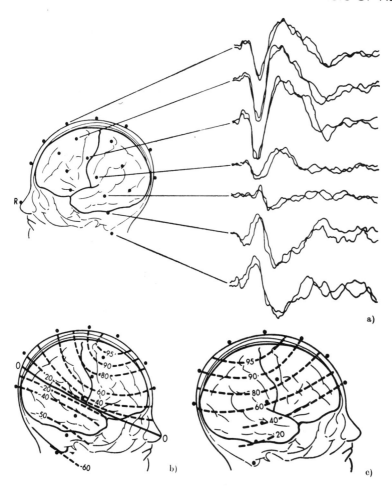

FIGURE 137. A, Recording of the slow auditory evoked potentials from intact skull of the adult human. B, Amplitude distribution of N_2 The numbers give the amplitude of N_2 in percent of the vertex potential. At the plane 00 a reversal of polarity occurs. C, Distribution of the amplitude of N_3 It shows no reversal of polarity. (According to Vaughan and Ritter [1173].)

Also, the latencies of the different components of the evoked potentials depend not only on the intensity of the stimulus but also on the rise time of the stimulus[993] and on the position of the recording electrode. Figure 138 shows the dependence of latency on intensity for ipsi- and contralateral stimulation that was studied in detail by Butler et al.[167]

At the end of the stimulus another evoked response occurs, the off response (Fig. 139). Thus, short stimuli (e.g. tone stimuli of 50 ms length) can lead to super-imposition of on- and off-response components.[1075] The off-response was studied by Onishi and Davis,[871] Keidel and Spreng,[609] Spreng,[1075] Gerian et al.,[394] Spychala et al.,[1095] Regan,[945] and Johannsen et al.[521]

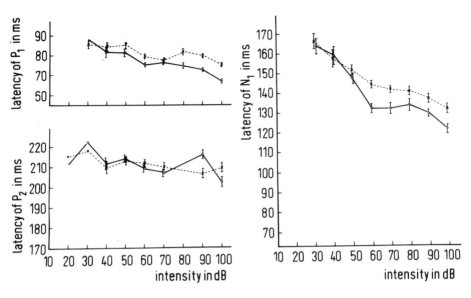

FIGURE 138. Latencies of the components P₁, N₁ and P₂ for ipsilateral (dashed curve) and contralateral (continuous curve) stimulation, recorded from the middle between the vertex and the mastoid. Stimuli: one-third-octave band filtered pure tones. (According to Spreng [1082].)

Aside from the on-responses and off-responses, there is a stimulus-related d.c. potential lasting the duration of the stimulus. If recorded directly from the cortex, this potential is called PSS (perstimulatory d.c. shift), if recorded from the intact skull it is called SPS (slow potential shift) (Fig. 140). This d.c. potential was studied in detail by Keidel* and by Finkenzeller.[338] Whereas upon visual stimulation the on-response is largest at the vertex, the SPS following visual stimuli is largest at the occiput. However, upon auditory stimulation, the SPS has its highest amplitude at the vertex. This indicates a specificity for sensory modalities. Interactions between visual and auditory evoked SPS were described by David et al.[223] These d.c. responses are not to be confused with the "contingent negative variation" described by Walter et al.[1183] (for details see Keidel[607]).

Based on the recordings of the d.c. potentials, Keidel and Finken-zeller[610, 614] and Finkenzeller and Keidel[339–341] tried to obtain an objective audiogram. They used tone bursts of 200 ms duration and gradually decreased the interstimulus interval from 8 s to zero (Fig. 141). In this way, all components of the auditory evoked potentials including the SPS could be recorded. By using an expanded time scale, the changes of N1 and P2 can be studied in detail. Thus, it became clear that N1 is composed of two

---

* References 585, 589, 594.

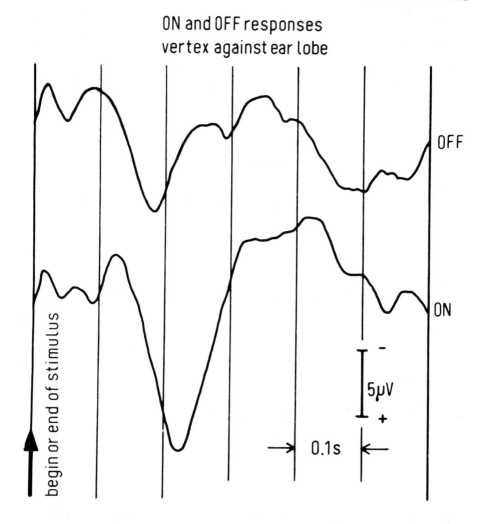

FIGURE 139. Similarity between On- and Off-response. Stimulus: 1200 Hz tones of 2 s duration each, rise time 2 ms, interstimulus interval 3 s. (According to Davis and Zerlin [245].)

components, N1a andN1b. Only N1a stays preserved from the second through the nth response (Fig. 141 right). With a higher stimulus repetition frequency, during the whole stimulus sequence, a SPS builds up reaching almost the height of N1.

Since for the evoked potentials changes of stimulus parameters are more effective than stable conditions (differential sensitivity), it is possible to obtain responses to step-like changes of intensity *and* frequency as on-effects and as SPS (Fig. 142).

The responses thus averaged over the whole audible frequency range for increasing intensities yield a new type of audiogram (Fig. 143). This

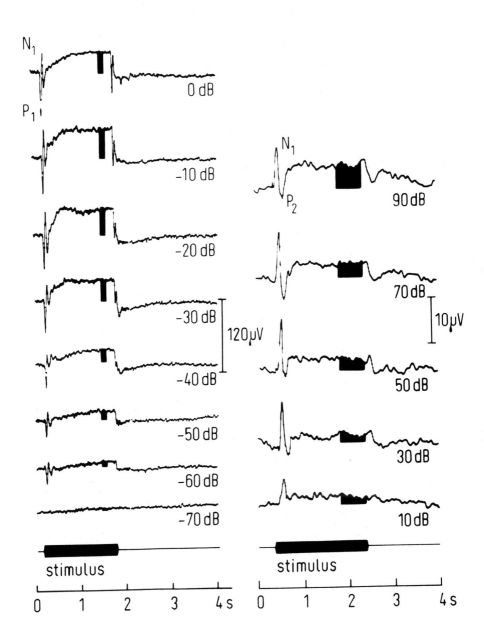

FIGURE 140. Left: PSS recorded from the awake cat; right: SPS recorded from the human. The black bars illustrate the dependence on intensity. (According to David et al. [221, 222].)

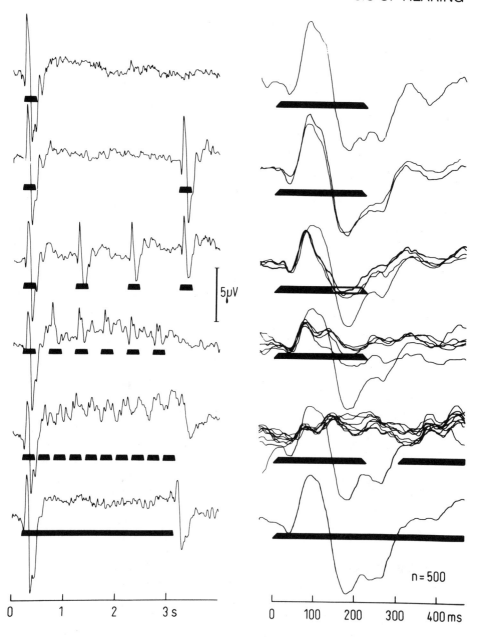

FIGURE 141. (Left) Averaged evoked potentials including the slow potential shift. The stimuli were 200 ms tones (1000 Hz, 80 dB SPL). The SPS increases with increasing stimulus repetition rate and, finally, reaches an amplitude comparable to that of N1. (Right) Superimposed responses to single stimuli on an enlarged time scale. The large P2 component appears following the first stimulus and disappears at the shorter stimulus intervals. The records were obtained from the vertex of the adult. (According to Finkenzeller and Keidel [340].)

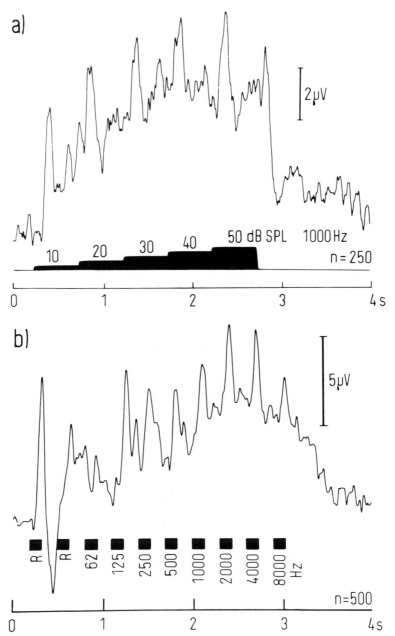

FIGURE 142. Averaged evoked potentials including the SPS upon stepwise change of the intensity and of the frequency. Stimulus repetition rate 1/8 s. A, Stepwise increase of the stimulus intensity (rise time about 15 ms). B, Stepwise increase of the stimulus frequency at 50 dB SPL. Two noise bursts (R) were presented before the tone series was offered. (According to Finkenzeller and Keidel [340].)

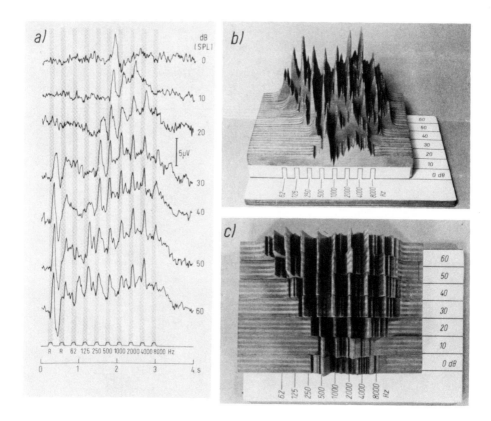

FIGURE 143. A, Averaged evoked potentials as in Fig. 142b obtained at different stimulus intensities. B and C, Front and top view of a three-dimensional model based on the recording shown in a. (According to Keidel and Finkenzeller [614].)

could form the basis of future threshold and suprathreshold audiometry. In addition, as a three-dimensional model (Fig. 143 c) it demonstrates the frequency and intensity dependence at one glance.

In recent years, the responses originating presumably from the brain stem and occurring with latencies between 6 and 30 ms have played an increasing role in ERA, especially since they are relatively stable and independent of wakefulness, attention, and anesthesia.*

---

* Clinical results were described by Starr and Achor (1102) and recently by Glasscock et al. (401).

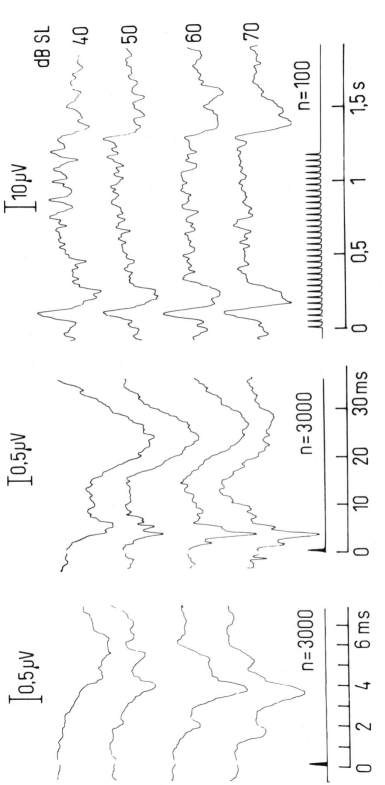

FIGURE 144. Simultaneous recording of ECoG, BERA, ERA and SPS at different stimulus intensities. For the 40 ms and the 2 s recordings dc-amplification was used (electrodes: vertex - mastoid), and the 8 ms recording broad-band (6 Hz to 6 kHz) ac-amplification was used (electrodes: mastoid - mastoid). (According to Keidel and Finkenzeller [614].)

Using a logarithmic time scale, Gestring et al.[398] described a method of simultaneously recording the early and late responses following auditory stimuli. Keidel proposed a method (1970 in Dundee "The Use of Fast Correlators in Electro-Cochleography," 1971 in Sirmione "Simultaneous Recording of Auditory Early, Late, and DC-Evoked Response in Man," and 1971 in Budapest "A New Technique for Simultaneous Recording of Auditory Early, Late, and DC-Evoked Response in Man") that enabled the simultaneous recording of these potentials using three different time scales (80 ms, 40 ms, and 2 s). The latest development was described by Keidel and Finkenzeller.[610] They used sequences of filtered clicks (0.5 ms). Each sequence consisted of 30 clicks with interstimulus intervals of 40 ms between the clicks. The pauses between the click sequences were 2 s in length. Such a sequence is experienced as *one* stimulus. Following each single click, the early response components occur and the whole sequence builds up the SPS (Fig. 144). Figure 145 shows original photographs taken from the scope of the computer.

Utilizing the method of running averages and of running correlation continued over hours, Keidel and Finkenzeller[610] were able to show that the running average value of N1 stays constant, whereas that of P2 decreases in time. After a break of 10 minutes, P2 shows an overshooting recovery. A corresponding behavior can be observed using the running correlation. This might offer an objective correlate for changes of vigilance in humans and is of interest not only for the ERA but also for clinical neurology. Finally, Figure 146 shows the electrophysiological correlate of the SISI-test.

With this short description of the auditory evoked potentials, their recording from the whole course of the auditory pathway and some references to future clinical applications, this review is brought to an end. A few topics being of some importance in this context were left out intentionally as, for example, general principles of information processing of the central nervous system, the unspecific reticular system, the phenomenon of loudness, and the effect of noise on the auditory system.

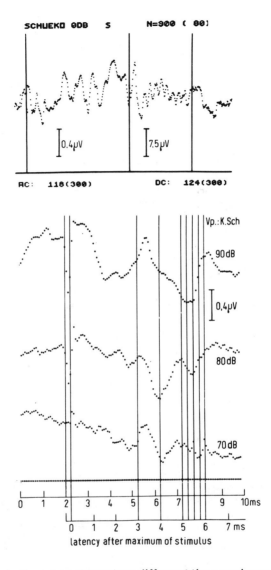

FIGURE 145. In the upper trace two different time scales were used for the same record (40 ms on the left, 2 s on the right). On the left of the first vertical line a short pre-stimulatory section and on the right of the third vertical line a short post-stimulatory section is shown. The 10 ms averaging carried out simultaneously is shown separately (below). (According to Finkenzeller and Keidel [341]. From Keidel [607].)

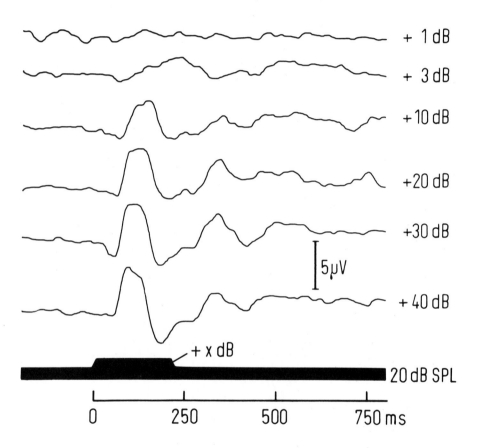

FIGURE 146. Objective SISI-test. According to the averaged potentials, the intensity difference threshold ranges between 1 and 3 dB and, thus, is in good agreement with the SISI-test results. (According to Finkenzeller and Keidel [341]. From Keidel [607].)

REFERENCES

1. Abbas, P.J. and Sachs, M.B.: Two-tone suppression in auditory-nerve fibers: Extension of a stimulus-response relationship. J. Acoust. Soc. Amer. *59*, 112-122 (1976)
2. Abel, S.M.: Discrimination of Temporal Gaps. J. Acoust. Soc. Amer *52*, 519-524 (1972)
3. Abeles, M. and Goldstein, M.H. Jr.: Functional architecture in cat primary auditory cortex: Columnar organization and organization according to depth. J. Neurophysiol. *33*, 172-187 (1970)
4. Abeles, M. and Goldstein, M.H. Jr.: Responses of single units in the primary auditory cortex of the cat to tones and to tone pairs. Brain Research *42*, 337-352 (1972)
5. Adams, J.C.: Crossed and descending projections to the inferior colliculus. Neuroscience Letters *19*, 1-5 (1980)
6. Adams, J.C. and Teas, D.C.: Organization of the Posterior Colliculus. J. Acoust. Soc. Amer. *53*, 361 (1973)
7. Ades, H.W.: A secondary acoustic area in the cerebral cortex of the cat. J. Neurophysiol. *6*, 59-63 (1943)
8. Ades, H.W. and Engström, H.: Anatomy of the Inner Ear In: Auditory System. Handbook of Sensory Physiology, Vol. V/1 Eds.: Keidel, W.D. and Neff, W.D. Springer-Verlag, Berlin-Heidelberg-New York 1974
9. Adrian, E.D.: The microphonic action of the cochlea: an interpretation of Wever and Bray's experiments. J. Physiol. *71*, 28-29 (1931)
10. Adrian, E.D.: Afferent discharges to the cerebral cortex from peripheral sense organs. J. Physiol. *100*, 159-191 (1941)
11. Adrian, E.D.: Rhythmic discharges from the thalamus. J. Physiol. *113*, 9P-10P (1951)
12. Adrian, H.O., Lifschitz, W.M., Tavitas, R.J. and Galli, F.P.: Activity of neural units in medial geniculate body of cat and rabbit. J. Neurophysiol. *29*, 1046-1060 (1966)
13. Aitkin, L.M.: Medial geniculate body of the cat: responses to tonal stimuli of neurons in medial division. J. Neurophysiol. *36*, 275-283 (1973)
14. Aitkin, L.M. and Dunlop, C.W.: Interplay of excitation and inhibition in the cat medial geniculate body. J. Neurophysiol. *31*, 44-61 (1968)
15. Aitkin, L.M. and Dunlop, C.W.: Inhibition in the medial geniculate body of the cat. Exp. Brain Res. *7*, 68-83 (1969)
16. Aitkin, L.M. and Webster, W.R.: Tonotopic organization in the medial geniculate body of the cat. Brain Research *26*, 402-405 (1971)
17. Aitkin, L.M. and Webster, W.R.: Medial geniculate body of the cat: organization and response to tonal stimuli of neurons in the ventral division. J. Neurophysiol. *35*, 365-380 (1972)

18. Aitkin, L.M. and Prain, S.M.: Medial Geniculate Body: Unit Responses in the Awake Cat. J. Neurophysiol. *37*, 512-521 (1974)
19. Aitkin, L.M. and Boyd, J.: Responses of single units in cerebellar vermis of the cat to monaural and binaural stimuli. J. Neurophysiol. *38*, 418-429 (1975)
20. Aitkin, L.M. and Moore, D.R.: Inferior Colliculus. II. Development of Tuning Characteristics and Tonotopic Organization in Central Nucleus of the Neonatal Cat. J. Neurophysiol. *38*, 1208-1216 (1975)
21. Aitkin, L.M., Dunlop, C.W. and Webster, W.R.: Click-evoked response patterns of single units in the medial geniculate body of the cat. J. Neurophysiol. *29*, 109-123 (1966)
22. Aitkin, L.M., Anderson, D.J. and Brugge, J.F.: Tonotopic organization and discharge characteristics of single neurons in nuclei of the lateral lemniscus of the cat. J. Neurophysiol. *33*, 421-440 (1970)
23. Aitkin, L.M., Fryman, S., Blake, D.W. and Webster, W.R.: Responses of neurones in the rabbit inferior colliculus. I. Frequency-specificity and topographic arrangement. Brain Research *47*, 77-90 (1972)
24. Aitkin, L.M., Blake, D.W., Fryman, S. and Bock, G.R.: Responses of neurones in the rabbit inferior colliculus. II. Influence of binaural tonal stimulation. Brain Research *47*, 91-101 (1972)
25. Aitkin, L.M., Webster, W.R., Veale, J.L. and Crosby, D.C.: Inferior colliculus. I. Comparison of response properties of neurons in central, pericentral, and external nuclei of adult cat. J. Neurophysiol. *38*, 1196-1207 (1975)
26. Aitkin, L.M., Bush, B.M.H. and Gates, G.R.: The auditory midbrain of a marsupial: The brush-tailed possum (Trichosurus vulpecula). Brain Res. *150*, 29-44 (1978)
27. Aitkin, L.M., Dickhaus, H., Schult, W. and Zimmermann, M.: External Nucleus of Inferior Colliculus: Auditory and Spinal Somatosensory Afferents and their Interactions. J. Neurophysiol. 41, 837-847 (1978)
28. Alkon, D.L. and Bak, A.: Hair cell Generator Potentials. J. Gen. Physiol. 61, 619-637 (1973)
29. Allen, J.B.: Two-dimension cochlear fluid model: New results. J. Acoust. Soc. Amer. *61*, 110-119 (1977)
30. Allen, J.B.: Cochlear micromechanics—a mechanism for transforming mechanical to neural tuning within the cochlea. J. Acoust. Soc. Amer. *62*, 930-939 (1977)
31. Altman, J. and Carpenter, M.B.: Fiber projections of the superior colliculus in the cat. J. comp. Neurol. *116*, 157-177 (1961)
32. Altman, J.A., Syka, J. and Shmigidina, G.N.: Neuronal activity in the medial geniculate body of the cat during monaural and binaural stimulation. Exp. Brain Res. *10*, 81-93 (1970)
33. Altman, J.A., Bechterev, N.N., Radionova, E.A., Shmigidina, G.N., Syka, J.: Electrical Responses of the Auditory Area of the Cerebellar Cortex to Acoustic Stimulation Exp. Brain Res. *26*, 285-298 (1976)
34. Amato, G., LaGrutta, V. and Enia, F.: The control of acoustic input in the medial geniculate body and inferior colliculus by auditory cortex. Experientia (Basel) *26*, 55-56 (1970)
35. Andersen, P.: Rhythmic 10/sec. activity in the thalamus. In: The Thalamus. Eds.: Purpura, D.P. and Yahr, M.D., Columbia University Press, New York and London 1966
36. Andersen, P. and Sears, T.A.: The role of inhibition in the phasing of spontaneous thalamocortical discharge. J. Physiol. *173*, 459-480 (1964)
37. Andersen, P., Brooks, C.M., Eccles, J.C. and Sears, T.A.: The ventro-basal nucleus of the thalamus: potential fields, synaptic transmission and excitability of both presynaptic and postsynaptic components. J. Physiol. *174*, 348-369 (1964)
38. Andersen, P., Eccles, J.C. and Sears, T.A.: The ventro-basal complex of the thalamus: types of cells, their responses and their functional organization. J. Physiol. *174*, 370-399 (1964)
39. Andersen, R.A., Knight, P.L. and Merzenich, M.M.: The Thalamocortical and Corticothalamic Connections of AI, AII, and the Anterior Auditory Field (AAF) in

the Cat: Evidence for Two Largely Segregated Systems of Connections. J. Comp. Neurol. *194*, 663-701 (1980)

40. Andersen, R.A., Roth, G.L., Aitkin, L.M. and Merzenich, M.M.: The Efferent Projections of the Central Nucleus and the Pericentral Nucleus of the Inferior Colliculus in the Cat. J. Comp. Neurol. *194*, 649-662 (1980)

41. Anderson, D.J., Rose, J.E., Hind, J.E. and Brugge, J.F.: Temporal position of discharges in single auditory nerve fibers within the cycle of a sine-wave stimulus: frequency and intensity effects. J. Acoust. Soc. Amer. *49*, 1131-1139 (1971)

42. Angelborg, C. and Engström, H.: Supporting Elements in the Organ of Corti. I. Fibrillar structures in the supporting cells of the organ of Corti of mammals. Acta Oto-Laryng. (Stockh.) Suppl. *301*, 49-60 (1972)

43. Angelborg, C. and Engström, H.: The normal organ of Corti. In: Basic Mechanisms in Hearing. Ed.: Møller, A.R., Academic Press, New York and London 1973

44. Antinoro, F. and Skinner, P.H.: The effects of frequency on the auditory evoked response. J. Aud. Res. *8*, 119-123 (1968)

45. Antinoro, F., Skinner, P.H. and Jones, J.J.: Relation between sound intensity and amplitude of the AER at different stimulus frequencies. J. Accoust. Soc. Amer. *46*, 1433-1436 (1969)

46. Aran, J.M.: The electrocochleogram: Recent results in children and in some pathological cases. Arch. klin. exp. Ohr.-, Nas.- u.Kehlk.Heilk. *198*, 128-143 (1971)

47. Aran, J.-M.: L'Electrocochléogramme. Les Cahiers de la C.F.A. *14*, 101-128 (1972)

48. Aran, J.M. and le Bert, G.: Les réponses nerveuses cochléaires chez l'homme: Image du fonctionnement de l'oreille et nouveau test d'audiométrie objective. Rev. de Laryng. (Bordeaux) *89*, 361-378 (1968)

49. Aran, J.M. and Portmann, M.: L'électrocochléogramme. J. Franc. ORL *21*, 211-221 (1972)

50. Aran, J.M. and Negrevergne, M.: Clinical study of some particular pathological patterns of eighth nerve responses in the human being. Audiology *12*, 488-503 (1973)

51. Aran, J.M., Portmann, Cl., Delaunay, J., Pelerin, J. and Lenoir, J. L'électrocochléogramme. Méthodes et premier résultats chez l'enfant. Rev. Laryngol (Bordeaux) *90*, 615-634 (1969)

52. Aran, J.M., Pelerin, J., Lenoir, J., Portmann, Cl. and Darrouzet, J.: Aspects theoretiques et pratiques des enregistrements électrocochleographiques selon la methode établie à Bordeaux. Rev. Laryngol. (Bordeaux) Suppl. *92*, 601-644 (1971)

53. Aran, J.M., Charlet de Sauvage, R. and Pelerin, J.: Comparaison des seuils électrocochléographiques et de l'audiogramme. Etude Statistique. Rev. Laryngol. (Bordeaux) *92*, 477-491 (1971)

54. Aran, J.M., Portmann, Cl. and Pelerin, J.: Electrocochléogramme chez l'adulte et chez l'enfant. Audiology *11*, 77 (1972)

55. Arezzo, J., Pickoff, A. and Vaughan, H.G. Jr.: The sources and intracerebral distribution of auditory evoked potentials in the alert rhesus monkey. Brain Research *90*, 57-73 (1975)

56. Arnesen, A.R. and Osen, K.K.: The Cochlear Nerve in the Cat: Topography, Cochleotopy and Fiber Spectrum. J. comp. Neurol. *178*, 661-678 (1978)

57. Arnesen, A.R., Osen, K.K. and Mugnaini, E.: Temporal and Spatial Sequence of Anterograde Degeneration in the Cochlear Nerve Fibers of the Cat. A Light Microscopic Study. J. comp. Neurol. *178*, 679-696 (1978)

58. Arthur, R.M., Pfeiffer, R.R. and Suga, N.: Properties of "two-tone inhibition" in primary auditory neurones. J. Physiol. *212*, 593-609 (1971)

59. Avanzini, G., Manicia, D. and Pellicioli, G.: Ascending and descending connections of the insular cortex of the cat. Arch. ital. Biol. *107*, 696-714 (1969)

60. Bárány, E.: A contribution to the physiology of bone conduction. Acta Oto-Laryng. Suppl. *26*, (1938)

61. Barnes, W.T., Magoun, H.W. and Ranson, S.W.: The ascending auditory pathway in the brain stem of the monkey. J. Comp. Neurol. *79*, 129-152 (1943)

62. Bast, T.H. and Anson, B.J.: The Temporal Bone and the Ear. Charles C. Thomas, Springfield, Ill., 1949

63. Bauch, H.: Die Schwingungsform der Basilarmembran bei Erregung durch Impulse und Geräusche, gemessen an einem elektrischen Modell des Innenohres. Frequenz *10*, 222-234 (1956)

64. Baylor, D.A. and Fuortes, M.G.F.: Electrical responses of single cones in the retina of the turtle. J. Physiol. (Lond.) *207*, 77-92 (1970)

65. Beagley, H.A. and Kellogg, S.E.: Amplitude of the auditory evoked response at high intensities. Sound *4*, 86-90 (1971)

66. Beaton, R. and Miller, J.M.: Single cell activity in the auditory cortex of the unanesthetized, behaving monkey: correlation with stimulus controlled behavior. Brain Research *100*, 543-562 (1975)

67. Beck, A.: Die Bestimmung der Lokalisation der Gehirn- und Rückenmarks-funktionen vermittelst der elektrischen Erscheinungen. Zbl. Physiol. *4*, 473-476 (1890)

68. Beck, A. und Cybulski, N.: Weitere Untersuchungen über die elektrischen Erschei-nungen in der Hirnrinde der Affen und Hunde. Zbl. Physiol. *6*, 90-91 (1892)

69. Beck, A. und Cybulski, N.: Weitere Untersuchungen über die elektrischen Erschei-nungen in der Hirnrinde der Affen und Hunde. Zbl. Physiol. *6*, 1-6 (1892)

70. von Békésy, G.: Zur Theorie des Hörens. Die Schwingungsform der Basilarmem-bran. Physik. Z. *29*, 793-810 (1928)

71. von Békésy, G.: Zur Theorie des Hörens. Über die Bestimmung des einem reinen Tonempfinden entsprechenden Erregungsgebietes der Basilarmembran vermittelst Ermüdungserscheinungen. Physik. Z. *30*, 115-125 (1929)

72. von Békésy, G.: Zur Theorie des Hörens bei der Schallaufnahme durch Knochen-leitung. Ann. Physik. V.F. *13*, 111-136 (1932)

73. von Békésy, G.: Über die Elastizitat der Schneckentrennwand des Ohres. Akust. Z. *6*, 265-278 (1941)

74. von Békésy, G.: Über die Schwingungen der Schneckentrennwand beim Präparat und Ohrenmodell. Akust. Z. *7*, 173-186 (1942)

75. von Békésy, G.: The Variation of Phase along the Basilar Membrane with Sinusoidal Vibrations. J. Acoust. Soc. Amer. *19*, 452-460 (1947)

76. von Békésy, G.: Vibrations of the head in a sound field and its role in hearing by bone conduction. J. Acoust. Soc. Amer. *20*, 749-760 (1948)

77. von Békésy, G.: DC-potentials and energy balance of the cochlear partition. J. Acoust. Soc. Amer. *23*, 576-582 (1951)

78. von Békésy, G.: The coarse pattern of the electrical resistance in the cochlea of the guinea pig (electro-anatomy of the cochlea). J. Acoust. Soc. Amer. *23*, 18-28 (1951)

79. von Békésy, G.: DC resting potentials inside the cochlear partition. J. Acoust. Soc. Amer. *24*, 72-76 (1952)

80. von Békésy, G.: Description of some mechanical properties of the organ of Corti. J. Acoust. Soc. Amer. *25*, 770-785 (1953)

81. von Békésy, G.: Shearing Microphonics Produced by Vibrations near the Inner and Outer Hair Cells. J. Acoust. Soc. Amer. *25*, 786-790 (1953)

82. von Békésy, G.: Some Electro-Mechanical Properties of the Organ of Corti. Ann. Otol. St. Louis *63*, 448 (1954)

83. von Békésy, G.: Paradoxical Direction of Wave-Travel along the Cochlear Partition. J. Acoust. Soc. Amer. *27*, 155-161 (1955)

84. von Békésy, G.: Beitrag zur Frage der Frequenzanalyse in der Schnecke. Arch. Ohr.-, Nas.- u.Kehlk.-Heilk. *167*, 238-255 (1955)

85. von Békésy, G.: Simplified Model to Demonstrate the Energy Flow and Formation of Traveling Waves Similar to those Found in the Cochlea. Proc. Nat. Acad. Sci. U.S., *42*, 930-944 (1956)

86. von Békésy, G.: Current Status of Theories of Hearing. Science *123*, 779-738 (1956)

87. von Békésy, G.: Preparatory and Air-Driven Micromanipulators for Electrophysi-ology. Rev. Sci. Instr. *27*, 690-692 (1956)

88. von Békésy, G.: The Ear. Scientific Amer. *197*, 66-78 (1957)

89. von Békésy, G.: Sensations on the Skin Similar to Directional Hearing, Beats and Harmonics of the Ear. J. Acoust. Soc. Amer. *29*, 489-501 (1957)

90. von Békésy, G.: Pendulums, Traveling Waves, and the Cochlea: Introduction and Script for a Motion Picture. Laryngoscope *68*, 317-327 (1958)
91. von Békésy, G.: Funneling Action in the Nervous System. J. Acoust. Soc. Amer. *30*, 399-412 (1958)
92. von Békésy, G.: Neural Funneling along the Skin and between the Inner and Outer Hair Cells of the Cochlea. J. Acoust. Soc. Amer. *31*, 1236-1249 (1959)
93. von Békésy, G.: Experiments in Hearing. McGraw Hill Book Comp., New York 1960
94. von Békésy, G.: Experimental Models of the Cochlea with and without Nerve Supply. In: Neural Mechanisms of the Auditory and Vestibular systems. Eds.: Rasmussen, G.L. and Windle, W.F., Charles C. Thomas Publ., Springfield/Ill. 1960
95. von Békésy, G.: Are Surgical Experiments on Human Subjects Necessary? Laryngoscope *71*, 367-376 (1961)
96. von Békésy, G.: Concerning the fundamental component of periodic pulse patterns and modulated vibrations observed in the cochlea model with nerve supply. J. Acoust. Soc. Amer. *33*, 888-896 (1961)
97. von Békésy, G.: Abweichung vom Ohmschen Gesetz der Frequenzauflösung beim Hören. Acustica, Acust. Beihefte 1, 241-244 (1961)
98. von Békésy, G.: Pitch Sensation and its Relation to the Periodicity of the Stimulus. Hearing and Skin Vibrations. J. Acoust. Soc. Amer. *33*, 341-348 (1961)
99. von Békésy, G.: Concerning the Pleasures of Observing and the Mechanics of the Inner Ear. Les prix Noble, Harvard Univ., Report XXVIII PNR-267 (1961)
100. von Békésy, G.: The gap between the hearing of external and internal sounds. J. exp. Biol., Harvard Univ., Report XXVIII PNR-258 (1961)
101. von Békésy, G.: Comments on the Measurement of the Relative Size of DC Potentials and Microphonics in the Cochlea. J. Acoust. Soc. Amer. *34*, 124 (1962)
102. von Békésy, G.: Wave Motion in an Inhomogeneous System: The Movements of the Basilar Membrane in the Cochlea. Script of a Motion Picture Film, Par-272, May 1962
103. von Békésy, G.: Enlarged mechanical model of the cochlea with nerve supply. In: Foundations of Modern Auditory Theory, Volume I. Ed.: Tobias, J.V., Academic Press, New York and London 1970
104. von Békésy, G.: The Early History of Hearing: Observations and Theories. J. Acoust. Soc. Amer. *20*, 727-748 (1948)
105. von Békésy, G. and Rosenblith, W.A.: The Mechanical Properties of the Ear. In: Handbook of Experimental Psychology. Ed.: Stevens, S. Wiley, New York 1951
106. Benevento, L.A. and Coleman, P.D.: Responses of single cells in cat inferior colliculus to binaural click stimuli: combinations of intensity levels, time differences, and intensity differences. Brain Research *17*, 387-405 (1970)
107. Benitez, L.D., Eldredge, D.H. and Templer, J.W.: Temporary threshold shifts in chinchilla: Electrophysiological correlates. J. Acoust. Soc. Amer. *52*, 1115-1123 (1972)
108. Bennett, M.V.L.: A Comparison of Electrically and Chemically Mediated Transmission. In: Structure and Function of Synapses. Eds.: Pappas, G.D. and Purpura, D.P. Raven, New York 1972
109. Benson, D.A. and Teas, D.C.: Single unit study of binaural interaction in the auditory cortex of the chinchilla. Brain Research *103*, 313-338 (1976)
110. Benson, D.A., Hienz, R.D. and Goldstein, M.H.Jr.: Single-unit activity in the auditory cortex of monkeys actively localizing sound sources: spatial tuning and behavioral dependency. Brain Res. *219*, 249-267 (1981)
111. Berlucchi, G., Munson, J.B. and Rizzolatti, G.: Changes in click-evoked responses in the auditory system and the cerebellum of free-moving cats during sleep and waking. Arch. ital. Biol. *105*, 118-135 (1967)
112. Berman, A.L.: The brain stem of the cat. A cytoarchitectonic atlas with stereotaxic coordinates. Univ. of Wisconsin Press, Madison 1968
113. Beyerl, B.D.: Afferent projections to the central nucleus of the inferior colliculus in the rat. Brain Res. *145*, 209-223 (1978)
114. Bignall, K.E.: Bilateral temporofrontal projections in the squirrel monkey: origin,

distribution, and pathways. Brain Res. *13*, 319-327 (1969)

115. Bignall, K.E. and Singer, P.: Auditory, somatic and visual input to association and motor cortex of the squirrel monkey. Exp. Neurol. *18*, 300-312 (1967)

116. Bignall, K.E. and Imbert, M.: Polysensory and cortico-cortical projections to frontal lobe of squirrel and rhesus monkeys. Electroenceph. clin. Neurophysiol. *26*, 206-215 (1969)

117. Blum, P.S., Abraham, L.D. and Gilman, S.: Vestibular, auditory and somatic input to the posterior thalamus of the cat. Exp. Brain Res. *34*, 1-9 (1979)

118. Bock, G.R. and Webster, W.R.: Spontaneous activity of single units in the inferior colliculus of anesthetized and unanesthetized cats. Brain Res. *76*, 150-154 (1974)

119. Bock, G.R. and Webster, W.R.: Coding of Spatial Location by Single Units in the Inferior Colliculus of the Alert Cat. Exp. Brain Res. *21*, 387-398 (1974)

120. Bock, G.R., Webster, W.R. and Aitkin, L.M.: Discharge Patterns of Single Units in Inferior Colliculus of the Alert Cat. J. Neurophysiol. *35*, 265-277 (1972)

121. Bodian, D.: The Generalized Vertebrate Neuron. Science *137*, 323-326 (1962)

122. de Boer, E.: On the "residue" in hearing. Academic thesis, Amsterdam 1956

123. de Boer, E.: Pitch of inharmonic signals. Nature (Lond.) *178*, 535-536 (1956)

124. de Boer, E.: On the "Residue" and Auditory Pitch Perception. In: Auditory System. Handbook of Sensory Physiology, Volume V/3 Eds.: Keidel, W.D. and Neff, W.D., Springer-Verlag, Berlin-Heidelberg-New York (1976)

125. Bogert, B.P.: Determination of the effects of dissipation in the cochlear partition by means of a network representing the basilar membrane. J. Acoust. Soc. Amer. *23*, 151-154 (1951)

126. Bordley, J.E., Ruben, R.J. and Lieberman, A.T.: Human cochlear potentials. Laryngoscope *74*, 463-479 (1964)

127. Bortoff, A.: Localization of slow potential responses in the Necturus retina. Vision Res. *4*, 627-635 (1964)

128. Bosher, S.K. and Warren, R.L.: Observations on the electrochemistry of the cochlear endolymph of the rat: a quantitative study of its electrical potential and ionic composition as determined by means of flame spectrophotometry. Proc.roy.Soc.B. *171*, 227-247 (1968)

129. Bosher, S.K. and Warren, R.L.: A study of the electrochemistry and osmotic relationships of the cochlear fluids in the neonatal rat at the time of the development of the endocochlear potential. J. Physiol. (Lond.) *212*, 739-761 (1971)

130. Bosher, S.K. and Warren, R.L.: Very low calcium content of cochlear endolymph, an extracellular fluid. Nature *273*, 377-378 (1978)

131. Boudreau, J.C. and Tsuchitani, C.: Binaural interaction in the cat superior olive S-segment. J. Neurophysiol. *31*, 442-454 (1968)

132. Boudreau, J.C. and Tsuchitani, C.: Cat Superior Olive S-segment Cell Discharge to Tonal Stimulation. In: Contributions to Sensory Physiology, Volume 4. Ed.: Neff, W.D. Academic Press, New York and London 1970

133. Bourk, T.R., Mielcarz, J.P. and Norris, B.E.: Tonotopic organization of the anteroventral cochlear nucleus of the cat. Hearing Research *4*, 215-241 (1981)

134. Bowsher, D.: Projection of the gracile and cuneate nuclei in Macaca mulatta. An experimental degeneration study. J. comp. Neurol. *110*, 135-155 (1968)

135. Bowsher, D.: The termination of secondary somatosensory nerve cells within the thalamus of Macaca mulatta. An experimental degeneration study. J. comp. Neurol. *117*, 213-222 (1961)

136. Brawer, J.R., Morest, D.K., Kane, E.C.: The neuronal architecture of the cochlear nucleus of the cat. J. comp. Neurol. *155*, 251-300 (1974)

137. Bredberg, G.: Cellular pattern and nerve supply of the human organ of Corti. Acta Oto-laryng. (Stockh.) Suppl. *236*, (1968)

138. Bredberg, G.: Scanning Electron Microscopy of the Nerves within the Organ of Corti. Arch. Oto-Rhino-Laryng. *217*, 321-330 (1977)

139. Bredberg, G.: The innervation of the organ of Corti. Acta Otolaryngol. (Stockh.) *83*, 71-78 (1977)

140. Bredberg, G., Lindeman, H., Ades, H.W., West, R. and Engström, H.: Scanning

electron microscopy of the organ of Corti. Science *170*, 861-863 (1970)

141. Bredberg, G. and Hunter-Duvar, I.M.: Behavioral Tests of Hearing and Inner Ear Damage. In: Auditory System. Handbook of Sensory Physiology, Volume V/2 Eds.: Keidel, W.D. and Neff, W.D. Springer-Verlag, Berlin-Heidelberg-New York 1975

142. Bredberg, G., Ades, H.W. and Engström, H.: Scanning Electron Microscopy of the Normal and Pathologically Altered Organ of Corti. Acta Otolaryng. Suppl. *301*, 3-48 (1972)

143. Bremer, F.: L'activité cérébrale au course du sommeil et de la narcose. Contribution à l'étude du méchanisme du sommeil. Bull. acad. med. Belg. *2*, 68-86 (1937)

144. Bremer, F.: Etude oscillographique des résponses sensorielles de l'aire acoustique corticale chez le chat. Arch. int. Physiol. *53*, 53-103 (1943)

145. Bremer, F.: Les aires auditives de l'écorce cérébrale. Cours International d-Audiologie Clinique, Mardo 12-Février 1952

146. Bremer, F.: Some Problems in Neurophysiology. Athlone Press, London 1953

147. Bremer, F. and Dow, R.S.: The acoustic area of the cerebral cortex in the cat. A combined oscillographic and cytoarchitectonic study. J. Neurophysiol. *2*, 308-318 (1939)

148. Bremer, F. and Bonnet, V.: Interprétation des réactions rhythmiques prolongées des aires sensorielles de l'écorce cérébrale. Electroenceph. clin. Neurophysiol. *2*, 389-400 (1959)

149. Britt, R.H.: Intracellular study of synaptic events related to phase-locking responses of cat cochlear nucleus cells to low frequency tones. Brain Res. *112*, 313-327 (1976)

150. Brown, J.C. and Howlett, B.: The olivocochlear tract in the rat and its hearing on the homologies of some constituent cell groups of the mammalian superior olivary complex: a thiocholine study. Acta Anat. *83*, 505-526 (1972)

151. Brugge, J.F. and Merzenich, M.M.: Representation of frequency in auditory cortex in the macaque monkey. In: Physiology of the Auditory System. Ed.: Sachs, M.B., National Educational Consultants, Inc., Baltimore/Maryland 1971

152. Brugge, J.F. and Merzenich, M.M.: Patterns of activity of single neurons of the auditory cortex in monkey. In: Basic Mechanisms in Hearing. Ed.: Møller, A.R. Academic Press, New York and London 1973

153. Brugge, J.F. and Merzenich, M.M.: Responses of Neurons in Auditory Cortex of the Macaque Monkey to Monaural and Binaural Stimulation. J. Neurophysiol. *36*, 1138-1158 (1973)

154. Brugge, J.F. and Imig, T.J.: Some relationships of binaural response patterns of single neurons to cortical columns and interhemispheric connections of auditory area AI of cat cerebral cortex. In: Evoked electrical activity in the auditory nervous system. Eds.: Naunton, R.F., Fernández, C. Academic Press, New York 1978

155. Brugge, J.F., Anderson, D.J., Hind, J.E. and Rose, J.E.: Time structure of discharges in single auditory nerve fibers of the squirrel monkey in response to complex periodic sounds. J. Neurophysiol. *32*, 386-401 (1969)

156. Brugge, J.F., Dubrovsky, N.A., Aitkin, L.M. and Anderson, D.J.: Sensitivity of single neurons in auditory cortex of cat to binaural tonal stimulation: effects of varying interaural time and intensity. J. Neurophysiol. *32*, 1005-1024 (1969)

157. Brugge, J.F., Anderson, D.J. and Aitkin, L.M.: Responses of neurons in the dorsal nucleus of the lateral lemniscus of cat to binaural tonal stimulation. J. Neurophysiol. *33*, 441-458 (1970)

158. Büchele, U. und Seiler, C.F.: Die reizkorrelierte Gleichspannungsantwort (RGA) akustisch evozierter Potentiale und ihre Abhängigkeit von Vigilanz und Aufmerksamkeit. H.N.O. (Berl.) *22*, 114-117 (1974)

159. Burke, W., and Sefton, A.J.: Discharge patterns of principal cells and interneurones in lateral geniculate nucleus of rat. J. Physiol. (Lond.) *187*, 201-212 (1966)

160. Burke, W. and Sefton, A.J.: Discharge patterns of principal cells and interneurones in lateral geniculate nucleus of rat. J. Physiol. *187*, 213-229 (1966)

161. Burke, W. and Sefton, A.J.: Inhibitory mechanisms in lateral geniculate nucleus of rat. J. Physiol. *187*, 231-246 (1966)

162. Butler, R.A.: Experimental observations on a negative dc-Resting Potential in the

Cochlea. J. Acoust. Soc. Amer. *36*, 1016 A (1964)

163. Butler, R.A.: Frequency specificity of the auditory evoked response to simultaneously and successively presented stimuli. Electroenceph. clin. Neurophysiol. *33*, 277-282 (1972)

164. Butler, R.A. and Honrubia, V.: Responses of cochlear potentials to changes in hydrostatic pressure. J. Acoust. Soc. Amer. *35*, 1188-1192 (1963)

165. Butler, R.A., Diamond, I.T. and Neff, W.D.: Role of auditory cortex in discrimination of changes in frequency. J. Neurophysiol. *20*, 108-120 (1957)

166. Butler, R.A., Gerstein, G.L. and Erulkar, S.D.: Inhibitory Phenomena in Cat Cochlear Nucleus. Fed. Proc. *26*, 543 (1967)

167. Butler, R.A., Keidel, W.D. and Spreng, M.: An investigation of the human cortical evoked potential under conditions of monaural and binaural stimulation. Acta otolaryng. (Stockh.) *68*, 317-326 (1969)

168. Butler, R.A., Spreng, M. and Keidel, W.D.: Stimulus repetition rate factors which influence the auditory evoked potential in man. Psychophysiol. *5*, 665-672 (1969)

169. Calford, M.B. and Webster, W.R.: Auditory Representation Within Principal Division of Cat Medial Geniculate Body: an Electrophysiological Study. J. Neurophysiol. *45*, 1013-1028 (1981)

170. Canzek, V. and Reubi, J.C.: The Effect of Cochlear Nerve Lesion on the Release of Glutamate, Aspartate, and GABA from Cat Cochlear Nucleus, in Vitro. Exp. Brain Res. *38*, 437-441 (1980)

171. Carey, C.L. and Webster, D.B.: The projections of the inferior colliculus in the kangaroo rat. Anat. Rec. *169*, 289 (1971)

172. Carlier, E. and Pujol, R.: Role of inner and outer hair cells in coding sound intensity: an ontogenetic approach. Brain Res. *147*, 174-176 (1978)

173. Carlier, E., Lenoir, M. and Pujol, R.: Development of cochlear frequency selectivity tested by compound action potential tuning curve. Hearing Research *1*, 197-201 (1979)

174. Carlson, R. and Grandström, B.: Perception of segmental duration. In: Structure and Process in Speech Perception. Communication and Cybernetics, Vol. 11. Eds.: Cohen, A. and Nooteboom, S.G., Springer-Verlag, Berlin-Heidelberg-New York 1975

175. Carpenter, M.B.: Lesions of the fastigial nuclei in the rhesus monkey. Amer. J. Anat. *104*, 1-33 (1959)

176. Carpenter, M.B.: Experimental anatomical-physiological studies of the vestibular nerve and cerebellar connections. In: Neural Mechanisms of the Auditory and Vestibular Systems. Eds.: Rasmussen, G.L. and Windle, W.F., Charles C. Thomas, Springfield/Ill. 1960

177. Carpenter, M.B., Brittin, G.M. and Pines, J.: Isolated lesions of the fastigial nuclei in the cat. J. comp. Neurol. *109*, 65-89 (1959)

178. Carpenter, M.B., Batton, R.B. III and Peter, P.: Transport of Radioactivity from Primary Auditory Neurons beyond the Cochlear Nuclei. J. comp. Neur. *179*, 517-534 (1978)

179. Caspary, D.M.: Stimulus coding and the cytoarchitecture of the cochlear nuclei of the kangaroo rat, Dipodomys spectabilis. Thesis, New York Univ., New York 1971

180. Caspary, D.M., Rupert, A.L. and Moushegian, G.: Neuronal Coding of Vowel Sounds in the Cochlear Nuclei. Exp. Neurol. *54*, 414-431 (1977)

181. Caspary, D.M., Havey, D.C. and Faingold, C.L.: Glutamate and aspartate: alteration of thresholds and response patterns of auditory neurons. Hearing Research *4*, 325-333 (1981)

182. Caspers, H. und Lerche, E.: Die Bedeutung der Retikulärformation des Hirnstammes für die Schallwahrnehmung. Z. Laryng. Rhinol. *38*, 36-41 (1959)

183. Caspers, H. und Lerche, E.: Über die Verwertbarkeit der corticalen Makroaktionspontentiale als Indicatoren einer corticopetalen Erregungsleitung. Pflügers Arch. ges. Physiol. *270*, 8 (1959)

184. Casseday, J.H. and Neff, W.D.: Auditory localization: role of auditory pathways in brainstem of the cat. J. Neurophysiol. *38*, 842-858 (1975)

185. Casseday, J.H., Diamond, I.T. and Harting, J.K.: Auditory pathways to the cortex in Tupaia glis. J. comp. Neur. *166*, 303-340 (1976)

186. Caton, R.: Interim report on investigation of the electric currents of the brain. Brit.Med.J.Suppl. *62*, 1 (1877)

187. Caton, R.: Researches on electrical phenomena of cerebral grey matter. Tr. Ninth Int. Med. Cong. *3*, 246 (1887)

188. Cazals, Y., Aran, J.-M., Erre, J.-P., Guilhaume, A. and Hawkins, J.E.Jr.: "Neural" Responses to Acoustic Stimulation after Destruction of Cochlear Hair Cells. Arch. Otorhinolaryngol. *224*, 61-70 (1979)

189. Chikamori, Y., Sasa, M., Fujimoto, S., Takaori, S. and Matsuoka, I.: Locus coeruleus-induced inhibition of dorsal cochlear nucleus neurons in comparison with lateral vestibular nucleus neurons. Brain Res. *194*, 53-63 (1980)

190. Chow, K.L.: Numerical estimates of the auditory central nervous system of the Rhesus monkey. J. Comp. Neurol. *95*, 159-175 (1951)

191. Citron, K., Exley, D. and Hallpike, C.S.: Formation, circulation, and chemical properties of labyrinthine fluids. Brit. Med. Bull. *12*, 101-104 (1956)

192. Citron, L., Exley, D. and Hallpike, C.S: Labyrinthine fluids. Brit. Med. J. *12*, 101-112 (1956)

193. Clopton, B.M. and Winfield, J.A.: Tonotopic organization in the inferior colliculus of the rat. Brain Research *56*, 355-358 (1973)

194. Coats, A.C.: Human auditory nerve action potentials and cochlear microphonics recorded nonsurgically. J. Acoust. Soc. Amer. *49*, 112-113 (1971)

195. Coats, A.C. and Dickery, J.R.: Non-surgical recording of human auditory nerve action potentials and cochlear microphonics. Ann. Otol. *79*, 844-852 (1970)

196. Coats, A.C. and Dickery, J.R.: Post masking recovery of human click action potentials and click loudness. J. Acoust. Soc. Amer. *52*, 1607-1612 (1972)

197. Cohen, A. and Nooteboom, S.G.: Structure and Process in Speech Perception. In: Communication and Cybernetics, Vol. 11. Eds.: Wolter, H. and Keidel, W.D. Springer-Verlag, Berlin-Heidelberg-New York 1975

198. Colavita, F.B.: Auditory cortical lesions and visual pattern discrimination in cat. Brain Research *39*, 437-447 (1972)

199. Colwell, S.A.: Corticothalamic projections from physiologically defined loci within primary auditory cortex in the cat: reciprocal structure in the medial geniculate body. Dissertation, University of California, San Francisco 1977

200. Commichau, R.: Adaptationszustand und Unterschiedsschwellenenergie fur Lichtblitze. Z. Biol. *108*, 145-160 (1955)

201. Coombs, J.S., Eccles, J.C. and Fatt, P.: The specific ionic conductances and the ionic movements across the motoneuronal membrane that produce the inhibitory postsynaptic potential. J. Physiol. (Lond.) *130*, 326-373 (1955)

202. Coombs, J.S., Eccles, J.C. and Fatt, P.: Excitatory synaptic action in motoneurones. J. Physiol. (Lond.) *130*, 374-395 (1955)

203. Crandall, W.E.: Diode pump cochlear audition theory. Intern. J. Neuroscience *6*, 203-213 (1975)

204. Cranford, J.L.: Polysensory cortex lesions and auditory frequency discrimination in the cat. Brain Research *148*, 499-503 (1978)

205. Cranford, J.L.: Auditory Cortex Lesions and Interaural Intensity and Phase-Angle Discrimination in Cats. J. Neurophysiol. *42*, 1518-1526 (1979)

206. Cranford, J.L., Igarashi, M. and Stramler, J.H.: Effect of Auditory Neocortex Ablation on Pitch Perception in the Cat. J. Neurophysiol. *39*, 143-152 (1976)

207. Crawford, A.C. and Fettiplace, R.: Ringing responses in cochlear hair cells of the turtle. J. Physiol. *284*, 120-122P (1978)

208. Crawford, A.C. and Fettiplace, R.: The frequency selectivity of auditory nerve fibres and hair cells in the cochlea of the turtle. J. Physiol. *306*, 79-125 (1980)

209. Crawford, A.C. and Fettiplace, R.: An electrical tuning mechanism in turtle cochlear hair cells. J. Physiol. *312*, 377-412 (1981)

210. Creutzfeldt, O. and Jung, R.: Neuronal discharge in the cat's motor cortex during sleep and arousal. In: The Nature of Sleep. Eds.: Wolstenholme, G.E.W. and

O'Conner, M., J. & A. Churchill Ltd., London 1961

211. Crow, G., Rupert, A.L., Moushegian, G.: Phase locking in monaural and binaural medullary neurons: Implications for binaural phenomena. J. Acoust. Soc. Amer. *64*, 493-501 (1978)

212. Cullen, J.K., Ellis, M.S., Berlin, C.I. and Lousteau, R.J.: Human acoustic nerve action potential recording from the tympanic membrane without anesthesia. Acta Otolaryng. (Stockholm) *74*, 15-22 (1972)

213. Dallos, P.: The auditory periphery. Biophysics and physiology. Academic Press, New York 1973

214. Dallos, P.: Cochlear potentials and cochlear mechanics. In: Basic Mechanisms of Hearing. Ed.: Møller, A.R., Academic Press, New York 1973

215. Dallos, P.: Electrical Correlates of Mechanical Events in the Cochlea. Audiology *14*, 408-418 (1975)

216. Dallos. P.: Cochlear Potentials. In: The Nervous System. Vol. 3: Human Communication and Its Disorders. Ed.: Tower, D.B., Raven Press, New York 1975

217. Dallos, P. and Harries, D.: Properties of Auditory Nerve Responses in Absence of Outer Hair Cells. J. Neurophysiol. *41*, 365-383 (1978)

218. David, E.: Elektronisches Analogmodell der Verarbeitung akustischer Information in Organismen. Habilitationsschrift, Erlangen 1972

219. David, E., Finkenzeller, P., Kallert, S. und Keidel, W.D.: Die mit Mikroelektroden ableitbare Reaktion einzelner Elemente des Colliculus inferior und des Corpus geniculatum mediale auf akustische Reize verschiedener Form und verschiedener Intensität. Pflügers Arch. ges. Physiol. *299*, 83-93 (1968)

220. David, E., Finkenzeller, P., Kallert, S. und Keidel, W.D.: Reizfrequenzkorrelierte "untersetzte" neuronale Entladungsperiodizitat im Colliculus inferior und im Corpus geniculatum mediale. Pflügers Arch. *309*, 11-20 (1969)

221. David, E., Finkenzeller, P., Kallert, S. und Keidel, W.D.: Akustischen Reizen zugeordnete Gleichspannungsänderungen am intakten Schädel des Menschen. Pflügers Arch. *309*, 362-367 (1969)

222. David, E., Finkenzeller, P., Kallert, S. und Keidel, W.D.: Reizkorrelierte Gleichspannungsänderungen der primären Hörrinde an der wachen Katze. Pflügers Arch. *306*, 281-289 (1969)

223. David, E., Finkenzeller, P., Kallert, S. und Keidel, W.D.: Beiträge höherer Hörbahnanteile der Katze zur Mustererkennung. In: Zeichenerkennung durch biologische und technische Systeme. Hrsg.: Grüsser, O.-J. und Klinke, R., Springer-Verlag, Berlin-Heidelberg-New York 1971

224. Davis, H.: Initiation of nerve in the cochlea and other mechanoreceptors. In: Physiological Triggers and Discontinuous Rate Process. Ed.: Bullock, T., Am. Physiol. Soc., Washington 1956

225. Davis, H.: Biophysics and physiology of the inner ear. Physiol. Rev. *37*, 1-49 (1957)

226. Davis, H.: A mechano-electrical theory of cochlear action. Ann. Otol. Rhin. *67*, 789-801 (1958)

227. Davis, H.: Excitation of auditory receptors. In: Handbook of Physiology. Section 1: Neurophysiology, Vol. I. Eds.: Field, J., Magoun, H.W. and Hall, V.E. American Physiological Society, Washington, D.C., 1959

228. Davis, H.: Mechanism of Excitation of Auditory Nerve Impulses. In: Neural Mechanisms of the Auditory and Vestibular Systems. Eds.: Rasmussen, G.L. and Windle, W.F. Charles C. Thomas Publ., Springfield/Ill. 1960

229. Davis, H.: Enhancement of evoked cortical potentials in humans related to a task requiring a decision. Science *145*, 182-183 (1964)

230. Davis, H.: A model for transducer action in the cochlea. Cold Spring Harbor Symp. Quant. Biol. *30*, 181-190 (1965)

231. Davis, H.: Validation of evoked-response audiometry (ERA) in deaf children. Int. Audiology—Audiologie Internationale *5*, 77-81 (1966)

232. Davis, H.: Mechanisms of the inner ear. Ann. Otol. (St. Louis) *77*, 644-655 (1968)

233. Davis, H.: Averaged-evoked-response EEG audiometry in North America. Acta otolaryng. (Stockh.) *65*, 79-85 (1968)

234. Davis, H.: Evoked response audiometry. Trans. Amer. Acad. Ophthal. Otolaryng. *74*, 1236-1237 (1970)

235. Davis, H.: Interactions of tactile and electric stimuli with auditory V potentials. Arch. klin. exp. Ohr.-, Nas.-u. Kehlk.Heilk. *198*, 108-109 (1971)

236. Davis, H.: Sedation of young children for ERA. ERA, 18th Issue, December 1971

237. Davis, H.: Is ERA ready for routine clinical use? Arch.klin.exp.Ohr.-,Nas.- u. Kehlk.Heilk. *198*, 2-8 (1971)

238. Davis, H.: Sedation of young children for electric response audiometry (ERA). (Summary of a symposium). Transactions, Released August 1972

239. Davis, H.: Sedation of young children for electric response audiometry (ERA). Summary of a symposium. Audiology *12*, 55-57 (1973)

240. Davis, H.: Classes of auditory evoked responses. Audiology *12*, 464-469 (1973)

241. Davis, H.: Relations of peripheral action potentials and cortical evoked potentials to the magnitude of sensation. In: Sensation and measurement. Eds.: Moskowitz, H.R., Scharf, B. and Stevens, J.C., D. Reidel Publ. Comp., Dordrecht/Holland—Boston, USA 1974

242. Davis, H.: Electric Response Audiometry, with Special Reference to the Vertex Potentials. In: Auditory System; Handbook of Sensory Physiology, Volume V/3, Eds.: Keidel, W.D. and Neff, W.D. Springer-Verlag, Berlin-Heidelberg-New York 1976

243. Davis, H. and Eldredge, D.H.: An interpretation of the mechanical detector action of the cochlea. Ann. Otol. Rhin. *68*, 665-674 (1959)

244. Davis, H. and Yoshie, N.: Human cortical response to auditory stimuli. Physiologist *6*, 164 (1963)

245. Davis, H. and Zerlin, S.: Acoustic relations of the human vertex potential. J. Acoust. Soc. Amer. *39*, 109-116 (1966)

246. Davis, H. and Niemoeller, A.F.: A system for clinical evoked response audiometry. J. Speech Dis. *33*, 33-37 (1968)

247. Davis, H., Davis, P.A., Loomis, A.L., Harvey, E.N. and Horbart, G.: Electrical reactions of the human brain to auditory stimulation during sleep. J. Neurophysiol. *2*, 500-514 (1939)

248. Davis, H., Gernandt, B.E. and Riesco-MacClure, J.S.: Threshold of action potentials in ear of guinea pig. J. Neurophysiol. *13*, 73-87 (1950)

249. Davis, H., Tasaki, I., Smith, C.A. and Deatherage, B.H.: Cochlear potentials after intra-cochlear injections and anoxia. Fed. Proc. *14*, 112 (1955)

250. Davis, H., Deatherage, B.H., Eldredge, D.H. and Smith, C.A.: Summating potentials of the cochlea. Amer. J. Physiol. *195*, 251-261 (1958)

251. Davis, H., Deatherage, B.H., Rosenblut, B., Fernández, C., Kimura, R. and Smith, C.A.: Modification of cochlear potentials produced by streptomycin poisoning and by extensive venous obstruction. Laryngoscope *68*, 596-627 (1958)

252. Davis, H., Engebretson, M., Lowell, E.L., Mast, T., Satterfield, J. and Yoshie, N.: Evoked responses to clicks recorded from the human scalp. Ann. N.Y. Acad. Sci. *112*, 224-225 (1964)

253. Davis, H., Mast, T., Yoshie, N. and Zerlin, S.: The slow response of the human cortex to auditory stimuli: recovery process. Electroenceph. clin. Neurophysiol. *21*, 105-113 (1966)

254. Davis, H., Hirsh, S.K., Shelnutt, J. and Bowers, C.: Further validation of evoked response audiometry (ERA). J. Speech Res. *10*, 717-732 (1967)

255. Davis, H., Osterhammel, P.A., Wier, C.C. and Gjerdingen, D.B.: Slow vertex potentials: interactions among auditory, tactile, electric, and visual stimuli. Electroenceph. clin. Neurophysiol. *33*, 537-545 (1972)

256. Deatherage, B.H., Eldredge, D.H. and Davis, H.: Latency of action potentials in the cochlea of the guinea pig. J. Acoust. Soc. Amer. *31*, 479-486 (1959)

257. Delgutte, B.: Representation of speech-like sounds in the discharge patterns of auditory-nerve fibers. J. Acoust. Soc. Amer. *68*, 843-857 (1980)

258. Denes, P.: Effect of Duration on the Perception of Voicing. J. Acoust. Soc. Amer. *27*, 761-764 (1955)

259. Derbyshire, A.J. and Davis, H.: The action potentials of the auditory nerve. Am. J. Physiol. *113*, 476-504 (1935)

260. Desmedt, J.E.: Auditory evoked potentials from cochlea to cortex as influenced by activation of efferent olivo-cochlear bundle. J. Acoust. Soc. Amer. *34*, 1478-1496 (1962)

261. Desmedt, J.E.: Physiological Studies of the Efferent Recurrent Auditory System. In: Auditory System. Handbook of Sensory Physiology, Vol. V/2, Eds.: Keidel, W.D. and Neff, W.D. Springer-Verlag, Berlin-Heidelberg-New York 1975

262. Diamond, I.T.: The sensory neocortex. In: Contributions to Sensory Physiology, Vol. 2, Ed.: Neff, W.D., Academic Press, New York and London 1967

263. Diamond, I.T.: The Auditory Cortex. In: Evoked electrical activity in the auditory nervous system. Eds.: Naunton, R.F., Fernández, C. Academic Press, New York 1978

264. Diamond, I.T. and Neff, W.D.: Ablation of temporal cortex and discrimination of auditory patterns. J. Neurophysiol. *20*, 300-315 (1957)

265. Diamond, I.T., Goldberg, J.M. and Neff, W.D.: Tonal discrimination after ablation of auditory cortex. J. Neurophysiol. *25*, 223-235 (1962)

266. Diamond, I.T., Jones, E.C. and Powell, T.P.S.: Interhemispheric fiber connections of auditory cortex of cat. Brain Res. *11*, 177-193 (1968)

267. Diamond, I.T., Jones, E.C. and Powell, T.P.S.: The association connections of auditory cortex in cat. Brain Res. *11*, 560-579 (1968)

268. Diamond, I.T., Jones, E.G. and Powell, T.P.S.: The projection of the auditory cortex upon the diencephalon and brain stem in the cat. Brain Res. *15*, 305-340 (1969)

269. Diestel, H.-G.: Akustische Messungen an einem mechanischen Modell des Innenohres. Acustica *4*, 489-499 (1954)

270. Disterhoft, J.F. and Stuart, D.K.: Trial Sequence of Changed Unit Activity in Auditory System of Alert Rat During Conditioned Response Acquisition and Extinction. J. Neurophysiol. *39*, 266-281 (1976)

271. Disterhoft, J.F., Perkins, R.D. and Evans, S.: Neuronal Morphology of the Rabbit Cochlear Nucleus. J. Comp. Neurol. *192*, 687-702 (1980)

272. Dowman, C.B.B., Woolsey, C.N. and Lende, R.A.: Auditory areas I, II and Ep: cochlear representation, afferent paths and interconnections. Bull. Johns Hopkins Hosp. *106*, 127-146 (1960)

273. Dunker, E. und Krämer, B.: Funktionskonzept fur die oberen Hörbahnabschnitte. HNO *20*, 351-362 (1972)

274. Dunlop, C.W., Itzkowic, D.J. and Aitkin, L.M.: Tone-burst response patterns of single units in the cat medial geniculate body. Brain Res. *16*, 149-164 (1969)

275. Duvall, J., Flock, A. and Wersäll, J.: The ultrastructure of the sensory hairs and associated organelles of the cochlear inner hair cells, with reference to directional sensitivity. J. cell. Biol. *29*, 497-505 (1966)

276. Eccles, J.C.: The physiology of nerve cells. Johns Hopkins Univ. Press, Baltimore 1957

277. Eccles, J.C.: Properties and functional organization of cells in the ventrobasal complex of the thalamus. In: The Thalamus. Eds.: Purpura, D.P. and Yahr, M.D. Columbia University Press, New York and London 1966

278. von Economo, C. and Horn, K.: Über Windungsrelief, Masse und Rindenarchitektonik der Supratemporalfläche, ihre individuellen und ihre Seitenunterschiede. Z. ges. Neurol. Psychiat. *130*, 678-757 (1930)

279. Eggermont, J.J.: Electrocochleography. In: Auditory System. Handbook of Sensory Physiology, Volume V/3. Eds.: Keidel, W.D. and Neff, W.D. Springer-Verlag, Berlin-Heidelberg-New York 1976

280. Eggermont, J.J. and Odenthal, D.W.: The clinical application of supraliminal electrocochleography: adaptation and masking of action potentials in response to short tone bursts. Audiology *11*, Suppl. 127 (1972)

281. Eggermont, J.J. and Odenthal, D.W.: Electrophysiological investigation of the human cochlea: recruitment, masking and adaptation. Audiology *13*, 1-22 (1974)

282. Eggermont, J.J. and Odenthal, D.W.: Action potentials and summating potentials in

the normal human cochlea. Acta oto-laryng. (Stockh.) Suppl. *316*, 39-61 (1974)

283. Eggermont, J.J. and Odenthal, D.W.: Frequency selective masking in electrocochleography. Rev. Laryngol. (Bordeaux) *95*, 489-496 (1974)

284. Eggermont, J.J., Odenthal, D.W., Schmidt, P.H. and Spoor, A.: Electrocochleography. Basic Principles and Clinical Application. Acta Otolaryng. Suppl. *316*, (1974)

285. Elberling, C. and Salomon, G.: Electrical potentials from the inner ear in man, in response to transient sounds generated in a closed acoustic system. Rev. Laryngol. (Bordeaux) Suppl. *92*, 691-708 (1971)

286. Elliott, D.N. and McGee, T.M.: Effects of cochlear lesions upon audiograms and intensity discrimination in cats. Ann. Otol. (St. Louis) *74*, 386-408 (1965)

287. Elliott, D.N. and Fraser, W.: Fatigue and Adaptation. In: Foundations of Modern Auditory Theory, Vol. I. Ed.: Tobias, J.V., Academic Press, New York and London 1970

288. Engebretson, A.M. and Eldredge, D.H.: Model for the nonlinear characteristics of cochlear potentials. J. Acoust. Soc. Amer. *44*, 548-554 (1968)

289. Engelstätter, R., Vater, M. and Neuweiler, G.: Processing of noise by single units of the inferior colliculus of the bat Rhinolophus ferrumequinum. Hearing Research *3*, 285-300 (1980)

290. Engström, B.: Scanning electron microscopy of the inner structure of the organ of Corti and its neural pathways. Acta Otolaryngol. (Stockh.) Suppl. *319*, 57-66 (1974)

291. Engström, H.: The cortilymph, the third lymph of the inner ear. Acta Morphol. Neerl. Scand. *3*, 195-204 (1960)

292. Engström, H.: Electron micrographic studies of the receptor cells of the organ of Corti. In: Neural Mechanisms of the Auditory and Vestibular Systems. Eds.: Rasmussen, G.L. and Windle, W.F. Charles C. Thomas Publ., Springfield/Ill. 1960

293. Engström, H. and Ades, H.W.: The ultrastructure of the ochlea. In: Ultrastructure of animal tissues and organs. Ed.: Friedmann, I., North-Holland Publ. Co., Amsterdam 1972

294. Engström, H. and Engström, B.: Structural and physiological features of the organ of Corti. Audiology *11*, 6-28 (1972)

295. Engström, H., Ades, H.W. and Hawkins, J.E.: Structure and function of the sensory hairs of the inner ear. J. Acoust. Soc. Amer. *34*, 1356-1363 (1962)

296. Engström, H., Ades, H.W. and Andersson, A.: Structural Pattern of the Organ of Corti. Almqvist & Wiksell, Stockholm 1966

297. Erulkar, S.D.: The responses of single units of the inferior colliculus of the cat to acoustic stimulation. Proc. roy. Soc. B *150*, 336-35 (1959)

298. Erulkar, S.D.: Physiological Studies of the Inferior Colliculus and Medial Geniculate Complex. In: Auditory System. Handbook of Sensory Physiology, Volume V/2. Eds.: Keidel, W.D. and Neff, W.D. Springer-Verlag, Berlin-Heidelberg-New York 1975

299. Erulkar, S.D., Rose, J.E. and Davies, P.W.: Single units activity in the auditory cortex of the cat. Bull. Johns Hopk. Hosp. *99*, 55-86 (1956)

300. Erulkar, S.D., Butler, R.A. and Gerstein, G.L.: Excitation and inhibition in cochlear nucleus. II. Frequency modulated tones. J. Neurophysiol. *31*, 537-548 (1968)

301. Erulkar, S.D., Nelson, P.G. and Bryan, J.S.: Experimental and Theoretical Approaches to Neural Processing in the Central Auditory Pathway. In: Contribution to Sensory Physiology, Vol. 3. Ed.: Neff, W.D. Academic Press, New York and London 1968

302. Evans, E.F.: Cortical representation. In: Hearing Mechanisms in Vertebrates. A Ciba Foundation Symposium. Eds.: de Reuck, A.V.S. and Knight, J., J. & A. Churchill Ltd. London 1968

303. Evans, E.F.: The frequency response and other properties of single fibers in the guinea-pig cochlear nerve. J. Physiol. *226*, 263-287 (1972)

304. Evans, E.F.: Auditory frequency selectivity and the cochlear nerve. In: Facts and Models in Hearing. Communication and Cybernetics, Vol. 8, Ed.: Zwicker, E. and Terhardt, E., Springer-Verlag, Berlin-Heidelberg-New York 1974

305. Evans, E.F., The effects of hypoxia on the tuning of single cochlear nerve fibers. J. Physiol. (Lond.) *238*, 65-67 P (1974)

306. Evans, E.F.: Neural processes for the detection of acoustic patterns and for sound localization. In: The Neurosciences: Third Study Program. Eds.: Schmitt, F.W. and Worden, F.G. MIT Press, Cambridge/Mass., USA 1974

307. Evans, E.F.: The Sharpening of Cochlear Frequency Selectivity in the Normal and Abnormal Cochlea. Audiology *14*, 419-442 (1975)

308. Evans, E.F.: Cochlear Nerve and Cochlear Nucleus. In: Auditory System. Handbook of Sensory Physiology, Vol. V/2. Eds.: Keidel, W.D. and Neff, W.D. Springer-Verlag, Berlin-Heidelberg-New York 1975

309. Evans, E.F.: Normal and abnormal functioning of the cochlear nerve. In: Sound Reception in Mammals. Symp. Zoo. Soc. London, Number 37. Eds.: Bench, R.J., Pye, A. and Pye, J.D., Academic Press, London 1975

310. Evans, E.F. and Whitfield, I.C.: Classification of unit responses in the auditory cortex of the unanesthetized and unrestrained cat. J. Physiol. *171* 476-493 (1964)

311. Evans, E.F., and Nelson, P.G., An intranuclear pathway to the dorsal division of the cochlear nucleus of the cat. J. Physiol. (Lond.) *196*, 76-78 (1968)

312. Evans, E.F. and Nelson, P.G., The responses of single neurones in the cochlear nucleus of the cat as a function of their location and the anesthetic state. Exp. Brain Res. *17*, 402-427 (1973)

313. Evans, E.F. and Nelson, P.G.: On the functional relationship between the dorsal and ventral divisions of the cochlear nucleus of the cat. Exp. Brain Res. *17*, 428-442 (1973)

314. Evans, E.F. and Klinke, R.: Reversible effects of cyanide and Furosemide on the tuning of single cochlear fibres. J. Physiol. (Lond.) *242*, 129-131 P (1974)

315. Evans, E.F. and Harrison, R.V.: Correlation between cochlear outer hair cell damage and deterioration of cochlear nerve tuning properties in the guinea-pig. J. Physiol. *256*, 43P-44P (1976)

316. Evans, E.F., Ross, H.F. and Whitfield, I.C.: The spatial distribution of unit characteristic frequency in the primary auditory cortex of the cat. J. Physiol. (Lond.) *171*, 238-247 (1965)

317. Evans, E.F., Rosenberg, J. and Wilson, J.P.: The effective bandwidth of cochlear nerve fibres. J. Physiol. (Lond.) 207, 62P-63P (1970)

318. Evarts, E.V.: Effects of sleep and waking on activity of single units in the unrestrained cat. In: The Nature of Sleep. Ed.: Wolstenholme, G.E.W. and O'Connor, M., J. & A. Churchill Ltd., London 1961

319. Evarts, E.V.: Activity of neurons in visual cortex of the cat during sleep with low voltage fast EEG activity. J. Neurophysiol. *25*, 812-816 (1962)

320. Evarts, E.V.: Temporal patterns of discharge of pyramidal tract neurons during sleep and waking in the monkey. J. Neurophysiol. *27*, 157-171 (1964)

321. Ewald. J.R.: Zur Physiologie des Labyrinths. VI. Mitteilung. Eine neue Hörtheorie. Pflügers Arch. Ges. Physiol. *76*, 147-188 (1899)

322. Ewald, J.R.: Zur Physiologie des Labyrinths. VII. Mitteilung. Die Erzeugung von Schallbildern in der Camera acustica. Pflügers Arch. Ges. Physiol. *93*, 485-500 (1903)

323. Fadiga, E. and Pupilli, G.C.: Teleceptive components of the cerebellar function. Physiol. Rev. *44*, 432-486 (1964)

324. Fant, G. and Tatham, M.A.A.: Auditory Analysis and Perception of Speech. Academic Press, London-New York-San Francisco 1975

325. Fatt, P.: Alterations produced in the post-junctional cell by the inhibitory transmitter. In: Inhibition in the nervous system and γ-aminobutyric acid. Ed.: Roberts, E., Pergamon Press, New York 1960

326. Fatt, P. and Katz, B.: An analysis of the end-plate potential recorded with an intra-cellular electrode. J. Physiol. (Lond.) *115*, 320-370 (1951)

327. Feldman, M.L. and Harrison, J.M.: The superior olivary complex in primates. Medical Primatology. S. Karger, Basel 1971

328. Fernald, R.D. and Gerstein, G.L.: A model of cochlear-nucleus neurons responding to complex stimuli. In: Physiology of the Auditory System. Eds.: Sachs, M.B. National Educational Consultants, Inc., Baltimore/Maryland 1971

329. Fernald, R.D. and Gerstein, G.L.: Response of cat cochlear nucleus neurons to frequency and amplitude modulated tones. Brain Res. *45*, 417-435 (1972)

330. Fernandez, C. and Karapas, F.: The course and termination of the stria of Monakow and Held in the cat. J. Comp. Neurol. *131*, 371-386 (1967)

331. Fettiplace, R. and Crawford, A.C.: The origin of tuning in turtle cochlear hair cells. Hearing Research *2*, 447-454 (1980)

332. Fetz, E.E.: Pyramidal tract effects on interneurons in the cat lumbar dorsal horn. J. Neurophysiol. *31*, 69-80 (1968)

333. Fex, J.: Augmentation of the cochlear microphonics by stimulation of efferent fibres to cochlea. Acta oto-laryng. (Stockh.) *50*, 540-541 (1959)

334. Fex, J.: Auditory activity in centrifugal and centripetal cochlear fibres in cat. A study of a feedback system. Acta physiol. scand. Suppl. *189*, 1-68 (1962)

335. Fex, J.: Neural Excitatory Processes of the Inner Ear. In: Auditory System. Handbook of Sensory Physiology, Vol. V/1 Eds.: Keidel, W.D. and Neff, W.D. Springer-Verlag, Berlin-Heidelberg-New York 1974

336. Finkenzeller, P.: Die Mitteilung von Reaktionspotentialen. Kybernetik *6*, 22-44 (1969)

337. Finkenzeller, P.: Hypothese zur Schallkodierung des Innenohres. Habilitationsschrift, Erlangen 1973

338. Finkenzeller, P.: Einzelaktivitäten und kortikale Gleichspannungsänderungen. In: Physiologie des Gehörs. Eds.: Keidel, W.D. Georg Thieme Verlag, Stuttgart 1975

339. Finkenzeller, P. und Keidel, W.D.: Eigenschaften akustisch evozierter Potentiale bei Gleichspannungsregistrierung. Arch. Ohr.-, Nas.- u. Kehlk.-Heilk. *207*, 508 (1974)

340. Finkenzeller, P. and Keidel, W.D.: Correlates of auditory perception in averaged perstimulatory EEG-DC recordings. In: Quantitative Analysis of the EEG. Methods and Applications. Proceedings of the 2nd Symposium of the Study Group for EEG-Methodology, Jongny sur Vevey, May 1975. (Printed by AEG-Telefunken, Konstanz.)

341. Finkenzeller, P. and Keidel, W.D.: Evoked potentials to evaluate the perception of complex sounds. IV. Biennial Symposium of the International ERA Study Group in London, 28.-30.7 1975.

342. Finkenzeller, P., David, E., Kallert, S. und Keidel, W.D.: Die Aussagekraft gemittelter Potentiale. Pflügers Arch. *307*, 136 (1969)

343. Fishman, M.C. and Michael, C.R.: Integration of auditory information in the cat's visual cortex. Vision Res. *13*, 1415-1419 (1973)

344. Fitzpatrick, K.A. and Imig, T.J.: Auditory Cortico-cortial Connections in the Owl Monkey. J. Comp. Neurol. *192*, 589-610 (1980)

345. Flammino, F. and Clopton, B.M.: Neural responses in the inferior colliculus of albino rat to binaural stimuli. J. Acoust. Soc. Amer. *57*, 692-695 (1975)

346. Flanagan, J.L.: Models for Approximating Basilar Membrane Displacement. Bell System Tech. J. *39*, 1163-1191 (1960)

347. Flanagan, J.L.: Models for Approximating Basilar Membrane Displacement. Bell System Tech. J. *41*, 959-1009 (1962)

348. Flanagan, J.L.: Computational model for basilar membrane displacement. J. Acoust. Soc. Amer. *34*, 1370-1376 (1962)

349. Flanagan, J.L.: Speech analysis synthesis and perception. In: Kommunikation und Kybernetik in Einzeldarstellungen, Bd. 3 Hrsg.: Wolter, H. und Keidel, W.D. Springer-Verlag, Berlin-Heidelberg-New York 1965

350. Flanagan, J.L.: Speech Analysis Synthesis and Perception. In: Kommunikation und Kybernetik in Einzeldarstellungen, Bd. 3, 2. Auflage Hrsg.: Wolter, H. und Keidel, W.D. Springer-Verlag, Berlin-Heidelberg-New York 1972

351. Fleischl v. Marxow, E.: Mittheilung, betreffend die Physiologie der Hirnrinde. Zbl. Physiol. *4*, 537-540 (1890)

352. Fletcher, H.: On the dynamics of the cochlea. J. Acoust. Soc. Amer. *23*, 673-645 (1951)

353. Fletcher, H. and Munson, W.A.: Loudness, its definition, measurement and calculation. J. Acoust. Soc. Amer. *5*, 82-108 (1933)

354. Flock, Å.: Electron microscopic and electrophysiological studies on the lateral line canal organ. Acta oto-laryng. (Stockh.) Suppl. *199*, 1-90 (1965)
355. Flock, Å.: Transducing mechanisms in the lateral line canal organ receptors. Cold Spr. Harb. Symp. quant. Biol. *30*, 133-144 (1965)
356. Flock, Å.: Sensory Transduction in Hair Cells. In: Principles of Receptor Physiology. Handbook of Sensory Physiology, Vol. I. Ed.: Loewenstein, W.R. Springer-Verlag, Berlin-Heidelberg-New York 1971
357. Flock, Å.: Neurobiology of hair cells and their synapses. In: Facts and Models in Hearing. Communication and Cybernetics, Vol. 8. Eds.: Zwicker, E. and Terhardt, E., Springer-Verlag, Berlin-Heidelberg-New York 1974
358. Flock, Å. and Wersäll, J.: A study of the orientation of the sensory hairs of the receptor cells in the lateral line organ of a fish with special reference to the function of the receptors. J. Cell. Biol. *15*, 19-27 (1962)
359. Flock, Å. and Russel, I.: Postsynaptic action of efferent fibres on hair cells. Nature, N.B. *243*, 89-91 (1973)
360. Flock, Å. and Russel, I.: Inhibition by efferent nerve fibres: action on hair cells and afferent synaptic transmission in the lateral line canal organ of the burbot Lota lota. J. Physiol. *257*, 45-62 (1976)
361. Flock, Å., Kimura, R., Lundquist, P.G. and Wersäll, J.: Morphological basis of directional sensitivity of the outer hair cells in the organ of Corti. J. acoust. Soc. Amer. *34*, 1351-1355 (1962)
362. Flock, Å., Jorgensen, M. and Russel, I.: The physiology of individual hair cells and their synapses. In: Basic Mechanisms in Hearing. Ed.: Møller, A.R. Academic Press, New York and London 1973
363. Flock, Å., Flock, B. and Murray, E.: Studies on the sensory hairs of receptor cells in the inner ear. Acta Otolaryngol. (Stockh.) *83*, 85-91 (1977)
364. Forbes, B. and Moskowitz, N.: The projections of the insular and opercular cortex of the squirrel monkey (Saimiri sciureus). Anat. Rec. *169*, 318 (1971)
365. Fourier, J.B.J.: Theorie du Mouvement de la Chaleur dans les Corps Solides. Mém. Acad. Sci. Inst. France *4*, 185-525 (1824)
366. Freeman, J.A.: Responses of cat cerebellar Purkinje cells to convergent inputs from cerebellar cortex and peripheral sensory system. J. Neurophysiol. *33*, 697-712 (1970)
367. Friedman, D., Simson, R., Ritter, W. and Rapin, I.: Cortical evoked potentials elicited by real speech words and human sounds. Electroenceph. clin. Neurophysiol. *38*, 13-19 (1975)
368. Frishkopf, L.S.: Excitation and inhibition of primary auditory neurones in the little brown bat. J. Acoust. Soc. Amer. *36*, 1016 A (1964)
369. Frishkopf, L.S. and Goldstein, M.H.: Responses to acoustic stimuli from units in the eighth nerve of the bullfrog. J. Acoust. Soc. Amer. *35*, 1219-1228 (1963)
370. Fromm, B., Nylen, C.O. and Zotterman, Y.: Studies in the mechanisms of the Wever and Bray effect. Acta Otolaryng. *22*, 477-486 (1935)
371. Fruhstorfer, H.: Habituation and dishabituation of the human vertex response. Electroenceph. Clin. Neurophysiol. *30*, 306-312 (1971)
372. Fruhstorfer, H. and Bergström, R.M.: Human vigilance and auditory evoked responses. Electroencephl. Clin. Neurophysiol. *27*, 346-355 (1969)
373. Fujisaki, H., Nakamura, K. and Imoto, T.: Auditory Perception of Duration of Speech and Non-Speech Stimuli. In: Auditory Analysis and Perception of Speech. Eds.: Fant, G. and Tatham, M.A.A. Academic Press, London 1975
374. Funkenstein, H.H. and Winter, P.: Responses to Acoustic Stimuli of Units in the Auditory Cortex of Awake Squirrel Monkeys. Exp. Brain Res. *18*, 464-488 (1973)
375. Funkenstein, H.H., Nelson, P.G., Winter, P., Wollberg, Z. and Newman, J.D.: Unit responses in auditory cortex of awake squirrel monkeys to vocal stimulation. In: Physiology of the Auditory System. Ed.: Sachs, M.B. National Educational Consultants, Inc., Baltimore/Maryland 1971
376. Fuortes, M.G.F.: Generation of Responses in Receptor. In: Principles of Receptor Physiology. Ed.: Loewenstein, W.R. Springer-Verlag, Berlin-Heidelberg-New York 1971

377. Fuortes, M.G.F., Frank, K. and Becker, M.C.: Steps in the Production of Motoneuron Spikes. J. gen. Physiol. *40*, 735-752 (1957)

378. Furman, G.G. and Frishkopf, L.S.: Model of neural inhibition in mammalian cochlea. J. Acoust. Soc. Amer. *36*, 2194-2201 (1964)

379. Furukawa, T. and Ishii, Y.: Neurophysiological studies on hearing in goldfish. J. Neurophysiol. *30*, 1377-1403 (1967)

380. Gacek, R.R.: Neuroanatomy of the Auditory System. In: Foundations of Modern Auditory Theory, Vol. II. Ed.: Tobias, J.V. Academic Press, New York and London 1972

381. Gacek, R.R. and Rasmussen, G.L.: Fiber analysis of the statoacoustic nerve of the guinea pig, cat, and monkey. Anat. Rec. *139*, 455-463 (1961)

382. Galaburda, A. and Sanides, F.: Cytoarchitectonic Organization of the Human Auditory Cortex. J. Comp. Neurol. *190*, 597-610 (1980)

383. Galambos, R.: Microelectrode studies on medial geniculate body of cat. III. Response to pure tones. J. Neurophysiol. *15*, 381-400 (1952)

384. Galambos, R.: Suppression of auditory nerve activity by stimulation of efferent fibers to cochlea. J. Neurophysiol. *19*, 424-437 (1956)

385. Galambos, R.: Electrical correlates of conditioned learning. In: The Central Nervous System and Behavior. Ed.: Brazier, M.A.B., Macy, New York 1958

386. Galambos, R. and Davis, H.: The response of single auditory nerve fibres to acoustic stimulation. J. Neurophysiol. *6*, 39-57 (1943)

387. Galambos, R., Rose, J.E., Bromiley, R.B. and Hughes, J.R.: Microelectrode studies on medial geniculate body of cat. II. Response to clicks. J. Neurophysiol. *15*, 359-380 (1952)

388. Galambos, R., Schwarztkopff, J., and Rupert, A. Microelectrode study of superior olivary nuclei. Amer. J. Physiol. *197*, 527-536 (1959)

389. Gannon, R.P., Eldredge, D.H., Smith, C.A. and Davis, H.: DC potentials in the semicircular canals. Physiologist *1*, 26-27 (1958)

390. Geisler, C.D.: Mathematical Models of the Mechanics of the Inner Ear. In: Auditory System. Handbook of Sensor Physiology, Volume V/3 Eds.: Keidel, W.D. and Neff, W.D. Springer-Verlag, Berlin-Heidelberg-New York 1976

391. Geisler, C.D. and Hubbard, A.E.: A hybrid-computer model of the cochlea. In: Physiology of the Auditory System. Ed.: Sachs, M.B. National Educational Consultants, Inc, Baltimore/Maryland 1971

392. Geisler, C.D., Rhode, W.S. and Hazelton, D.W.: Responses of inferior colliculus neurons in the cat to binaural acoustic stimuli having wide-band spectra. J. Neurophysiol. *32*, 960-974 (1969)

393. Geniec, P. and Morest, D.K.: The neuronal architecture of the human posterior colliculus: a study with the Golgi method. Acta oto-laryng. (Stockh.) Suppl. *295*, 1-33 (1971)

394. Gerin, P., Morgon, A., Charachon, D., Munier, F., Pernier, J., Arnal, D. et Lebreton, M.F.: Une methode d'audiometrie objective - l'audiometrie electroencephalographique. J. franc. Oto-rhino-laryng. *17*, 547-595 (1968)

395. Gernandt, B.: Midbrain activity in response to vestibular stimulation. Acta physiol. scand. *21*, 73-81 (1950)

396. Gerstein, G.L. and Kiang, N.Y.-S.: Responses of single units in the auditory cortex. Exp. Neurol. *10*, 1-18 (1964)

397. Gerstein, G.L., Butler, R.A. and Erulkar, S.D.: Excitation and inhibition in cochlear nucleus. I. Tone-burst stimulation. J. Neurophysiol. *31*, 526-536 (1968)

398. Gestring, G.F., Burian, K. and Innitzer, J.: Computer sweep-splitting for simultaneous ECOG and ERA display. IIIrd Symposium of the International Electric Response Audiometry Study Group in Bordeaux, 10.-12.9. 1973

399. van Gisbergen, J.A.M., Grashuis, J.L., Johannesma, P.I.M. and Vendrik, A.J.H.: Neurons in the Cochlear Nucleus Investigated with Tone and Noise Stimuli. Exp. Brain Res. *23*, 387-406 (1975)

400. Gisselsson, L., Sørensen, H.: Auditory adaptation and fatigue in cochlear potentials. Acta otolaryng. (Stockh.) *50*, 391-405 (1959)

401. Glasscock, E., Jackson, C.G. and Josey, A.F.: Brain Stem Electric Response Audiometry. Thieme-Stratton Inc., New York 1981
402. Goblick, T.J.Jr. and Pfeiffer, R.R.: Time domain measurements in cochlear nonlinearities using combination click stimuli. J. Acoust. Soc. Amer. *46*, 924-938 (1969)
403. Godfrey, D.A., Kiang, N.Y.-S. and Norris, B.E.: Single Unit Activity in the Dorsal Cochlear Nucleus of the Cat. J. comp. Neur. *162*, 269-284 (1975)
404. Godfrey, D.A., Kiang, N.Y.-S. and Norris, B.E.: Single Unit Activity in the Posteroventral Cochlear Nucleus of the Cat. J. comp. Neur. *162*, 247-268 (1975)
405. Godfrey, D.A., Williams, A.D., Matschinsky, F.M.: Quantitative histochemical mapping of enzymes of the cholinergic system in cat cochlear nucleus. J. Histochem. Cytochem. *25*, 397-416 (1977)
406. Godfrey, D.A., Carter, J.A., Berger, S.J., Lowry, O.H. and Matschinsky, F.M.: Quantitative histochemical mapping of candidate transmitter amino acids in cat cochlear nucleus. J. Histochem. Cytochem. *25*, 417-431 (1977)
407. Godfrey, D.A., Carter, J.A., Lowry, O.H. and Matschinsky, F.M.: Distribution of gamma-aminobutyric acid, glycine, glutamate and aspartate in the cochlear nucleus of the rat. J. Histochem. Cytochem. *26*, 118-126 (1978)
408. Goldberg, J.M.: Physiological Studies of Auditory Nuclei of the Pons. In: Auditory System. Handbook of Sensory Physiology, Volume V/2 Eds.: Keidel, W.D. and Neff, W.D. Springer-Verlag, Berlin-Heidelberg-New York 1975
409. Goldberg, J.M. and Neff, W.D.: Frequency discrimination after bilateral section of the brachium of the inferior colliculus. J. comp. Neurol. *116* 265-290 (1961)
410. Goldberg, J.M. and Neff, W.D.: Frequency discrimination after bilateral ablation of cortical auditory areas. J. Neurophysiol. *24*, 119-128 (1961)
411. Goldberg, J.M. and Greenwood, D.D.: Response of neurons of the dorsal and posteroventral cochlear nuclei of the cat to acoustic stimuli of long duration. J. Neurophysiol. *29*, 72-93 (1966)
412. Goldberg, J.M. and Moore, R.Y.: Ascending projections of the lateral lemniscus in the cat and the monkey. J. Comp. Neurol. *129*, 143-155 (1967)
413. Goldberg, J.M. and Brown, P.B.: Functional organization of the dog superior olivary complex: An anatomical and electrophysiological study. J. Neurophysiol. *31*, 639-656 (1968)
414. Goldberg, J.M. and Brown, P.B.: Response of binaural neurons of dog superior olivary complex to dicotic tonal stimuli: some physiological mechanisms of sound localization. J. Neurophysiol. *32*, 613-636 (1969)
415. Goldberg, J.M. and Brownell, W.E.: Discharge characteristics of neurons in anteroventral and dorsal cochlear nuclei of cat. Brain Res. *64*, 35-64 (1973)
416. Goldberg, J.M., Smith, F.D. and Adrian, H.O.: Response of single units of the superior olivary complex of the cat to acoustic stimuli: laterality of afferent projections. Anat. Rec. *145*, 232 (1963)
417. Goldberg, J.M., Adrian, H.O. and Smith, F.D.: Response of neurons of the superior olivary complex of the cat to acoustic stimuli of long duration. J. Neurophysiol. *27*, 706-749 (1964)
418. Goldberg, J.M., Brownell, W.E. and Lavine, R.A.: Discharge characteristics of single units of the anteroventral and dorsal cochlear nuclei. In: Physiology of the Auditory System. Ed.: Sachs, M.B. National Educational Consultants, Inc., Baltimore/Maryland 1971
419. Goldstein, J.L.: Aural Combination Tones. In: Frequency Analysis and Periodicity Detection in Hearing. Eds.: Plomp, R. and Smoorenburg, G.F. A.W. Sijthoff, Leiden 1970
420. Goldstein, J.L. and Kiang, N.Y.-S. Neural correlates of the aural combination tone 2f1-f2. Proc. IEEE *56*, 981-992 (1968)
421. Goldstein, M.H.Jr. and Abeles, M.: Single Unit Activity of the Auditory Cortex. In: Auditory System. Handbook of Sensory Physiology, Vol. V/2. Eds.: Keidel, W.D. and Neff, W.D. Springer-Verlag, Berlin-Heidelberg-New York 1975
422. Goldstein, M.H.Jr., Hall, J.L. II and Butterfield, B.O.: Single-unit activity in the

primary auditory cortex of unanesthetized cats. J. Acoust. Soc. Amer. *43*, 444-455 (1968)

423. Goldstein, M.H.Jr., Abeles, M., Daly, R.L. and McIntosh, J.: Functional architecture in cat primary auditory cortex: Tonotopic organization. J. Neurophysiol. *33*, 188-197 (1970)

424. Goldstein, M.H.Jr., de Ribaupierre, R. and Yeni-Komshian, G.H.: Cortical coding of periodicity pitch. In: Physiology of the Auditory System. Ed.: Sachs, M.B. National Educational Consultants, Inc., Baltimore/Maryland 1971

425. Green, D.M. and Yost, W.A.: Binaural Analysis. In: Auditory System. Handbook of Sensory Physiology, Vol. V/2. Eds.: Keidel, W.D. and Neff, W.D. Springer-Verlag, Berlin-Heidelberg-New York 1975

426. Greenwood, D.D. and Maruyama, N.: Excitatory inhibitory response areas of auditory neurons in the cochlear nucleus. J. Neurophysiol. *28*, 863-892 (1965)

427. Grinnell, A.D.: The neurophysiology of audition in bats: intensity and frequency parameters. J. Physiol. *167*, 38-66 (1963)

428. Grinnell, A.D.: The neurophysiology of audition in bats: temporal parameters. J. Physiol. *167*, 67-96 (1963)

429. Grinnell, A.D.: The neurophysiology of audition in bats: directional localization and binaural interaction. J. Physiol. *167*, 97-113 (1963)

430. Groen, J.J.: The value of the Weber test. In: Internat. Symp. on Otosclerosis. Ed.: Schuknecht, H. Little Brown, Boston 1962

431. Gross, N.B. and Anderson, D.J.: Single unit responses recorded from the first order neuron of the pigeon auditory system. Brain Res. *101*, 209-222 (1976)

432. Gross, N.B., Lifschitz, W.S. and Anderson, D.J.: The tonotopic organization of the auditory thalamus of the squirrel monkey (Saimiri sciureus). Brain Res. *65*, 323-332 (1974)

433. Grundfest, H.: Electrical inexcitability of synapses and some of its consequences in the central nervous system. Physiol. Rev. *37*, 337-361 (1957)

434. Grundfest, H.: Electrophysiology and pharmacology of different components of bioelectric transducers. Cold Spr. Harb. Symp. quant. Biol. *30*, 1-14 (1965)

435. Grundfest, H.: The General Electrophysiology of Input Membrane in Electrogenic Excitable Cells. In: Principles of Receptor Physiology. Handbook of Sensory Physiology, Vol. I. Ed.: Loewenstein, W.R. Springer-Verlag, Berlin-Heidelberg-New York 1971

436. Guild, S.R.: Correlations of the histological observations and the acuity of hearing. Acta Oto-Laryngol. *17*, 207-249 (1932)

437. Guinan, J.J.Jr.: Firing patterns and locations of single auditory neurons in the brainstem (Superior olivary complex) of anesthetized cats. Sc.D. Thesis, Mass. Inst. Technol. 1968

438. Guinan, J.J.Jr., Norris, B.E. and Guinan, S.S.: Single auditory units in the superior olivary complex II: Locations of unit categories and tonotopic organization. Int.J.Neurosci. *4*, 147-166 (1972)

439. Gulick, W.L.: Hearing. Physiology and Psychophysics. Oxford University Press, New York-London-Toronto 1971

440. Gulley, R.L., Landis, D.M.D. and Reese, T.S.: Internal Organization of Membranes at End Bulbs of Held in the Anteroventral Cochlear Nucleus. J. comp. Neurol. *180*, 707-742 (1948)

441. Hafter, E.R. and Jeffress, L.A.: Two-image lateralization of tones and clicks. J. Acoust. Soc. Amer. *44*, 563-569 (1968)

442. Hafter, E.R. and De Maio, J.: Difference thresholds for interaural delay. J. Acoust. Soc. Amer. *57*, 181-187 (1975)

443. Hall, J.G.: Hearing and Primary Auditory Centers of the Whales. Acta Oto-Laryngol. Suppl. *224*, 244-250 (1967)

444. Hall, J.L. II: Binaural interaction in the accessory superior-olivary nucleus of the cat. J. Acoust. Soc. Amer. *37*, 814-823 (1965)

445. Hall, J.L.: Two-tone distortion products in a nonlinear model of the basilar membrane. J. Acoust. Soc. Amer. *56*, 1818-1828 (1974)

446. Hall, J.L. II and Goldstein, M.H. Jr.: Representation of binaural stimuli by single units in primary auditory cortex of unanesthetized cats. J. Acoust. Soc. Amer. *43*, 456-461 (1968)
447. Hall, R.D.: Habituation of evoked potentials in the rat under conditions of behavioral control. Electroenceph. clin. Neurophysiol. *24*, 155-165 (1968)
448. Hansson, E., Jarlstedt, J. and Sellstrom, A.: Sound-stimulated C-glutamate release from the nucleus cochlearis. Experientia *36*, 576-577 (1980)
449. Harris, G.G. and Milne, D.C.: Input-output characteristics of the lateral-line organs of Xenopus laevis. J. Acoust. Soc. Amer. *40*, 32-42 (1966)
450. Harris, G.G., Flanagan, J.L. and Watson, B.J.: Binaural interaction of a click with a click pair. J. Acoust. Soc. Amer. *35*, 672-678 (1963)
451. Harris, G.G., Frishkopf, L. and Flock, Å.: Receptor potentials in the hair cells of mudpuppy lateral line. J. Acoust. Soc. Amer. *45*, 300-301 (1969)
452. Harris, G.G., Frishkopf, L. and Flock, Å.: Receptor potentials from hair cells of the lateral line. Science *167*, 76-79 (1970)
453. Harris, J.D.: Pitch discrimination. J. Acoust. Soc. Amer. *24*, 750-755 (1952)
454. Harrison, J.M. and Irving, R.: Nucleus of the trapezoid body: Dual afferent innervation. Science *143*, 473-474 (1964)
455. Harrison, J.M. and Irving, R.: The anterior ventral . Amer. *24*, 750-755 (1952)
456. Harrison, J.M. and Irving, R.: Organization of the posterior ventral cochlear nucleus in the rat. J. comp. Neurol. *126*, 391-403 (1966)
457. Harrison, J.M. and Irving, R.: Visual and non-visual auditory systems in mammals. Science *154*, 738-742 (1966)
458. Harrison, J.M. and Irving, R.: Ascending connections of the anterior ventral cochlear nucleus in the rat. J. comp. Neurol. *126*, 51-64 (1966)
459. Harrison, J.M. and Feldman, M.L.: Anatomical aspects of the cochlear nucleus and superior olivary complex. In: Contributions to Sensory Physiology, Vol. 4. Ed.: Neff, W.D. Academic Press, New York 1970
460. Harrison, J.M. and Howe, M.E.: Anatomy of the Afferent Auditory Nervous System of Mammals. In: Auditory System. Handbook of Sensory Physiology, Vol. V/1. Eds.: Keidel, W.D. and Neff, W.D. Springer-Verlag, Berlin-Heidelberg-New York 1974
461. Harrison, J.M. and Warr, B.: The cochlear nucleus and ascending auditory pathways of the medulla. J. comp. Neurol. *119*, 341-380 (1962)
462. Hawkins, J.E.jr.: Cochlear signs of streptomycin intoxication. J. Pharmacol. & Exper. Therap. *100*, 38-44 (1950)
463. Hawkins, J.E.jr.: The Ototoxicity of Hydrostreptomycin. Streptom. Conf. Fulton County, Med. Soc., Atlanta Georgia 1951
464. Hawkins, J.E.jr.: Antibiotics and the inner ear. Trans. Am. Acad. Ophthal. Otolaryng., Rochester 1959
465. Hawkins, J.E.jr.: Ototoxicity of Kanamycin. Ann. Otol. Rhinol. Laryngol. *68*, 698-715 (1959)
466. Hawkins, J.E.jr.: Comparative otopathology: aging, noise and ototoxic drugs. Advanc. Oto-rhino-laryng. *20*, 125-141 (1973)
467. Hawkins, J.E.jr.: Ototoxic mechanisms: a working hypothesis. Audiology *12*, 383-393 (1973)
468. Hawkins, J.E.jr.: Drug Ototoxicity. In: Auditory System. Handbook of Sensory Physiology, Vol. V/3. Eds.: Keidel, W.D. and Neff, W.D. Springer-Verlag, Berlin-Heidelberg-New York 1976
469. Hawkins, J.E.jr. and Urie, M.H.: The ototoxicity of streptomycin. Ann. Otol. Rhin. & Laryng. *61*, 789-809 (1952)
470. Hawkins, J.E.jr. and Engström, H.: Effect of kanamycin on cochlear cytoarchitecture. Acta oto-laryng. (Stockhl.) Suppl. *188*, 100-106 (1964)
471. Heath, C.J. and Jones, E.G.: An experimental study of ascending connections from posterior group of thalamic nuclei in the cat. J. comp. Neurol. *141*, 397-426 (1971)
472. Heffner, H.: Effect of Auditory Cortex Ablation on Localization and Discrimination of Brief Sounds. J. Neurophysiol. *41*, 963-976 (1978)

473. Heffner, H. and Masterton, B.: Contribution of Auditory Cortex to Sound Localization in the Monkey (Macaca mulatta). J. Neurophysiol. *38*, 1340-1358 (1975)
474. Heffner, H. and Whitfield, I.C.: Perception of the missing fundamental by cats. J. Acoust. Soc. Amer. *59*, 915-919 (1976)
475. Held, H.: Die centrale Gehörleitung. Arch. Anat. Physiol. anat. Abt. 201-248 (1893)
476. Held, H.: Die Cochlea der Säuger and der Vögel, ihre Entwicklung und ihr Bau. In: Handbuch der normalen und pathologischen Physiologie. Band 11: Receptionsorgane I. Hrsg.: Bethe, A., v. Bergmann, G., Embden, G. und Ellinger, A. Verlag von Julius Springer, Berlin 1926
477. Helle, R.: Selektivitätssteigerung in einem hydromechanischen Innenohrmodell mit Basilar- und Deckmembran. Acoustica *30*, 301-312 (1974)
478. Helle, R.: Enlarged hydromechansponses of the cerebellar vermis to binaural auditory stimulation. Brain Res. *10*, 470-473 (1968)
479. v. Helmholtz, H.L.F.: Über physikalische Ursache der Harmonie und Disharmonie. Gesellsch. dtsch.Naturf.u.Aerzte, Amtl. Ber. *34*, 157 (1859)
480. v. Helmholtz, H.L.F.: Die Lehre von den Tonempfindungen als physiologische Grundlage für die Theorie der Musik. F. Vieweg & Sohn, Braunschweig 1863
481. Herzog, H.: Das Knochenleitungsproblem. Theoretische Erwägungen. Z. Hals-Nasen-Ohrenheilkunde *15*, 300-306 (1926)
482. Highstein, S. Coleman, P.D.: Responses of the cerebellar vermis to binaural auditory stimulation. Brain Res. *10*, 470-473 (1968)
483. Hilding, A.C.: Studies on the otic labyrinth. I. On the origin and insertion of the tectorial membrane. Ann.Otol.Rhinol.Laryngol. *61*, 354-370 (1952)
484. Hind, J.E., Rose, J.E., Davies, P.W., Woolsey, C.N., Benjamin, R.M., Welker, W.I. and Thompson, R.F.: Unit activity in the auditory cortex. In: Neural mechanisms of the auditory and vestibular systems. Eds.: Rasmussen, G.L. and Windle, W., Charles C. Thomas, Springfield/Ill. 1960
485. Hind, J.E., Goldberg, J.M., Greenwood, D.D. and Rose, J.E.: Some discharge characteristics of single neurons in the inferior colliculus of the cat. II. Timing of the discharge and observations on binaural stimulation. J. Neurophysiol. *26*, 321-341 (1963)
486. Hind, J.E., Anderson, D.J., Brugge, J.F. and Rose, J.E.: Coding of information pertaining to paired low-frequency tones in single auditory nerve fibers of the squirrel monkey. J. Neurophysiol. *30*, 794-816 (1967)
487. Hind, J.E., Rose, J.E., Brugge, J.F. and Anderson, D.J.: Two tone masking effects in squirrel monkey auditory nerve fibers. In: Frequency Analysis and Periodicity Detection in Hearing. Eds.: Plomp, R. and Smoorenburg, G.F. A.W. Sijthoff, Leiden 1970
488. Hind, J.E., Rose, J.E., Brugge, J.F. and Anderson, D.J.: Some effects of intensity on the discharge of auditory-nerve fibers. In: Physiology of the Auditory System. Ed.: Sachs, M.B., National Educational Consultants, Inc., Baltimore/Maryland USA 1971
489. Hocherman, S., Benson, D.A., Goldstein, M.H.jr., Heffner, H.E. and Hienz, R.D.: Evoked unit activity in auditory cortex of monkeys performing a selective attention task. Brain. Res. *117*, 51-68 (1976)
490. Hodgkin, A.L. and Huxley, A.F.: A quantitative description of membrane current and its application to conduction and excitation in nerve. J. Physiol. (Lond.) *117*, 500-544 (1952)
491. Hoke, M.: Über den Nachweis der Mikrofonpotentiale beim Menschen. Methodik-Ergebnisse-Bedeutung. Habilitationsschrift, Münster 1972
492. Hoke, M., Landwehr, F.J. and Lerche, E.: Über die Nichtlinearitat der Innenohrmechanik. Arch. klin. exp. Ohr.-, Nas- u. Kehlkopfheilk. *191*, 577-581 (1968)
493. Holstein, S.B., Buchwald, J.S. and Schwafel, J.A.: Tone response of the auditory nuclei during normal wakefulness, paralysis and anesthesia. Brain Res. *15*, 483-499 (1969)
494. Holstein, S.B., Buchwald, J.S. and Schwafel, J.A.: Progressive changes in auditory

response patterns to repeated tone during normal wakefulness and paralysis. Brain Res. *16*, 133-148 (1969)

495. Honrubia, V. and Ward, P.H.: Longitudinal distributions of the cochlear microphonics inside the cochlear duct (guinea pig). J. Acoust. Soc. Amer. *44*, 951-958 (1968)

496. Honrubia, V. and Ward, P.H.: Temporal and spatial distribution of the CM and SP of the cochlea. In: Frequency Analysis and Periodicity Detection in Hearing. Eds.: Plomp, R. and Smoorenburg, G.F., A.W. Sijthoff, Leiden 1970

497. Honrubia, V. Strelioff, D., Sitko, S.T.: Physiological basis of cochlear transduction and sensitivity. Ann.Otol. Rhinol. Laryngol. *85*, 697-710 (1976)

498. Horenstein, S. and Yamamoto, T.: The relationship of the feline temporal cortex to the medial geniculate body. 5. Meeting of the Neuroscience Society, New York 1975

499. Hoshino, T.: Relationship of the tectorial membrane to the organ of Corti. A scanning electron microscope study of cats and guinea pigs. Arch. Histol. Jap. *37*, 25-39 (1974).

500. Hoshino, T.: Attachment of the inner sensory cell hairs to the tectorial membrane: A scanning electron microscopic study. ORL *38*, 11-18 (1976)

501. Hoshino, T.: Contact between the tectorial membrane and the cochlear sensory hairs in the human and the monkey. Arch. Oto-Rhino-Laryng. *217*, 53-60 (1977)

502. Hubbard, A.E. and Geisler, C.D.: A hybrid computer model of the cochlear partition. J. Acoust. Soc.Amer. *51*, 1885-1894 (1972)

503. Hubel, D.H. and Wiesel, T.N.: Receptive fields, binocular interaction and functional architecture in the cat's visual cortex. J. Physiol. (Lond.) *160*, 106-154 (1962)

504. Huggins, A.W.F.: The Perception of Timing in Natural Speech I: Compensation Within the Syllable. Language and Speech *11*, 1-11 (1968)

505. Huggins, A.W.F.: How Accurately Must a Speaker Time His Articulations? IEEE Tran.Audio and Electroacoustics, *AU-16*, 112-117 (1968)

506. Huggins, A.W.F.: Just Noticeable Differences for Segment Duration in Natural Speech. J. Acoust. Soc. Amer. *51*, 1270-1278 (1972)

507. Huggins, A.W.F.: On the Perception of Temporal Phenomena in Speech. J. Acoust. Soc. Amer. *51*, 1279-1290 (1972)

508. Hui, G.S. and Disterhoft, J.F.: Cochlear Nucleus Unit Responses to Pure Tones in the Unanesthetized Rabbit. Exp. Neurol. *69*, 576-588 (1980)

509. Imig, T.J. and Reale, R.A.: Patterns of Cortico-cortical Connections Related to Tonotopic Maps in Cat Auditory Cortex. J. Comp. Neurol. *192*, 293-332 (1980)

510. Inselberg, A. and von Foerster, H.: A mathematical model of the basilar membrane. Math. Biosciences *7*, 341-363 (1970)

511. Irvine, D.R.F., H. Huebner: Acoustic Response Characteristics of Neurons in Nonspecific Areas of Cat Cerebral Cortex. J. Neurophysiol. *42*, 107-122 (1979)

512. Irving, R. and Harrison, J.M.: Superior olivary complex and audition: A comparative study. J. Comp. Neurol. *130*, 77-86 (1967)

513. Ishii, Y., Matsura, S. and Furukawa, T.: Quantal nature of transmission at the synapse between hair cells and eighth nerve fibers. Japan.J. Physiol. *21*, 79-89 (1971)

514. Ishii, Y., Matsuura, S. and Furukawa, T.: An input-output relation at the synapse between hair cells and eighth nerve fibers in goldfish. Japan.J.Physiol. *21*, 91-98 (1971)

515. Iurato, S.: Efferent fibers to the sensory cells of Corti's organ. Exp. Cell. Res. *27*, 162-164 (1962)

516. Iurato, S.: Fibre efferenti dirette e crociate alle cellule acustiche dell'organo del Corti. Monit.Zool.It. Suppl. *72*, 62-63 (1964)

517. Iurato, S.: Submicroscopic structure of the inner ear. Pergamon Press, London 1967

518. Jaffe, S.L., Bourlier, P.F. and Hagamen, W.D.: Adaptation of evoked auditory potentials: A midbrain through frontal lobe map in the unanesthetized cat. Brain Res. *15*, 121-136 (1969)

519. Jeffress, L.A.: Localization of Sound. In: Auditory Handbook of Sensory Physiology, Vol. V/2. Eds.: Keidel, W.D. and Neff, W.D. Springer-Verlag, Berlin-Heidelberg-New York 1975

520. Jielof, R., Spoor, A. and de Fries, H.: The microphonic activity of the lateral line. J. Physiol. *116*, 137-157 (1952)

521. Johannsen, H.S., Keidel, W.D. und Spreng, M.: Der Einfluß von Intensität und Dauer der Beschallung auf den Off-Effekt des akustisch evozierten Potentials. Arch.klin.exp.Ohr.-,Nas.- u.Kehlk.Heilk. *201*, 208-221 (1972)

522. Johnstone, B.M. and Boyle, A.J.F.: Basilar membrane vibration examined with the Mössbauer technique. Science *158*, 389-390 (1967)

523. Johnstone, B.M. and Taylor, K.J.: Mechanical aspects of cochlear function. In: Frequency Analysis and Periodicity Detection in Hearing. Eds.: Plomp, R. and Smoorenburg, C.F. A.W. Sijthoff. Leiden 1970

524. Johnstone, B.M., Taylor, K.J. and Boyle, A.: Mechanics of the guinea pig cochlea. J. Acoust. Soc. Amer. *47*, 504-509 (1970)

525. Johnstone, B.M. and Taylor, K.J.: Physiology of the middle ear transmission system. J. Oto-Laryngol. Soc. Aust. *3*, 226-228 (1971)

526. Johnstone, B.M. and Yates, G.K.: Basilar membrane tuning curves in the guinea pig. J.Acoust.Soc.Amer. *55*, 584-587 (1974)

527. Johnstone, J.R. and Johnstone, B.M.: Origin of summating potential. J.Acoust. Soc.Amer. *40*, 1405-1413 (1966)

528. Jones, D.R. and Casseday, J.H.: Projections of auditory nerve in the cat as seen by anterograde transport methods. Neuroscience *4*, 1299-1313 (1979)

529. Jones, E.C. and Powell, T.P.S.: An anatomical study of converging sensory pathways within the cerebral cortex of the monkey. Brain *93*, 793-820 (1970)

530. Jones, E.C. and Rockel, A.J.: The synaptic organization in the medial geniculate body of afferent fibres ascending from inferior colliculus. Zeitschr.f.Zellf. *113*, 44-66 (1971)

531. Jürgens, U. and Ploog, D.: Cerebral representation of vocalization in the squirrel monkey. Exp. Brain Res. *10*, 532-554 (1970)

532. Kallert, S.: Über die Reizantwort einzelner Zellen im Corpus geniculatum mediale der Katze bei Untersuchung mit Mikroelektroden. Dissertation, Erlangen 1972

533. Kallert, S.: Periodizitäten bei der zentralnervösen Informationsverarbeitung. In: Mechanismen und Bedeutung schwingender Systeme. Hrsg.: Rensing, K. und Birukow, G., Vandenhoeck & Ruprecht, Göttingen 1972

534. Kallert, S.: Telemetrische Mikroelektrodenuntersuchungen am Corpus geniculatum mediale der wachen Katze. Habilitationsschrift, Erlangen 1974

535. Kallert, S.: Einzelzellverhalten in den verschiedenen Hörbahnteilen. In: Physiologie des Gehörs. Hrsg.: Keidel, W.D. Georg Thieme Verlag, Stuttgart 1975

536. Kallert, S. und Kroha, E.: Reversible Kälteblockade der primären Hörrinde bei der wachen Katze. Naturwissenschaften *65*, 211 (1978)

537. Kallert, S. und Wünsche, B.: Einfluß reversibler Kälteblockade der primären Hörrinde auf die Erkennung von zeitabhängigen Schallreizmustern. Naturwissenschaften *69*, 97-99 (1982)

538. Kallert, S., David, E., Finkenzeller, P. and Keidel, W.D.: Two different neuronal discharge periodicities in the acoustical channel. In: Frequency Analysis and Periodicity Detection in Hearing. Eds.: Plomp, R. and Smoorenburg, G.F. A.W. Sijthoff, Leiden 1970

539. Kane, E.C.: Synaptic Organization in the Dorsal Cochlear Nucleus of the Cat: A Light and Electron Microscopic Study. J. Comp. Neurol. *155*, 301-330 (1974)

540. Kane, E.S.: Primary afferents and the cochlear nucleus. In: Evoked electrical activity in the auditory nervous system. Eds.: Naunton, R.F., Fernández, C., Academic Press, New York 1978

541. Kane, E.S. and Barone, L.M.: The Dorsal Nucleus of the Lateral Lemniscus in the Cat: Neuronal Types and Their Distributions. J. Comp. Neurol. *192*, 797-826 (1980)

542. Kaneko, A. and Hashimoto, H.: Recording site of the single cone response determined by an electrode marking technique. Vision Res. *7*, 847-851 (1967)

543. Karlan, M.S., Tonndorf, J. and Khanna, S.M.: Cochlear microphonic, the resultant of two separate sets of generators. J. Acoust. Soc. Amer. *51*, 104 (A) (1972)

544. Katsuki, Y.: Integrative organization in the thalamic and cortical auditory centers.

In: The Thalamus. Eds.: Purpura, D.P. and Yahr, M.D., Columbia University Press, New York 1966

545. Katsuki, Y., Sumi, T., Uchiyama, H. and Watanabe, T.: Electric responses of auditory neurons in cat to sound stimulation J. Neurophysiol. *21*, 569-588 (1958)

546. Katsuki, Y. Watanabe, T. and Suga, N.: Interaction of auditory neurons in response to two sound stimuli in cat. J. Neurophysiol. *22*, 603-623 (1959)

547. Katsuki, Y., Watanabe, T. and Maruyama, N.: Activity of auditory neurons in upper levels of brain of cat. J. Neurophysiol. *22*, 343-359 (1959)

548. Katsuki, Y., Kanno, Y., Suga, N. and Mannen, M.: Primary auditory neurons of monkey. Jap. J. Physiol. *11*, 678-683 (1961)

549. Katsuki, Y., Suga, N. and Kanno, Y.: Neural mechanism of the peripheral and central auditory system in monkeys. J. Acoust. Soc. Amer. *34*, 1396-1410 (1962)

550. Katz, B. and Miledi, R.: A study of synaptic transmission in the absence of nerve impulses. J. Physiol. (Lond.) *192*, 407-436 (1967)

551. Kay, R.H.: The Physiology of Auditory Frequency Analysis. In: Progress in Biophysics and Molecular Biology, Vol. 28. Eds.: Butler, J.A.V. and Noble, D., Pergamon Press, Oxford-New York-Toronto-Sydney-Braunschweig 1974.

552. Keidel, W.D.: Aktionspotentiale des N. dorsocutaneous bei niederfrequenter Vibration der Froschrückenhaut. Pflügers Arch. ges. Physiol. *260*, 416-436 (1955)

553. Keidel, W.D.: Vibrationsreception. Der Erschütterungssinn des Menschen. Erlanger Forschungen Bd. 2, Reihe B: Naturwissenschaften, Universitätsbund Erlangen e.V., 1956

554. Keidel, W.D.: Periphere und corticale Komponenten der Adaptation bei Reizung des Ohres und der Haut der Katze mit Impulsfolgen. Pflügers Arch. ges. Physiol. *268*, 34-35 (1958)

555. Keidel, W.D.: Codierung, Signalleitung und Decodierung in der Sinnesphysiologie. In: Aufnahme und Verarbeitung von Nachrichten durch Organismen. Hrsg.: Nachrichtentechn. Gesellschaft im VDE-Fachausschuß "Informations- und System-theorie"; S. Hirzel Verlag, Stuttgart 1961

556. Keidel, W.D.: Otto F. Ranke. Ergebn. Physiol. , 21-37 (1961)

557. Keidel, W.D.: Rankes Adaptationstheorie. Z. Biol. *112*, 411-425 (1961)

558. Keidel, W.D.: Grundprinzipien der akustischen und taktilen Informationsverar-beitung. Ergebn. Biol. *24*, 213-246 (1961)

559. Keidel, W.D.: Elektronisch gemittelte langsame Rindenpotentiale des Menschen bei akustischer Reizung. Collegium ORLAS in Athen, 16.-21.9. 1962

560. Keidel, W.D.: Physiologie der Hautsinne. In: Ergänzungswerk zum Handbuch der Haut- und Geschlechtskrankheiten, Bd. I/3 Hrsg.: Jadassohn, J., Springer-Verlag, Berlin-Heidelberg-Göttingen 1963

561. Keidel. W.D.: Kybernetische Systeme des menschlichen Organismus. Hrsg.: Ar-beitsgemeinschaft für Forschung des Landes Nordrhein/Westf., Westdeutscher Verlag, Köln und Opladen *118*, 31-71 (1963)

562. Keidel, W.D.: Tuning between central auditory pathways and the ear. IEEE Transactions on Military Electronics MIL-7, 131-143 (1963)

563. Keidel, W.D.: Rindenpotentiale beim Menschen und Hörvermögen. Tagung der Deutschen Audiologen in Bremen, 5.-8.3. 1964

564. Keidel, W.D.: Audiometric aspects and multisensory power functions of electroni-cally averaged slow evoked cortical responses in man. Tagung des Collegium ORLAS. Wurzburg, 30.8.-3.9. 1964

565. Keidel, W.D.: Objective audiometry in man. 7th International Congress of Audiology in Copenhagen, 25.-28.8. 1964

566. Keidel, W.D.: Biophysical aspects of auditory information processing. International Biophysics Meeting at Paris, June 1964

567. Keidel, W.D.: Kybernetische Leistungen des menschlichen Organismus. Elektro-techn. Z. *24*, 769-808 (1964)

568. Keidel, W.D.: Die Physiologie der Informationsverarbeitung. Pflügers Arch. ges. Physiol. *281*, 5-7 (1964)

569. Keidel, W.D.: Physiologie des Innenohres. In: Hals-Nasen-Ohren-Heilkunde. Ein

kurzgefaßtes Handbuch in drei Bänden. Band III/Teil 1. Hrsg.: Berendes, J., Link, R. und Zöllner, R., George Thieme Verlag, Stuttgart 1965

570. Keidel, W.D.: Neuere Ergebnisse der Physiologie des Hörens. Arch.Ohr.-,Nas.- u. Kehlk.Heilk. *185*, 548-575 (1965)

571. Keidel, W.D.: Objektive Audiometrie. Arbeitstagung Deutscher Audiologen in Erlangen am 9.-10.4. 1965

572. Keidel, W.D.: Das räumliche Hören. In: Handbuch der Psychologie in 12 Bd., Bd 1: Wahrnehmung und Bewußtsein. Hrsg.: Metzger, W., Verlag für Psychologie, Dr. C.J. Hogrefe, Göttingen 1966

573. Keidel, W.D.: Kurzgefaßtes Lehrbuch der Physiologie. Georg Thieme Verlag, Stuttgart 1967

574. Keidel, W.D.: Electrophysiology of vibratory perception. In: Contributions to Sensory Physiology, Vol. 3. Ed.: Neff, W.D. Academic Press, New York and London 1968

575. Keidel, W.D.: Informationsphysiologische Aspekte des Hörens. Studium Generale *22*, 49-82 (1969)

576. Keidel, W.D.: Neuere Ergebnisse der akustischen Informationsverarbeitung. Erg. Exp. Med. *3*, 167-193 (1969)

577. Keidel, W.D.: Biophysics, Mechanics and Electrophysiology of the Human Cochlea. In: Frequency Analysis and Periodicity Detection in Hearing. Eds.: Plomp, R. and Smoorenburg, G.F., A.W. Sijthoff, Leiden 1970

578. Keidel, W.D.: Der Mensch, ein kybernetisches Wesen. Naturwiss. Rundschau *23*, 401-409 (1970)

579. Keidel, W.D.: Optische und akustische Zeichenerkennung beim Menschen. Naturwiss. Rundschau *23*, 491-498 (1970)

580. Keidel, W.D.: Neuere Ergebnisse der akustischen Informationsverarbeitung. In: Ergebnisse der experimentellen Medizin, Band 3. Hrsg: Präsidium der Deutschen Gesellschaft für experimentelle Medizin. VEB Verlag Volk und Gesundheit, Berlin 1970

581. Keidel, W.D.: Kybernetische Deutung menschlichen Lebens. Festvortrag; gehalten am 7.5 1970 in Regensburg anläßlich der 44. Fortbildungstagung fur Ärzte.

582. Keidel, W.D.: Neuere Ergebnisse der akustischen Informationsverarbeitung. In: Forschungsbericht 1970 des I. Physiologischen Institutes Erlangen

583. Keidel, W.D.: The use of quick correlators in electro-cochleography both in oto-audiography (OAG) and in neuro-audiography (NAG). Revue de Laryngologie, Supplement 1971 Ed.: Portmann, G., Bordeaux

584. Keidel, W.D.: Sinnesphysiologie. Teil I: Allgemeine Sinnesphysiologie, Visuelles System. Heidelberger Taschenbücher, Band 97. Springer-Verlag, Berlin-Heidelberg-New York 1971

585. Keidel, W.D.: What Do We Know about the Human Cortical Evoked Potential after All? Arch.klin.exp.Ohr.-, Nas.- u.Kehlk.Heilk. *198*, 9-37 (1971)

586. Keidel, W.D.: Information processing in the higher parts of the auditory pathway. In: Proc. of the International Union of Physiological Sciences, Volume VIII: XXV International Congress, Munich 1971 Ed.: German Physiological Society, Munich 1971

587. Keidel, W.D.: Neuere Ergebnisse der akustischen Informationsverarbeitung. Naturwiss. Rundschau *24*, 461-471 (1971)

588. Keidel, W.D.: Physiologische Grundlagen zum Bild des Menschen. (Der Beitrag der Biokybernetik zum Bild des Menschen). Acta Teilhardiana, Supplementa II, Evolutive Anthropologie, München 1971

589. Keidel, W.D.: D.C.-Potentials in the auditory evoked response in man. Acta otolaryng. (Stockh.) *71*, 242-248 (1971)

590. Keidel, W.D.: Temporal and Spatial Aspects of Sensory Pattern Recognition in Man. Paper given at the International Symposium: Neurophysiological Mechanisms of Mental Activity. 2.-5. July 1972 in Leningrad

591. Keidel, W.D.: Human Biocybernetics. Paper given at the International Congress of Cybernetics and Systems from 28. August to 3. September 1972 in Oxford

592. Keidel, W.D.: Codierung, Informationsfluß und Decodierung im Organismus. Nova Acta Leopoldina *37*, 225-250 (1972)
593. Keidel, W.D.: Biokybernetik des Menschen. Ärztl. Forschung *26*, 73-86 (1972)
594. Keidel, W.D.: The dc-potential in the human cortical evoked response, a new contribution to the objective audiometry. J. franc. Oto-rhino-laryng. *21*, 153-158 (1972)
595. Keidel, W.D.: Intermodale Spezifitat elektrophysiologischer Reizkorrelate. In: Schmerz. Grundlagen - Pharmakologie - Therapie. Hrsg.: Janzen, R., Keidel, W.D., Herz, A. und Steichele, C. George Thieme Verlag, Stuttgart 1972
596. Keidel, W.D.: The Use of Fast Correlators in Electro-Cochleography in Man. In: Disorders of Auditory Function. Ed.: Taylor, W., Academic Press, London-New York 1973
597. Keidel, W.D.: Elektronenmaschinelle Darstellung der heutigen Vorstellung über die Schwingungsform der Basilarmembran mit kritischem Vergleich der klassischen und neuesten Gleichungsätze. In: Funktion und Therapie des Innenohrs. Hals-, Nas-. u. Ohrenheilkunde, Heft 23. Hrsg.: Jakobi, H. und Lotz, P. Johann Ambrosius Barth, Leipzig 1973
598. Keidel, W.D.: Zeitliche und räumliche Aspekte der menschlichen Zeichenerkennung. In: Nova Acta Leopoldina Nr. 211, Bd. 38, "Festschrift fur Bernd Lueken". Hrsg.: Motnes, K. und Scharf, J.-H., Deutsche Akademie der Naturforscher, Leopoldina, Halle/Saale 1973
599. Keidel, W.D.: Recent advances in information processing within the auditory system. In: Kybernetik und Bionik - Cybernetics and Bionics. Hrsg.: Keidel, W.D., Händler, W. und Spreng, M., R. Oldenbourg Verlag, München-Wien 1974
600. Keidel, W.D.: Information Processing in the Higher Parts of the Auditory Pathway. In: Psychophysical Models and Physiological Facts in Hearing. Communication and Cybernetics, Vol. 8. Eds.: Zwicker, E. and Terhardt, E., Springer-Verlag, Berlin-Heidelberg-New York 1974
601. Keidel, W.D.: Kurzgefaßtes Lehrbuch der Physiologie. Georg Thieme Verlag, Stuttgart 1975
602. Keidel, W.D.: Physiologie des Gehörs. Georg Thieme Verlag, Stuttgart 1975
603. Keidel, W.D.: Anatomische und kommunikationstheoretische Grundlagen des Gehörs. In: Physiologie des Gehörs. Hrsg.: Keidel, W.D. Georg Thieme Verlag, Stuttgart 1975
604. Keidel, W.D.: Bedeutung des Zentralnervensystems für die Physiologie des Hörens. HNO *24*, 1-13 (1976)
605. Keidel, W.D.: Der Harmoniebegriff des Pythagoras aus sinnesphysiologischer Sicht. In: Musik und Zahl, Interdisziplinare Beiträge zum Grenzbereich zwischen Musik und Mathematik. Hrsg.: Schnitzler, G. Verlag fur systematische Musikwissenschaft GmbH Bonn-Bad Godesberg 1976
606. Keidel, W.D.: Sensory-Neuronal Encoding and Decoding Processes in Higher Organized Organisms with Emphasis upon Speech Information Processing. Arbeitsberichte des IMMD, Band 9, Heft 8 163-192 (1976)
607. Keidel, W.D.: The Physiological Background of the Electric Response Audiometry. In: Auditory System. Handbook of Sensory Physiology, Vol. V/3. Eds.: Keidel, W.D. and Neff, W.D. Springer-Verlag, Berlin-Heidelberg-New York 1976
608. Keidel, W.D. and Sick, L.: Die objektive Hörschwelle im Frequenzbereich 2 bis 57, 5 kHz am Meerschweinchen und Katze. Z. Biol. *105*, 443-453 (1953)
609. Keidel, W.D. und Spreng, M.: Elektronisch gemittelte langsame Rindenpotentiale des Menschen bei akustischer Reizung. Acta oto-laryng. (Stockh.) *56*, 318-328 (1963)
610. Keidel, W.D. and Finkenzeller, P.: Simultaneous computation of ECG, early response and ERA. IV. Biennial Symposium of the International ERA Study Group in London, 28.-30.7. 1965
611. Keidel, W.D. and Spreng, M.: Neurophysiological evidence for the Stevens power function in man. J. Acoust. Soc. Amer. *38*, 191-195 (1965)
612. Keidel, W.D. and Spreng, M.: Computed audio-encephalograms in man (a technique of objective audiometry). Int. Audiology *4*, 56-60 (1965)

613. Keidel, W.D. and Spreng, M.: Recent status results and problems of objective audiometry in man. 1st Part. J. franc. Oto-rhino-laryng. *14*, 45-53 (1970)

614. Keidel, W.D. et Finkenzeller, P.: Manifestations électriques du fonctionnement de l'ensemble de la voie auditive chez l'homme. Revue de Laryngologie *97*, 563-572 (1976)

615. Keidel, W.D. and Finkenzeller, P.: Electric signs of the activity of the whole auditory system in man. Paper given at the European Symposium on Neurophysiology of Hearing. Interpretation of Human Electrophysiological Data. Bordeaux: 20-22.5. 1976

616. Keidel, W.D. and Kallert, S.: Auditory Nervous System. In: Scientific Foundations of Otolaryngology. Eds.: Hinchcliffe, R. and Harrison, D. William Heinemann Medical Books Ltd., London 1976

617. Keidel, W.D., Keidel, U.O. and Kiang, N.Y.-S: Cortical and peripheral responses to vibratory stimulation of the cat's whiskers. Quarterly Progress Report, Massachusetts Institute of Technology, RLE July 1957, 135-139

618. Keidel, W.D., Keidel, U.O., Kiang, N.Y.-S. and Frishkopf, L.S.: Time course of adaptation of evoked responses from the cat's somesthetic and auditory system. Quart. Progr. Rep. Massachusetts Inst. Technol. RLE *48*, 121-124 (1958)

619. Keidel, W.D., Keidel, U.O. and Kiang, N.Y.-S.: Cortical and peripheral responses to vibratory stimulation of the cat's vibrissae. Arch.int.Physiol.Biochim. *68*, 241-262 (1960)

620. Keidel, W.D., Keidel, U.O. und Wigand, M.E.: Adaptation: Loss or gain of sensory information. In: Sensory Communication. Ed.: Rosenblith, W.A., J. Wiley & Sons, New York and London 1961

621. Keidel, W.D., Breuing, G. und Wiegand, H.P.: Zur Frage der intermodalen Gleichzeitigkeitsempfindung, ein Beitrag zur Messung des "physiologischen Augenblickes". Annals Academiae Scientiarum Fennicae, Series A, V. Medica *143*, 3-8 (1969)

622. Keidel, W.D., Innitzer, J., Neuhäuser, G. and Plattig, K.-H.: Electroencephalographical audiometry of the new-born. J.franc. Oto-rhino-laryng. *22*, 671-683 (1973)

623. Kelly, J.B.: Polysensory cortical lesions and auditory temporal pattern discriminations in the cat. Brain Res. *80*, 317-327 (1974)

624. Kelly, J.B.: Effects of Auditory Cortical Lesions on Sound Localization by the Rat. J. Neurophysiol. *44*, 1161-1174 (1980)

625. Kelly, J.B. and Whitfield, I.C.: Effects of auditory cortical lesions on discriminations of rising and falling frequency-modulated tones. J. Neurophysiol. *34*, 802-816 (1971)

626. Kelly, J.B. and Glazier, S.J.: Auditory cortex lesions and discrimination of spatial location by the rat. Brain Res. *145*, 315-321 (1978)

627. Kelly, J.P. and Wong, D.: Laminar connections of the cat's auditory cortex. Brain Res. *212*, 1-15 (1981)

628. Kelly, J.P. Hudspeth, A.J., Kennedy, S.: Transneuronal transport in the auditory system of the cat. Brain Res. *158*, 207-212 (1978)

629. Kern, E.: Der Bereich der Unterschiedsempfindlichkeit des Auges bei festgehaltenem Adaptationszustand. Z. Biol. *105*, 237-245 (1952)

630. Kiang, N.Y.-S.: An electrophysiological study of cat auditory cortex. Thesis (No. 3028), Univ. Chicago 1955

631. Kiang, N.Y.-S.: A survey of recent developments in the study of auditory physiology. Ann. Otol., (St. Louis) *77*, 656-676 (1968)

632. Kiang, N.Y.-S.: Stimulus Representation in the Discharge Patterns of Auditory Neurons. In: The Nervous System. Vol. 3: Human Communication and its Disorder. Ed: Eagles, E.L., Raven Peess, New York 1975

633. Kiang, N.Y.S.: Processing of speech by the auditory nervous system. J. Acoust. Soc. Am. *68*, 830-835 (1980)

634. Kiang, N.Y.-S. and Moxon E.C.: Physiological considerations in artificial stimulation of the inner ear. Ann.Otol. (St. Louis) *81*, 714-730 (1972)

635. Kiang, N.Y.-S. and Moxon, E.C.: Tails of tuning curves of auditory-nerve fibers. J. Acoust. Soc. Amer. *55*, 620-630 (1974)

636. Kiang, N.Y.-S. Watanabe, T., Thomas, E.C. and Clark, L.F.: Discharge Patterns of Single Fibers in the Cat's Auditory Nerve. Research Monograph No. 35, M.I.T. Press, Cambridge, Mass. 1965

637. Kiang, N.Y.-S., Pfeiffer, R.R., Warr, W.B. and Backus, A.S.N.: Stimulus coding in the cochlear nucleus. Ann.Otol.Rhinol.Laryng. 74, 463-485 (1965)

638. Kiang, N.Y.-S., Sachs, M.B. and Peake, W.T.: Shapes of tuning-curves for single auditory-nerve fibers. J.Acoust.Soc.Amer. 42, 1341-1342 (1967)

639. Kiang, N.Y.-S., Baer, T., Marr, E.M. and Demont, D.: Discharge rates of single auditory nerve fibers as functions of tone level. J.Acoust.Soc.Amer. 46, 106 (1969)

640. Kiang, N.Y.-S., Moxon, E.C. and Levine, R.A.: Auditory-nerve activity in cats with normal and abnormal cochleas. In: Sensorineural hearing loss. Ciba Symp. J. & A. Churchill, London 1970

641. Kiang, N.Y.-S., Morest, D.K. Godfrey, D.A., Guinan, J.J. Jr. and Kane, E.C.: Stimulus coding at caudal levels of the cat's auditory nervous system: I. Response characteristics of single units. In: Basic Mechanisms in Hearing. Ed.: Møller, A.R., Academic Press, New York London 1973

642. Kim, D.O. and Molnar, C.E.: A Population Study of Cochlear Nerve Fibers: Comparison of Spatial Distributions of Average-Rate and Phase-Locking Measures of Responses to Single Tones. J. Neurophysiol. 42, 16-30 (1979)

643. Kim, D.O., Molnar, C.E. and Pfeiffer, R.R.: A system of Nonlinear Differential Equations Modeling Basilar-Membrane Motion. J. Acoust. Soc.Amer. 54, 1517-1529 (1973)

644. Kimura, R.S.: Hairs of the cochlear sensory cells and their attachment to the tectorial membrane. Acta oto-laryng. (Stockh.) 61, 55-72 (1965)

645. Kimura, R.S. and Wersall, J.: Termination of the olivo-cochlear bundle in relation to the outer hair cells of the organ of Corti in guinea pig. Acta Otolaryngol. (Stockh.) 55, 11-32 (1962)

646. Kitzes, M. and Buchwald, J.: Progressive alterations in cochlear nucleus, inferior colliculus and medial geniculate responses during acoustic habituation. Exp. Neurol. 25, 85-105 (1969)

647. Kitzes, L.M., Farley, G.R. and Starr, A.: Modulation of Auditory Cortex Unit Activity during the Performance of a Conditioned Response. Exp. Neurol. 62, 678-697 (1978)

648. Kitzes, L.M., Gibson, M.M., Rose, J.E. and Hind, J.E.: Initial Discharge Latency and Threshold Considerations for Some Neurons in Cochlear Nuclear Complex of the Cat. J. Neurophysiol. 41, 1165-1182 (1978)

649. Klatt, D.H.: Voice onset time, frication and aspiration in word-initial consonant clusters. M.I.T. Research Laboratory of Electronics, Quarterly Progress Report No. 109, 124-136 (1973)

650. Klatt, D.H.: The Duration of (s) in English Words. J. Speech and Hearing Research 17, 51-63 (1974)

651. Klatt, D.H.: Vowel Lengthening is Syntactically Determined in a Connected Discourse. J. Phonetics 3, 161-172 (1975)

652. Klatt, D.H. and Cooper, W.D.: Perception of Segment Duration in Sentence Contexts. In: Structure and Process in Speech Perception. Communication and Cybernetics 11. Eds.: Cohen, A. and Nooteboom, S.G., Springer-Verlag, Berlin-Heidelberg-New York 1975

653. Klinger, K.-P.: Amplitudenvariationen akustisch evozierter Potentiale in Abhangigkeit von der Signalinformation und belastungsbedingter Ermudung. Int. Z. angew. Physiol. 31, 269-278 (1973)

654. Klinke, R.: Frequency analysis in the inner ear of mammals in comparison to other vertebrates. Verh. Dtsch. Zool. Ges., pp. 1-15, 1978 Fischer, Stuttgart 1978

655. Klinke, R.: Basic Mechanisms of Auditory Processing in the Cochlea. In: Hearing Mechanisms and Speech. Experimental Brain Research, Supplementum II. Eds.: Creutzfeldt, O., Scheich, H. and Schreiner, Chr., Springer-Verlag, Berlin-Heidelberg 1979

656. Klinke, R. and Galley, N.: Efferent Innervation of Vestibular and Auditory

Receptors. Physiol. Reviews *54*, 316-357 (1974)

657. Klinke, R. and Pause, M.: Discharge Properties of Primary Auditory Fibres in Caiman Crocodilus: Comparisons and Contrasts to the Mammalian Auditory Nerve. Exp. Brain Res. *38*, 137-150 (1980)

658. Knight, P.L.: Representation of the cochlea within the anterior auditory field (AAF) of the cat. Brain Res. *130*, 447-467 (1977)

659. Knudsen, E.I. and Konishi, M.: Space and Frequency are Represented Separately in Auditory Midbrain of the Owl. J. Neurophysiol. *41*, 870-884 (1978)

660. Knudsen, E.I. and Konishi, M.: Center-Surround Organization of Auditory Receptive Fields in the Owl. Science *202*, 778-780 (1978)

661. Knudsen, E.I. and Konishi, M.: A Neural Map of Auditory Space in the Owl. Science *200*, 795-797 (1978)

662. Knudsen, E.I. and Konishi, M.: Monaural occlusion shifts receptive-field locations of auditory midbrain units in the owl. J. Neurophysiol. *44*, 687-695 (1980)

663. Kobal, G., Wandhoefer, A. and Plattig, K.-H.: EEG power spectra and auditory evoked potentials in transcendental meditation (TM). Pflügers Arch. *359*, R 96 (1975)

664. Koerber, K.L., Pfeiffer, R.R., Warr, W.B. and Kiang, N.Y.-S.: Spontaneous spike discharges from single units in the cochlear nucleus after destruction of the cochlea. Exp. Neurol. *16*, 119-130 (1966)

665. Kohllöffel, L.U.E.: Cochlear microphonics distribution and spatial filtering. In: Frequency Analysis and Periodicity Detection in Hearing. Eds.: Plomp, R. and Smoorenburg, G.F., A.W. Sijthoff, Leiden 1970

666. Kohllöffel, L.U.E.: Longitudinal amplitude and phase distribution of the cochlear microphonic (Guinea pig) and spatial filtering. J. Sound Vib. *11*, 325-334 (1970)

667. Kohllöffel, L.U.E.: Studies of the Distribution of Cochlear Potentials Along the Basilar Membrane. Acta Oto-Laryngologica, Suppl. 288 (1971)

668. Kohllöffel, L.U.E.: A study of Basilar Membrane Vibrations I. Fuzziness-Detection: A New Method for the Analysis of Microvibrations with Laser Light. Acustica *27*, 49-65 (1972)

669. Kohllöffel, L.U.E.: A Study of Basilar Membrane Vibrations II. The Vibratory Amplitude and Phase Pattern Along the Basilar Membrane (Post-Mortem). Acustica *27*, 66-81 (1972)

670. Kohllöffel, L.U.E.: A Study of Basilar Membrane Vibrations III. The Basilar Membrane Frequency Response Curve in the Living Guinea Pig. Acustica *27*, 82-89 (1972)

671. Kohllöffel, L.U.E.: Observations of the mechanical disturbances along the basilar membrane with laser illumination. In: Basic Mechanisms in Hearing. Ed.: Møller, A.R., Academic Press, New York 1973

672. Kohllöffel, L.U.E.: Recordings from spiral ganglion neurones. In: Psychophysical Models and Physical Facts in Hearing. Eds.: Zwicker, E. and Terhardt, E., Springer-Verlag, Berlin-Heidelberg-New York 1974

673. Kohllöffel, L.U.E.: A Study of Neurons Activity in the Spiral Ganglion of the Cat's Basal Turn. Arch. Oto-Rhino-Laryng. *209*, 179-202 (1975)

674. Kohllöffel, L.U.E.: Personal Communication 1976

675. Kohllöffel, L.U.E.: On the Connection Membrana Corti - Organ of Corti. In: Inner Ear Biology Eds.: Postmann, M. and Aran, J.-M. Inserm. Paris 15-24 (1977)

676. König, E.: Pitch discrimination and age. Acta oto-laryng., Stockh. *48*, 475-489 (1957)

677. Konigsmark, B.W.: Neuronal population of the ventral cochlear nucleus in man. Anat. Rec. *163*, 213 (1969)

678. Konigsmark, B.W.: Cellular organization of the cochlear nuclei in man. J. Neuropath. exp. Neurol. *32*, 153-154 (1973)

679. Konigsmark, B.W.: Neuroanatomy of the auditory system. Arch. Otolaryngol. *98*, 397-413 (1973)

680. Konishi, M.: Comparative neurophysiological studies of hearing and vocalizations in songbirds. Z. vergl. Physiol. *66*, 257-272 (1970)

681. Konishi, T. and Yasuno, T.: Summating potential of the cochlea of the guinea pig. J.

Acoust. Soc. Amer. *35*, 1448-1452 (1963)

682. Konishi, T. and Kelsey, E.: Effect of sodium deficiency on cochlear potentials. J. Acoust. Soc. Amer. *43*, 462-472 (1968)

683. Konishi, T. and Kelsey, E.: Effect of calcium deficiency on cochlear potentials. J. Acoust. Soc. Amer. *47*, 1055-1062 (1970)

684. Konishi, T. and Mendelsohn, M.: Effect of ouabain on cochlear potentials and endolymph composition in guinea pigs. Acta Otolaryngol. (Stockh.) *69*, 192-199 (1970)

685. Konishi, T. and Kelsey, E.: Effect of potassium deficiency on cochlear potentials and cation contents of the endolymph. Acta Otolaryngol (Stockh.) *76*, 410-418 (1973)

686. Konishi, T., Kelsey, E. and Singleton, G.T.: Effect of chemical alteration in the endolymph on cochlear potentials. Acta Otolaryngol. (Stockh.) *62*, 393-404 (1966)

687. Konishi, T., Hamrick, P.E. and Walsh, P.J.: Ion transport in guinea pig cochlea. I. Potassium and sodium transport. Acta Otolaryngol. *86*, 22-34 (1978)

688. Kormüller, A.E.: Bioelektrische Erscheinungen architektonischer Felder. Eine Methode der Lokalisation auf der Großhirnrinde. Dtsch. Z. Nervenheilk. *130*, 44-60 (1933)

689. Kozhevnikov, V.A. and Chistovich, L.A.: Speech Articulation and Perception. JPRS 30, 543. Washington: U.S. Department of Commerce, 1965

690. Krainz, W.: Das Knochenleitungsproblem. Experimentelle Ergebnisse. Z. Hals-Nasen-Ohrenheilkunde *15*, 306-313 (1926)

691. Kraus, N. and Disterhoft, J.F.: Location of rabbit auditory cortex and description of single unit activity. Brain Res. *214*, 275-286 (1981)

692. Kromer, L.F. and Moore, R.Y.: Cochlear nucleus innervation by central norepinephrine neurons in the rat. Brain Res. *118*, 531-537 (1976)

693. Kromer, L.F. and Moore, R.Y.: Norepinephrine Innervation of the Cochlear Nuclei by Locus Coeruleus Neurons in the Rat. Anat. Embryol. *158*, 227-244 (1980)

694. Kudo, M.: Projections of the nuclei of the lateral lemniscus in the cat: an autoradiographic study. Brain Res. *221*, 57-69 (1981)

695. Kudo, M., Niimi, K.: Ascending projections of the inferior colliculus onto the medial geniculate body in the cat studied by anterograde and retrograde tracing techniques. Brain Res. *155*, 113-117 (1978)

696. Kudo, M. and Niimi, K.: Ascending Projections of the Inferior Colliculus in the Cat: An Autoradiographic Study. J. Comp. Neurol. *191*, 545-556 (1980)

697. Kuijpers, W. and Bonting, S.L.: The Cochlear Potentials. I. The Effect of Ouabain on the Cochlear Potentials of the Guinea Pig. Pflügers Arch. *320*, 348-358 (1970)

698. Kuijpers, W. and Bonting, S.L.: The cochlear potentials II. The nature of the cochlear endolymphatic resting potential. Pflügers Arch. *320*, 359-372 (1970)

699. Kuiper, J.W.: The microphonic effect of the lateral line organ. Publ. Biophys. Group "Natuurkundig. laboratorium," Groningen, 1-159 (1956)

700. La Grutta, V., Giammanco, S. and Amato, G.: Azione inibitoria del nucleo caudato. II. Alcune caratteristiche dell'azione inibitoria del nucleo caudato sull-area auditiva primaria e sul corpo genicolato mediale. Boll. Soc. ital. Biol. sper.*44*, 1810-1812 (1968)

701. Lavine, R.A.: Phase-locking in response of single neurons in cochlear nuclear complex of the cat to low-frequency tonal stimuli. J. Neurophysiol. *34*, 467-483 (1971)

702. Lawrence, M.: Dynamic range of the cochlear transducer. Cold Spr. Harb. Symp. quant. Biol. *30*, 159-167 (1965)

703. Lawrence, M.: Electric polarization of the tectorial membrane. Ann. Otol. (St. Louis) *76*, 287-312 (1967)

704. Lawrence, M.: Resting Potentials in the Inner Sulcus and Tunnel of Corti. Acta Otolaryngol. *79*, 304-309 (1975)

705. Lawrence, M. and Nuttall, A.L.: Electrophysiology of the Organ of Corti. In: Biochemical mechanism in hearing and deafness. Ed.: Paparella, M.M. Charles C. Thomas, Springfield/Ill. 1970

706. Lawrence, M., Nuttall, A.L. and Clapper, M.P.: Electrical potentials and fluid

boundaries within the organ of Corti. J. Acoust. Soc. Amer. *55*, 122-138 (1974)

707. Legouix, J.-P., Remond, M.-C. and Greenbaum, H.B.: Interference and two-tone inhibition. J. Acoust. Soc. Amer. *53*, 409-419 (1973)

708. Legouix, J.P., Teas, D.C., Beagley, H.A. and Remond, M.C.: Relation between the waveform of the cochlear whole nerve action potential and its intensity function. Acta Otolaryngol. *85*, 177-183 (1978)

709. Lehnhardt, E.: Die überschwellige Audiometrie in der Hand des praktischen HNO-Arztes. Arch. Oto-Rhino-Laryng. *210*, 327-342 (1975)

710. Lenoir, M., Shnerson, A. and Pujol, R.: Cochlear Receptor Development in the Rat with Emphasis on Synaptogenesis. Anat. Embryol. *160*, 253-262 (1980)

711. Leppelsack, H.-J.: Funktionelle Eigenschaften der Hörbahn im Feld L des Neostriatum caudale des Staren (Sturnus vulgaris L., Aves). J. comp. Physiol. *88*, 271-320 (1974)

712. Leppelsack, H.-J. und Schwartzkopff, J.: Eigenschaften von akustischen Neuronen im kaudalen Neostriatum von Vögeln. J. comp. Physiol. *80*, 137-140 (1972)

713. Leppelsack, H.-J. and Vogt, M.: Responses of Auditory Neurons in the Forebrain of a Songbird to Stimulation with Species-specific Sounds. J. comp. Physiol. *107*, 263-274 (1976)

714. Lesser, M.B. and Berkley, D.A.: Fluid Mechanics of the Cochlea. Part 1. J. Fluid Mech. *51*, 497-512 (1972)

715. Lev, A. and Sohmer, H.: Sources of averaged neural responses recorded in animal and human subjects during cochlear audiometry (electrocochleogram). Arch.klin. exp.Ohr.-,Nas.-u.Kehlk,Heilk. *201*, 79-90 (1972)

716. Lewy, F.H. and Kobrak, H.: The neural projections of the cochlear spirals on the primary acoustic centers. Arch. Neurol. Psychiat. *35*, 839-852 (1936)

717. Lhermitte, F., Chain, F. Escourolle, R., Ducarne, B., Pillon, B. et Chedru, G.: Etude des troubles perceptifs auditifs dans les lesions temporales bilaterales. Rev. Neurol. *124*, 329-351 (1971)

718. Licklider, J.C.R.: Basic correlates of the auditory stimulus. In: Handbook of Experimental Psychology. Ed.: Stevens, S.S., Wiley, New York 1951

719. Licklider, J.C.R.: "Periodicity pitch" and "place pitch." J. Acoust. Soc. Amer. *26*, 945 (A) (1954)

720. Licklider, J.C.R.: Auditory frequency analysis. Proceedings Third London Symposium on Information Theory 1955

721. Lien, M.D. and Cox, J.R.: A Mathematical Model of the Mechanics of the Cochlea. Ph.D dissertation (Sever Institute of Washington University, St. Louis, MO) (unpublished) 1973

722. Liff, H.J. and Goldstein, M.H. Jr.: Peripheral inhibition in auditory fibres in the frog. J. Acoust. Soc. Amer. *47*, 1538-1547 (1970)

723. Lilly, J.C. and Cherry, R.B.: Surface movements of click responses from acoustic cerebral cortex of cat: leading and trailing edges of a response figure. J. Neurophysiol. *17*, 521-532 (1954)

724. Lim, D.: Morphological relationship between the tectorial membrane and the organ of Corti. - Scanning and transmission electron microscopy. J. Acoust. Soc. Amer. *50*, 92 (A) (1971)

725. Lim, D.J.: Fine morphology of the tectorial membrane. Its relationship to the organ of Corti. Arch. Otolaryngol. *96*, 199-215 (1972)

726. Lim, D.J.: Cochlear anatomy related to cochlear micromechanics. A review. J. Acoust. Soc. Amer. *67*, 1686-1695 (1980)

727. Lindblom, B. and Rapp. K.: Some Temporal Regularities of Spoken Swedish. Papers from the Institute of Linguistics, University of Stockholm, Publication 21 (1973)

728. Lindeman, H.H. and Bredberg, G.: Scanning Electron Microscopy of the Organ of Corti after Intense Auditory Stimulation: Effects on Stereocilia and Cuticular Surface of Hair Cells. Arch.klin.exp.Ohr.-,Nas.-u.Kehlk,Heilk. *203*, 1-15 (1972)

729. Lindeman, H.H., Ades, H.W., Bredberg, G. and Engström, H.: The sensory hairs and the tectorial membrane in the development of the cat's organ of Corti. Acta oto-

laryng. (Stockh.) *72*, 229-242 (1971)

730. von Loewenich, V.: Methodische Voraussetzungen zur diagnostischen Verwertung auditorisch evozierter Potentiale bei Kleinkindern und Säuglingen. Pädiat. Fortbildk. Praxis *34*, 39-48 (1972)

731. Lorente de No, R.: Anatomy of the eighth nerve. The central projection of the nerve endings of the inner ear. Laryngoscope (St. Louis) *43*, 1-38 (1933)

732. Lorente de No, R.: Anatomy of the eighth nerve. III. General plan and strukture of the primary cochlear nuclei. Laryngoscope (St. Louis) *43*, 327-350 (1933)

733. Love, J.A. and Scott, J.W.: Some response characteristics of cells of the magnocellular division of the medial geniculate body of the cat. Can. J. Physiol. Pharmacol. *47*, 881-888 (1969)

734. Lowenstein, O. and Wersäll, J.: A functional interpretation of the electron microscopic structure of the sensory hairs in the cristae of the eleasmobranch Raja clavata in terms of directional sensitivity. Nature (Lond.) *184*, 1807-1810 (1959)

735. Lowy, K.: Some experimental evidence for peripheral auditory masking. J. Acoust. Soc. Amer. *16*, 197-202 (1945)

736. Lowy, K., Hirota, N.: Effect of peripheral auditory stimulation on unit activity in the vermis cerebelli of cats. Fed. Proc. *27*, n.2, 517 (A) (1968)

737. Lullies, H.: Physiologie der Stimme und Sprache. In: Lehrbuch der Physiologie. Hrsg.: Trendelenburg, W. und Schütz, E., Springer-Verlag, Berlin-Heidelberg-Göttingen 1953

738. Lynn, P.A. and Sayers, B.McA.: Cochlear innervation, signal processing, and their relation to auditory time-intensity effects. J. Acoust. Soc. Amer. *47*, 525-533 (1970)

739. Magoun, H.W.: The Waking Brain. Thomas Springfield/Ill. 1960

740. Majorossy, K., Réthelyi, M.: Synaptic Architecture in the Medial Geniculate Body (Ventral Division). Exp. Brain Res. *6*, 306-323 (1968)

741. Majorossy, K., Kiss, A.: Specific Patterns of Neuron Arrangement and of Synaptic Articulation in the Medial Geniculate Body. Exp. Brain Res. *26*, 1-17 (1976)

742. Majorossy, K. and Kiss, A.: Types of Interneurons and their Participation in the Neuronal Network of the Medial Geniculate Body. Exp. Brain Res. *26*, 19-37 (1976)

743. Manley, G.A.: Frequency sensitivity of auditory neurons in the caiman cochlear nucleus. Z. vergl. Physiol. *66*, 251-256 (1970)

744. Manley, G.A. and Robertson, D.: Analysis of spontaneous activity of auditory neurones in the spiral ganglion of the guinea-pig cochlea. J. Physiol. (Lond.) *258*, 323-336 (1976)

745. Manley, J.A. and Müller-Preuß, P.: Response variability of auditory cortex cells in the squirrel monkey to constant acoustic stimuli. Exp. Brain Res. *32*, 171-180 (1978)

746. Marsh, J.T. and Worden, F.G.: Sound evoked frequency-following responses in the central auditory pathway. Laryngoscope *78*, 1149-1163 (1968)

747. Maruyama, N.P. and Kawasaki, T.: Unitary responses to tone stimulation recorded from the cerebellar cortex of the cat. In: XXIII Int. Congr. Physiol. Sci., Abstr. Tokio 1965, P. 372

748. Mast, T.E.: Binaural interaction and contralateral inhibition in dorsal cochlear nucleus of chinchilla. J. Neurophysiol. *33*, 108-115 (1970)

749. Mast, T.E.: Study of single units of the cochlear nucleus of the chinchilla. J. Acoust. Soc. Amer. *48*, 505-512 (1970)

750. Mast, T.E.: Binaural interaction in the dorsal cochlear nucleus of the chinchilla. In: Physiology of the Auditory System. Ed.: Sachs, M.B., National Educational Consultants, Inc., Baltimore/Maryland 1971

751. Masterton, R.B. and Diamond, I.T.: Effects of auditory cortex ablation on discrimination of small binaural time differences. J. Neurophysiol. *27*, 15-36 (1964)

752. Masterton, B. and Diamond, I.T.: The medial superior olive and sound localization. Science *155*, 1696-1697 (1967)

753. Masterton, B., Thompson, G.C., Bechtold, J.K. and Robards, J.: Neuroanatomical basis of binaural phase-difference analysis for sound localization: a comparative study. J. comp. physiol. Psychol. *89*, 379-386 (1975)

754. Matsumiya, Y., Tagliasco, V., Lombroso, C.T. and Goodglass, H.: Auditory Evoked

Response: Meaningfulness of Stimuli and Interhemispheric Asymmetry. Science *175*, 790-792 (1972)

755. Mehler, W.R., Feferman, M.E. and Nauta, W.J.H.: Ascending axon degeneration following anterolateral cordotomy. An experimental study in the monkey. Brain *83*, 718-750 (1960)

756. Mendelsohn, M. and Konishi, T.: The effect of local anoxia on the cation content of the endolymph. Ann. oto-rhino-laryngol. *78*, 65-75 (1969)

757. Merzenich, M.M. and Brugge, J.F.: Representation of the cochlear partition on the superior temporal plane of the macaque monkey. Brain Res. *50*, 275-296 (1973)

758. Merzenich, M.M. and Reid. M.D.: Representation of the cochlea within the inferior colliculus of the cat. Brain Res. *77*, 397-415 (1974)

759. Merzenich, M.M., Knight, P.L. and Roth, G.L.: Cochleotopic organization of primary auditory cortex in the cat. Brain Res. *63*, 343-346 (1973)

760. Merzenich, M.M., Knight, P.L. and Roth, G.L.: Representation of cochlea within primary auditory cortex in the cat. J. Neurophysiol. *38*, 231-249 (1975)

761. Mesulam, M.-M. and Pandya, D.N.: The projections of the medial geniculate complex within the sylvian fissure of the rhesus monkey. Brain Res. *60*, 315-333 (1973)

762. Mettler, F.A.: Connections of the auditory cortex of the cat. J. Comp. Physiol. *55*, 139-183 (1932)

763. Meyer, D.R. and Woolsey, C.N.: Effects of localized cortical destruction on auditory discriminative conditioning in the cat. J. Neurophysiol. *15*, 149-162 (1952)

764. Meyer, M.F.: The hydraulic principles governing the function of the cochlea. J. Gen. Psychol. *1*, 239-265 (1928)

765. Meyer zum Gottesberge, A.: Zur Physiologie der Haarzellen. Arch.Ohr.-,Nas.-u.Kehlk,Heilk. *155*, 308-314 (1948)

766. Mickle, W.A. and Ades, H.W.: Rostral projection pathway of the vestibular system. Amer. J. Physiol. *176*, 243-246 (1954)

767. Middlebrooks, J.C., Dykes, R.W. and Merzenich, M.M.: Binaural response-specific bands in primary auditory cortex (AI) of the cat: topographical organization orthogonal to isofrequency contours. Brain Res. *181*, 31-48 (1980)

768. Miller, J.M.: Single unit discharges in behaving monkeys. In: Physiology of the Auditory System. Ed.: Sachs, M.B. National Educational Consultants, Inc., Baltimore/Maryland 1971

769. Miller, J.M., Sutton, D., Pfingst, B., Ryan, A., Beaton, R. and Gourevitch, G.: Single cell activity in the cortex of rhesus monkeys: behavioral dependency. Science *177*, 449-451 (1972)

770. Miller, J.M., Beaton, R.D., O'Connor, T. and Pfingst, B.E.: Response pattern complexity of auditory cells in the cortex of unanesthetized monkeys. Brain Res. *69*, 101-113 (1974)

771. Misrahy, G.A., Hildreth, K.M., Shinabarger, E.W. and Gannon, W.J.: Electrical properties of wall of endolymphatic space of the cochlea (guinea pig). Amer. J. Physiol. *194*, 396-402 (1958)

772. Møller, A.R.: Unit responses in the cochlear nucleus of the rat to pure tones. Acta physiol. scand. *75*, 530-541 (1969)

773. Møller, A.R.: Unit responses in the cochlear nucleus of the rat to sweep tones. Acta physiol. scand. *76*, 503-512 (1969)

774. Møller, A.R.: Unit Responses in the Rat Cochlear Nucleus to Repetitive, Transient Sounds. Acta physiol. scand. *75*, 542-551 (1969)

775. Møller, A.R.: Studies of the Damped Oscillatory Response of the Auditory Frequency Analyzer. Acta physiol. scand. *78*, 299-314 (1970)

776. Møller, A.R.: Periodicity Coding in the Peripheral Auditory System. In: Excitatory Synaptic Mechanisms. Proceeding of the Fifth International Meeting of Neurobiologists. Eds.: Andersen, P. and Jansen, J.K.S. Universitetsforlaget, Oslo 1970

777. Møller, A.R.: Two different types of frequency selective neurons in the cochlear nucleus of the rat. In: Frequency Analysis and Periodicity Detection in Hearing. Eds.: Plomp, R. and Smoorenburg, G.F. A.W. Sijthoff, Leiden 1970

778. Møller, A.R.: Unit Responses in the Cochlear Nucleus of the Rat to Noise and Tones. Acta physiol. scand. *78*, 289-298 (1970)
779. Møller, A.R.: Unit responses in the rat cochlear nucleus to tones of rapidly varying frequency and amplitude. Acta physiol. scand. *81*, 540-556 (1971)
780. Møller, A.R.: Coding of sounds in lower levels of the auditory system. Quarterly Reviews of Biophysics *5*, 59-155 (1972)
781. Møller, A.R.: Coding of amplitude and frequency modulated sounds in the cochlear nucleus of the rat. Acta physiol. scand. *86*, 223-238 (1972)
782. Møller, A.R.: Coding of amplitude modulated sounds in the cochlear nucleus of the rat. In: Basic Mechanisms in Hearing. Ed.: Møller, A.R., Academic Press, New York and London 1973
783. Møller, A.R.: Statistical evaluation of the dynamic properties of cochlear nucleus units using stimuli modulated with pseudorandom noise. Brain Res. *57*, 443-456 (1973)
784. Møller, A.R.: Responses of Units in the Cochlear Nucleus to Sinusoidally Amplitude-Modulated Tones. Exp. Neurol. *45*, 104-117 (1974)
785. Møller, A.R.: Coding of sounds with rapidly varying spectrum in the cochlear nucleus. J. Acoust. Soc. Amer. *55*, 631-640 (1974)
786. Møller, A.R.: Coding of Amplitude and Frequency Modulated Sounds in the Cochlear Nucleus. Acustica *31*, 292-299 (1974)
787. Møller, A.R.: Latency of unit responses in cochlear nucleus determined in two different ways. J. Neurophysiol. *38*, 812-821 (1975)
788. Møller, A.R.: Dynamic Properties of Excitation and Inhibition in the Cochlear Nucleus. Acta physiol. scand. *93*, 442-454 (1975)
789. Møller, A.R.: Dynamic Properties of Primary Auditory Fibers Compared with Cells in the Cochlear Nucleus. Acta physiol. scand. *98*, 157-167 (1976)
790. Møller, A.R.: Dynamic Properties of Excitation and Two-tone inhibition in the Cochlear Nucleus Studied Using Amplitude-Modulated Tones. Exp. Brain Res. *25*, 307-321 (1976)
791. Møller, A.R.: Dynamic Properties of the Responses of Single Neurones in the Cochlear Nucleus of the Rat. J. Physiol. *259*, 63-82 (1976)
792. Møller, A.R.: Frequency selectivity of single auditory-nerve fibers in response to broadband noise stimuli. J. Acoust. Soc. Amer. *62*, 135-142 (1977)
793. Møller, A.R.: Frequency selectivity of the peripheral auditory analyzer studied using broad band noise. Acta physiol. scand. *104*, 24-32 (1978)
794. Møller, A.R.: Responses of auditory nerve fibres to noise stimuli show cochlear nonlinearities. Acta Otolaryngol. *86*, 1-8 (1978)
795. Møller, A.R.: Frequency analysis in the peripheral auditory system. In: Kybernetik '77. Hrsg.: Hauske, G. und Butenandt, E. Oldenbourg, München 1978
796. Møller, A.R.: Coding of time-varying sounds in the cochlear nucleus. Audiology *17*, 446-468 (1978)
797. Møller, A.R.: Coding of Complex Sounds in the Auditory Nervous System. In: Hearing Mechanisms and Speech. Eds.: Creutzfeldt, O., Scheich, H. and Schreiner, Chr., Springer-Verlag, Berlin-Heidelberg-New York; Experimental Brain Research, Supplementum II, 1979
798. Möller, J., Neuweiler, G. and Zöller, H.: Response characteristics of inferior colliculus neurons of the awake CF-FM bat, Rhinolophus ferrumequinum. I. Single-tone stimulation. J. comp. Physiol. *125*, 217-225 (1978)
799. Molnar, C.E. and Pfeiffer, R.R.: Interpretation of spontaneous spike discharge patterns in the Cochlear nucleus. Proc. IEEE *56*, 993-1004 (1968)
800. Monakow, C.: Weitere Mitteilungen über einige durch Exstirpation circumscripter Hirnrindenregionen bedingte Entwicklungshemmungen des Kaninshengehirns. Arch. Psychiat. Nervenkr. *12*, 535-544 (1882)
801. Moore, C.N., Casseday, J.H. and Neff, W.D.: Sound localization: the role of the commissural pathways of the auditory system of the cat. Brain Res. *82*, 13-26 (1974)
802. Moore, E.J. II and Rose, D.E.: Variability of latency and amplitude of acoustically evoked responses to pure tones of moderate to high intensity. Int. Audiol. *8*, 172-181

(1969)

803. Moore, J.K. and Osen, K.K.: The Cochlear Nuclei in Man. Am. J. Anat. *154*, 393-418 (1979)

804. Moore, J.K. and Osen, K.K.: The Human Cochlear Nuclei. Exp. Brain Res. Suppl. 2, 36-44 (1979)

805. Moore, R.Y. and Goldberg, J.M.: Midbrain auditory connections in the cat. Anat. Record *139*, 256 (1961)

806. Moore, R.Y. and Goldberg, J.M.: Ascending projections of the inferior colliculus in the cat. J. comp. Neurol. *121*, 109-135 (1963)

807. Moore, R.Y. and Goldberg, J.M.: Projections of the inferior colliculus in the monkey. Exp. Neurol. *14*, 429-438 (1966)

808. Moore, T.J. and Cashin, J.L. Jr.: Response patterns of cochlear nucleus neurons to excerpts from sustained vowels. J. Acoust. Soc. Amer. *56*, 1565-1576 (1974)

809. Morest, D.K.: The laminar structure of the inferior colliculus of the cat. Anat. Rec. *148*, 314 (1964)

810. Morest, D.K.: The neuronal architecture of the medial geniculate body of the cat. J. Anat. (Lond.) *98*, 611-630 (1964)

811. Morest, D.K.: The probable significance of synaptic and dendritic patterns of the thalamic and midbrain auditory system. Anat. Rec. *148*, 390-391 (1964)

812. Morest, D.K.: The laminar structure of the medial geniculate body of the cat. J. Anat. (Lond.) *99*, 148-160 (1965)

813. Morest, D.K.: The lateral tegmental system of the midbrain and the medial geniculated body: study with Golgy and Nauta methods in cat. J. Anat. (Lond.) *99*, 611-634 (1965)

814. Morest, D.K.: The cortical structure of the inferior quadrigeminal lamina of the cat. Anat. Rec. *154*, 389-390 (1966)

815. Morest, D.K.: The non-cortical neuronal architecture of the inferior colliculus of the cat. Anat. Rec. *154*, 477 (1966)

816. Morest, D.K.: The collateral system of the medial nucleus of the trapezoid body of the cat, its neuronal architecture and relation to the olivo-cochlear bundle. Brain Res. *9*, 288-311 (1968)

817. Morest, D.K.: Dendrodendritic synapses of cells that have axons: The fine structure of the Golgi type II cells in the medial geniculate body of the cat. Z. Anat. Entwickl.-Gesch. *133*, 216-246 (1971)

818. Morest, D.K.: Synaptic Relationships of Golgy Type II Cells in the Medial Geniculate Body of the Cat. J. comp. Neur. *162*, 157-194 (1975)

819. Morest, D.K., Kiang, N.Y.-S., Kane, E.C., Guinan, J.J.Jr. and Godfrey, D.A.: Stimulus coding at caudal levels of the cat's auditory nervous system: II. Patterns of synaptic organization. In: Basic Mechanisms in Hearing. Ed.: Møller, A.R., Academic Press, Inc., New York and London 1973

820. Morrell, L.K. and Salamy, J.G.: Hemispheric Asymmetry of Electrocortical Responses to Speech Stimuli. Science *174*, 164-166 (1971)

821. Mortimer, J.A.: Cerebellar responses to teleceptive stimuli in alert monkeys. Brain Res. *83*, 369-390 (1975)

822. Moskowitz, N. and Jung-Ching Liu: Central projection of the spiral ganglion of the squirrel monkey. J. comp. Neurol. *144*, 335-344 (1972)

823. Moushegian, G. and Rupert, A.L.: Response diversity of neurons in ventral cochlear nucleus of kangaroo rat to low-frequency tones. J. Neurophysiol. *33*, 351-364 (1970)

824. Moushegian, G., Rupert, A. and Galambos, R.: Microelectrode study of ventral cochlear nucleus of the cat. J. Neurophysiol. *25*, 515-529 (1962)

825. Moushegian, G., Rupert, A. and Whitcomb, M.A.: Medial superior-olivary-unit response patterns to monaural and binaural clicks. J. Acoust. Soc. Amer. *36*, 196-202 (1964)

826. Moushegian, G., Rupert, A. and Whitcomb, M.A.: Brain-stem neuronal response patterns to monaural and binaural tones. J. Neurophysiol. *27*, 1174-1191 (1964)

827. Moushegian, G., Rupert, A.L. and Langford, T.L.: Stimulus coding by medial superior olivary neurons. J. Neurophysiol. *30*, 1239-1261 (1967)

828. Moushegian, G., Stillman, R.D. and Rupert, A.L.: Characteristic delays in superior olive and inferior colliculus. In: Physiology of the Auditory System. Ed.: Sachs, M.B. National Educational Consultants, Inc., Baltimore/Maryland 1971

829. Moushegian, G., Rupert, A.L. and Gidda, J.S.: Functional Characteristics of Superior Olivary Neurons to Binaural Stimuli. J. Neurophysiol. 38, 1037-1048 (1975)

830. Müller, J.: Handbuch der Physiologie des Mehschen. II. Band. Verlag von J. Holscher, Coblenz 1840

831. Müller-Preuss, P. and Ploog, D.: Inhibition of auditory cortical neurons during phonation. Brain Res. 215, 61-76 (1981)

832. Mulroy, M.J., Altmann, D.W., Weiss T.F. and Peake, W.T.: Intracellular electric responses to sound in a vertebrate cochlea. Nature 249, 482-485 (1974)

833. Mundie, J.R.: Neurophysiological principles of auditory information processing. In: Principles and Practice of Bionics, AGARD Conference Proceedings No. 44. Eds.: von Gierke, H.E., Keidel, W.D. and Oestreicher, H.L., Technivision Services Slough, England 1970

834. Murata, K. and Kameda, K.: The activity of single cortical neurons of unrestrained cats during sleep and wakefulness. Arch.ital.Biol. 101, 306-331 (1963)

835. Naftalin, L.: Some new proposals regarding acoustic transmission and transduction. Cold Spring Harbor Symp. Quant. Biol. 30, 169-180 (1965)

836. Nauta, W.J.H.: The problem of the frontal lobe: a re-interpretation. J. psychiat. Res. 8, 167-187 (1971)

837. Nauta, W.J.H.: Connections of the frontal lobe with the limbic system. In: Surgical approaches in psychiatry. Eds.: Laitinen, L.V. and Livingstone, K.E., University Park Press, Baltimore/Maryland 1973

838. Necker, R.: Zur Entstehung der Cochleopotentiale von Vögeln: Verhalten bei O_2-Mangel, Cyanidvergiftung und Unterkühlung sowie Beobachtungen über die räumliche Verteilung. Z. Vergl. Physiol. 69, 367-425 (1970)

839. Necker, R. and Schwarztkopff, J.: Entstehungsort und räumliche Verteilung der Mikrophon- und Summationspotentiale im Vogelohr. Naturwiss. 56, 92 (1969)

840. Neff, W.D.: Neural mechanisms of auditory discrimination. In: Sensory Communication. Ed.: Rosenblith, W.A., M.I.T. Press, Cambridge, Mass. 1961

841. Neff, W.D. and Casseday, J.H.: Effects of Unilateral Ablation of Auditory Cortex on Monaural Cat's Ability to Localize Sound. J. Neurophysiol. 40, 44-52 (1977)

842. Neff, W.D., Casseday, J.H. and Cranford, J.L.: The medial geniculate body and associated thalamic cell groups: behavioral studies. Brain, Behav. Evol. 6, 302-210 (1972)

843. Neff, W.D., Diamond, I.T. and Casseday, J.H.: Behavioral Studies of Auditory Discrimination: Central Nervous System. In: Auditory System. Handbook of Sensory Physiology, Vol. V/2. Eds.: Keidel, W.D. and Neff, W.D. Springer-Verlag, Berlin-Heidelberg-New York 1975

844. Nelson, C.N. and Bignall, K.E.: Interactions of sensory and nonspecific thalamic inputs to cortical polysensory units in the squirrel monkey. Exp. Neurol. 40, 189-206 (1973)

845. Nelson, P.G. and Evans, E.F.: Relationship between dorsal and ventral cochlear nuclei. In: Physiology of the Auditory System. Ed.: Sachs, M.B., National Educational Consultants, Inc., Baltimore/Maryland 1971

846. Nelson, P.G., Erulkar, S.D. and Bryan, J.S.: Responses of units of the inferior colliculus to time-varying acoustic stimuli. J. Neurophysiol. 29, 834-860 (1966)

847. Neubert, K.: Innere Haarzellen des Cortischen Organs und Schallanalyse. Naturwissenschaften 47, 526-527 (1960)

848. Newman, J.D. and Wollberg, Z.: Multiple coding of species-specific vocalizations in the auditory cortex of squirrel monkeys. Brain Res. 54, 287-304 (1973)

849. Newman, J.D. and Wollberg, Z.: Responses of single neurons in the auditory cortex of squirrel monkeys to variants of a single call type. Exp. Neurol. 40, 821-824 (1973)

850. Newman, J.D. and Lindsley, D.F.: Single Unit Analysis of Auditory Processing in Squirrel Monkey Frontal Cortex. Exp. Brain Res. 25, 169-181 (1976)

851. Niemer, W.T. and Cheng, S.K.: The ascending auditory system. A study of

retrograde degeneration. Anat. Rec. *103*, 490 (1949)

852. Nienhuys, T.G.W. and Clark, G.M.: Frequency Discrimination Following the Selective Destruction of Cochlear Inner and Outer Hair Cells. Science *199*, 1356-1357 (1978)

853. Niimi, K. and Naito, F.: Cortical Projections of the Medial Geniculate Body in the Cat. Exp. Brain Res. *19*, 326-342 (1974)

854. Niimi, K. and Matsuoka, H.: Thalamocortical Organization of the Auditory System in the Cat Studied by Retrograde Axonal Transport of Horseradish Peroxidase. Advances in Anatomy, Embryology and Cell Biology, Vol. 57. Springer Verlag, Berlin 1979

855. Nilsson, H.G.: A Comparison of Models for Sharpening of the Frequency Selectivity in the Cochlea. Biol. Cybernetics *28*, 177-181 (1978)

856. Noda, H. and Adey, W.R.: Neuronal activity in the association cortex of the cat during sleep, wakefulness, and anesthesia. Brain Res. *54*, 243-259 (1973)

857. Nomoto, M.: Discharge Patterns of the Primary Auditory Cortex in Cats. Jap. J. Physiol. *30*, 427-442 (1980)

858. Nomoto, M., Suga, N. and Katsuki, Y.: Discharge pattern and inhibition of primary auditory nerve fibers in the monkey. J. Neurophysiol. *27*, 768-787 (1964)

859. van Noort, J.: The structure and connections of the inferior colliculus. An investigation of the lower auditory system. Van Corcum, Leiden 1969

860. Nooteboom, S.G.: The Perceptual Reality of Some Prosodic Durations. J. Phonetics *1*, 25-45 (1973)

861. Nooteboom, S.G.: Contextual Variation and the Perception of Phonemic Vowel Length. Proc. Speech Communication Seminar, Stockholm, Vol. *3*, 149-154, Almqvist and Wiksell, Upsalla (1974)

862. Nuttall, A.L., Brown, M.C., Masta, R.I. and Lawrence, M.: Inner hair cell responses to the velocity of basilar membrane motion in the guinea pig. Brain Res. *211*, 171-174 (1981)

863. Odenthal, D.W. and Eggermont, J.J.: Amplitude-latency relations for cochlear action potentials in man and animal in recruiting and non-recruiting hearing loss. Audiology *11*, Suppl. 128 (1972)

864. Ohm, G.S.: Uber die Definition des Tones, nebst daran geknüpfter Theorie der Sirene und ähnlicher tonbildender Vorrichtungen. Ann. Phys. Chem. *59*, 513-565 (1843)

865. Ohm, G.S.: Noch ein Paar Worte über die Definition des Tones. Ann. Phys. Chem. *62*, 1-18 (1844)

866. Oliver, D.L. and Hall, W.C.: The Medial Geniculate body of the Tree Shrew, Tupaia glis. I. Cytoarchitecture and Midbrain Connections. J. comp. Neurol. *182*, 423-458 (1978)

867. Oliver, D.L. and Hall, W.C.: The Medial Geniculate Body of the Tree Shrew, Tupaia glis. II. Connections with the neocortex. J. Comp. Neurol. *182*, 459-494 (1978)

868. Oller, D.K.: The Duration of Speech Segments: The Effect of Position in Utterance and Word Length. J. Acoust. Soc. Amer. *54*, 1235-1247 (1973)

869. O'Malley, M.H., Kloker, D.R. and Dara-Abrams, D.: Recoveirng Parentheses from Spoken Algebraic Expressions. IEEE Trans. Audio and Electroacoustics AU-21, 217-220 (1973)

870. Onishi, S. and Katsuki, Y.: Functional organization and integrative mechanism in the auditory cortex of the cat. Jap. J. Physiol. *15*, 342-365 (1965)

871. Onishi, S. and Davis, H.: Effects of duration and rise time of tone bursts on evoked V potentials. J. Acoust. Soc. Amer. *44*, 582-591 (1968)

872. Ornitz, E.M., Ritvo, E.R., Carr, E.M., Panman, L.M. and Walter, R.D.: The variability of the auditory averaged evoked response during sleep and dreaming in children and adults. Electroenceph. clin. Neurophysiol. *22*, 514-524 (1967)

873. Ornitz, E.M., Ritvo, E.R., Tanguay, P.E. and Walter, R.D.: EEG spikes and the averaged evoked response to clicks and flashes. Electroenceph. clin. Neurophysiol. *27*, 387-391 (1969)

874. Osen, K.K.: Cytoarchitecture of the cochlear nucleus in cat. J. comp. Neurol. *136*,

453-483 (1969)

875. Osen, K.K.: Course and termination of primary afferents in the cochlear nucleus of cat: An experimental anatomical study. Arch. ital. Biol. *108*, 21-51 (1970)

876. Osen, K.K.: Projection of the cochlear nuclei on the inferior colliculus in the cat. J. Comp. Neurol. *144*, 355-372 (1972)

877. Osterhammel, P.A., Davis, H., Wir, C.C. and Hirsh, S.K.: Adult auditory evoked vertex potentials in sleep. Audiology *12*, 116-128 (1973)

878. Ozdamar, O. and Dallos, P.: Input-output functions of cochlear whole-nerve action potentials: Interpretation in terms of one population of neurons. J. Acoust. Soc. Amer. *59*, 143-147 (1976)

879. Panayiotopoulos, C.P. and Stopp, P.E.: The characteristics of the cochlear after-potential studied in the guinea pig by perfusion and stimulation. J. Physiol. (Lond.) *210*, 495-505 (1970)

880. Pandya, D.N. and Kuypers, H.G.J.M.: Corticocortical connections in rhesus monkey. Brain Res. *13*, 13-36 (1969)

881. Pandya, D.N., Hallett, M. and Mukherjee, S.K.: Inter- and intrahemispheric connections of the neocortical auditory system in the rhesus monkey. Brain Res. *14*, 49-65 (1969)

882. Peake, W.T., Sohmer, H.S. and Weiss, T.F.: Microelectrode recordings of intracochlear potentials. Quarterly Progress Report, MIT Research Laboratory of Electronics. Cambridge, Massachusetts, No. 94, 293-304 (1969)

883. Perkins, R.E. and Morest, D.K.: A Study of Cochlear Innervation Patterns in Cats and Rats with the Golgi Method and Nomarski Optics. J. Comp. Neurol. *163*, 129-158 (1975)

884. Pestalozza, G. and Davis, H.: Electric responses of the guinea pig ear to high audio frequencies. Am. J. Physiol. *185*, 595-600 (1956)

885. Peterson, L.C. and Bogert, B.P.: A dynamical theory of the cochlea. J. Acoust. Soc. Amer. *22*, 369-381 (1950)

886. Pfeiffer, R.R.: Response characteristics of some single units in the cochlear nucleus to tone-burst stimulation. J. Acoust. Soc. Amer. *36*, 1017A (1964)

887. Pfeiffer, R.R.: Classification of response patterns of spike discharges for units in the cochlear nucleus: tone-burst stimulation. Exp. Brain Res. *1*, 220-235 (1966)

888. Pfeiffer, R.R. and Kiang, N.Y.-S.: Spike discharge patterns of spontaneously and continuously stimulated activity in the cochlear nucleus of anaesthetized cats. Biophys. J. *5*, 301-316 (1965)

889. Pfeiffer, R.R. and Molnar, C.E.: Cochlear nerve fiber discharge patterns: relationship to the cochlear microphonic. Science *167*, 1614-1616 (1970)

890. Pfeiffer, R.R. and Kim, D.O.: Response patterns of single cochlear nerve fibers to click stimuli: descriptions for cat. J. Acoust. Soc. Amer. *52*, 1669-1677 (1972)

891. Pfeiffer, R.R. and Kim, D.O.: Cochlear nerve fiber responses: Distribution along the cochlear partition. J. Acoust. Soc. Amer. *58*, 867-869 (1975)

892. Pfingst, B.E., O'Connor, T.A., Miller, J.M.: Response plasticity of neurons in auditory cortex of the rhesus monkey. Exp. Brain Res. *29*, 393-404 (1977)

893. Pfingst, B.E. and O'Connor, T.A.: Characteristics of Neurons in Auditory Cortex of Monkeys Performing a Simple Auditory Task. J. Neurophysiol. *45*, 16-34 (1981)

894. Pfurtscheller, G.: Änderungen in der evozierten und spontanen Hirnaktivitat des Menschen bei extracranialer Polarisation. Z. ges. exp. Med. *152*, 284-293 (1970)

895. Phillips, D.P. and Irvine, D.R.F.: Responses of single Neurons in Physiologically Defined Primary Auditory Cortex (AI) of the Cat: Frequency Tuning and Responses to Intensity. J. Neurophysiol. *45*, 48-58 (1981)

896. Phillips, D.P. and Irvine, D.R.F.: Responses of single neurons in physiologically defined area AI of cat cerebral cortex: sensitivity to interaural intensity differences. Hearing Research *4*, 299-307 (1981)

897. Picton, T.W. and Hillyard, S.A.: Human auditory evoked potentials. Part II: Effects of attention. Electroenceph. clin. Neurophysiol. *36*, 191-199 (1974)

898. Picton, T.W., Hillyard, S.A., Krausz, H.I. and Galambos, R.: Human auditory evoked potentials. Part I: Evaluation of components. Electroenceph. clin. Neuro-

physiol. *36*, 179-190 (1974)

899. Picton, T.W., Hillyard, S.A. and Galambos, R.: Habituation and Attention in the Auditory System. In: Auditory System. Handbook of Sensory Physiology, Vol. V/3. Eds.: Keidel, W.D. and Neff, W.D. Springer-Verlag, Berlin-Heidelberg-New York 1976

900. Pirsig, W.: Regionen, Zelltypen und Synapsen im ventralen Nucleus cochlearis des Meerschweinchens. Arch.klin.exp. Ohr.-,Nas.-u.Kehlk.Heilk. *192*, 333-350 (1968)

901. Pirsig, W.: Tonotope Organisation der Hörbahn: Morphologische und funktionelle Befunde. HNO *22*, 309-316 (1974)

902. Piggio, G.F. and Mountcastle, V.B.: On the nature of a second thalamic relay subserving some forms of somatic sensibility. Fed. Proc. *18*, 121 (1959)

903. Ploog, D.: Kommunikation in Affengesellschaften und deren Bedeutung für die Verständigungsweisen des Menschen. In: Neue Anthroplogie, Band 2 Biologische Anthropologie, zweiter Teil. Hrsg.: Gadamer, H.-G., Vogler, P., Thieme Verlag, Stuttgart 1972

904. Pollak, G. and Schuller, G.: Tonotopic organization and response patterns to frequency modulated signals in the inferior colliculus of Horseshoe bats. Soc. Neurosci. Abstr. *4*, 9 (1978)

905. Pollak, G.D., Marsh, D.S., Bodenhamer, R. and Souther, A.: A Single-Unit Analysis of Inferior Colliculus in Unanesthetized Bats: Response Patterns and Spike-Count Functions Generated by Constant-Frequency and Frequency-Modulated Sounds. J. Neurophysiol. *41*, 677-691 (1978)

906. Pontes, C., Reis, F.F. and Sousa-Pinto, A.: The auditory cortical projections onto the medial geniculate body in the cat. An experimental anatomical study with silver and autoradiographic methods. Brain Res. *91*, 43-63 (1975)

907. Portmann, M.: Discussion to H. Spoendlin: In: Innervation densities of the cochlea. Acta Oto-Rhino-Laryng. *73*, 235-248 (1972)

908. Portmann, M. and Aran, J.M.: Electrocochléographie sur le nourrisson et le jeune enfant. Méthode de l'audiometrie objective. Acta Otolaryng. *71*, 253-261 (1971)

909. Portmann, M. and Aran, J.M.: Electrocochleography. Laryngoscope *81*, 899-910 (1971)

910. Portmann, M. and Aran, J.M.: Relation entre "patterns" électrocochléographique et pathologie rétro-labyrinthique. Acta Otolaryng. *73*, 190-196 (1972)

911. Portmann, M., le Bert, G. and Aran, J.M.: Potentials cochléaires obtenues chez l'homme en dehors de toute intervention chirurgicale. Rev. Laryngol. (Bordeaux) *88*, 157-164 (1967)

912. Powell, E.W. and Hatton, J.B.: Projections of the inferior colliculus in cat. J. comp. Neurol. *136*, 183-192 (1969)

913. Powell, E.W., Furlong, L.D. and Hatton, J.B.: Influence of the septum and inferior colliculus on medial geniculate body units. Electroenceph. clin. Neurophysiol. *29*, 74-82 (1970)

914. Pujol, R.: Development of tone-burst responses along the auditory pathway in the cat. Acta oto-laryng. (Stockh.) *74*, 383-391 (1972)

915. Pujol, R., Hilding, D.: Anatomy and physiology of the onset of auditory function. Acta oto-laryng. (Stockh.) *76*, 1-10 (1973)

916. Pujol, R., Abonnenc, M.: Receptor maturation and synaptogenesis in the golden hamster cochlea. Arch. Oto-Rhino-Laryng. *217*, 1-12 (1977)

917. Pujol, R., Carlier, E. and Devigne, C.: Different Patterns of Cochlear Innervation during the Development of the Kitten. J. Comp. Neurol. *177*, 529-536 (1978)

918. Pujol, R., Carlier, E. and Lenoir, M.: Ontogenetic approach to inner and outer hair cell function. Hearing Research *2*, 423-430 (1980)

919. Raczkowksi, D. and Winer, J.: Auditory thalamo-cortical projections in the cat: a study using retrograde transport of horseradish perioxidase. 5. Meeting of the Neuroscience Society, New York 1975

920. Raczkowski, D., Diamond, I.T. and Winer, J.: Organization of thalamocortical auditory system in the cat studied with horseradish perioxidase. Brain Res. *101*, 345-354 (1975)

921. Ramón y Cajal, S.: Histologie de système nerveux de l'homme et des vertébrés, Vol. I + II. Inst. Ramón y Cajal, Madrid 1952; Reprints of papers of 1902, 1909 and 1911
922. Ranke, O.F.: Die Gleichrichter-Resonanztheorie. Habilitationsschrift, München 1931
923. Ranke, O.F.: Das Massenverhaltnis zwischen Membran und Flüssigkeit im Innenohr. Akust. Z. 7, 1-11 (1942)
924. Ranke, O.F.: Hydrodynamik der Schneckenflüssigkeit. Z. Biol. 103, 409-434 (1950)
925. Ranke, O.F.: Theory of Operation of the Cochlea: A contribution to the Hydrodynamics of the Cochlea. J. Acoust. Soc. Amer. 22, 772-777 (1950)
926. Ranke, O.F.: Die Knochenleitung nach Fensterungsoperation. Arch. Ohr.-, Nas.-u. Kehlk.Heilk. 161, 534-537 (1952)
927. Ranke, O.F.: Physiologie des Gehörs. In: Lehrbuch der Physiologie. Hrsg.: Trendelenburg, W. und Schütz E., Springer-Verlag, Berlin-Heidelberg-Göttingen 1953
928. Ranke, O.F.: Die optische Simultanschwelle. Z. Biol. 105, 224-231 (1953)
929. Ranke, O.F.: Das Wesen des Rekruitment. In: Audiologie Hrsg.: Zöllner, R., Georg Thieme Verlag, Stuttgart 1954
930. Ranke, O.F.: Die Fortentwicklung der Hörtheorie und ihre klinische Bedeutung. Arch. Ohr.-, Nas.-u. Kehlk.Heilk. 167, 1-15 (1955)
931. Ranke, O.F.: Sinnesorgane. In: Handbuch der gesamten Arbeitsmedizin, Band I. Hrsg.: Lehmann, G., Urban & Schwarzenberg, München-Berlin 1961
932. Ranke, O.F., Keidel, W.D. und Weschke, H.G.: Die zeitlichen Beziehungen zwischen Reiz und Reizfolgestrom (Cochleaeffekt) des Meerschweinchens. Zeitschrift fur Biologie 105, 380-392 (1953)
933. Ranke, O.F., Keidel, W.D. und Wigand, M.E.: Die Funktion der Sinneszelle beim Hören. Pflügers Arch. ges. Physiol. 272, 90 (1960)
934. Raphael, L.J.: Preceding Vowel Duration as a Cue to the Voicing Characteristics of Word-Final Consonants in English. J. Acoust. Soc. Amer. 51, 1296-1303 (1972)
935. Rasmussen, A.T.: Studies of the eighth cranial nerve of man. Laryngoscope (St. Louis) 50, 67-83 (1940)
936. Rasmussen, G.L.: The olivary peduncle and other fiber projections of the superior olivary complex. J. Comp. Neurol. 84, 141-220 (1946)
937. Rasmussen, G.L.: Efferent fibres of the cochlear nerve and cochlear nucleus. In: Neural mechanisms of the auditory and vestibular systems. Eds.: Rasmussen, G.L. and Windle, W.F., Charles C. Thomas Publ., Springfield/Ill. 1960
938. Rasmussen, G.L.: Distribution of fibers originating from the inferior colliculus. Anat. Rec. 139, 266 (1961)
939. Rasmussen, G.L.: Efferent connections of the cochlear nucleus. In: Sensorineural hearing processes and disorders. Ed.: Graham, A.B., Little, Brown and Cie, Boston 1967
940. Rau, R.M.: Über die Abhängigkeit der objektiven ermittelten Intensitatsfunktion des menschlichen Gehörs von der Tonfolgefrequenz. Arch.klin.exo.Ohr.-,Nas.-u.Kehlk.Heilk. 190, 133-145 (1968)
941. Rauch, S.: Biochemie des Hörorgans. Georg Thieme Verlag, Stuttgart 1964
942. Rauch, S. and Kostlin, A.: Aspects chimiques de l'endolymphe et de la périlymph. Pract.oto-rhino-laryng. (Basel) 20, 287-296 (1958)
943. Ravizza, J.C., Diamond, I.T. and Whitfield, I.C.: Unilateral ablation of the auditory cortex in the cat impairs complex sound localization. Science 172, 286-288 (1971)
944. Reale, R.A. and Imig, T.J.: Tonotopic Organization in Auditory Cortex of the Cat. J. Comp. Neurol. 192, 265-291 (1980)
945. Regan, D.: Evoked potentials in psychology, sensory physiology and clinical medicine. Chapman and Hall Ltd., London 1972
946. Reichardt, W.: Grundlagen der technischen Akustik. Akademische Verlagsgesellschaft Geest & Portig K.-G., Leipzig 1968
947. Rejto, A.: Beiträge zur Physiologie der Knochenleitung. Verh. Dt. Otol. Ges. 23, 268-285 (1914)
948. Rhode, W.S.: The measurement of the amplitude and phase of vibration of the

basilar membrane using the Mössbauer effect. Doctoral Dissertation, University of Wisconsin, Madison, Wis. 1970

949. Rhode, W.S.: Vibration of the basilar membrane observed with the Mössbauer technique. In: Physiology of the Auditory System. Ed.: Sachs, M.B., National Educational Consultants, Inc., Baltimore, Maryland 1971

950. Rhode, W.S.: Observations of the vibration of the basilar membrane in squirrel monkey using the Mössbauer technique. J. Acoust. Soc. Amer. 49, 1218-1231 (1971)

951. Rhode, W.S.: An investigation of cochlear mechanics using the Mössbauer effect. In: Basic Mechanisms in Hearing. Ed.: Møller, A.R., Academic Press, New York 1973

952. Rhode, W.S.: Some observations on cochlear mechanics. J. Acoust. Soc. Amer. 64, (1) 158-176 (1978)

953. Rhode, W.S. and Robles, L.: Evidence from Mössbauer experiments for nonlinear vibration in the cochlea. J. Acoust. Soc. Amer. 55, 588-596 (1974)

954. Ribaupierre, R. de, Goldstein, M.H. Jr. and Yeni-Komshian, G.: Intracellular study of the cat's primary auditory cortex. Brain Res. 48, 185-204 (1972)

955. Ribaupierre, F. de, Goldstein, M.H. Jr. and Yeni-Komshian, G.: Cortical coding of repetitive acoustic pulses. Brain Res. 48, 205-225 (1972)

956. Ribaupierre, F. de, Rouiller, E., Toros, A. and de Ribaupierre, Y.: Transmission delay of phase-locked cells in the medial geniculate body. Hearing Research 3, 65-77 (1980)

957. Rigby, D.C., Ross, H.F. and Whitfield, I.C.: Frequency organization in the second auditory area (AII) of the cat. J. Physiol. (Lond.) 194, 67P-68P (1968)

958. Rinsdorf, G.: Ohrfunktionstheorien, Mathematik der Basilarmembran. In: Physiologie des Gehörs. Hrsg.: Keidel, W.D. Georg Thieme Verlag, Stuttgart 1975

959. Rioch, D.M.: Studies on the diencephalon of carnivora. I. Nuclear configuration of thalamus, epithalamus, and hypothalamus of dog and cat. J. comp. Neurol. 49, 1-94 (1929)

960. Robertson, D.: Possible relation between structure and spike shapes of neurones in guinea pig cochlear ganglion. Brain Res. 109, 487-496 (1976)

961. Robertson, R.T., Mayers, K.S., Teyler, T.J., Bettinger, L.A., Birch, H., Davis, J.L., Phillips, D.S. and Thompson, R.F.: Unit Activity in Posterior Association Cortex of Cat. J. Neurophysiol. 38, 780-794 (1975)

962. Robinson, D.W. and Dadson, R.S.: Threshold of Hearing and Equal Loudness Relations of Pure Tones, and the Loudness Function. J. Acoust. Soc. Amer. 29, 1284-1288 (1957)

963. Robles, L., Rhode, W.S. and Geisler, C.D.: Transient response of the basilar membrane measured in squirrel monkeys using the Mössbauer effect. J. Acoust. Soc. Amer. 59, 926-939 (1976)

964. Rockel, A.J.: Observations on the inferior colliculus of the adult cat stained by the Golgi technique. Brain Res. 30, 407-410 (1971)

965. Rockel, A.J. and Jones, E.G.: The neuronal organization of the inferior colliculus of the adult cat. J. comp. Neurol. 147, 11-60 (1973)

966. Rockel, A.J. and Jones, E.G.: Observations on the fine structure of the central nucleus of the inferior colliculus of the cat. J. comp. Neurol. 147, 61-92 (1973)

967. Rockel, A.J. and Jones, E.G.: The neuronal organization of the inferior colliculus of the adult cat. II. The pericentral nucleus J. comp. Neurol. 149, 301-333 (1973)

968. Romand, R.: Survey of intracellular recording in the cochlear nucleus of the cat. Brain Res. 148, 43-65 (1978)

969. Romand, R.: Intracellular recording of 'chopper responses' in the cochlear nucleus of the cat. Hearing Research 1, 95-99 (1979)

970. Ronis, B.J. Cochlear potentials in otosclerosis. Laryngoscope 76, 212-231 (1966)

971. Rose, J.E.: Organization of frequency sensitive neurons in the cochlear nucleus complex of the cat. In: Neural Mechanisms of the Auditory and Vestibular Systems. Eds.: Rasmussen, G.L. and Windle, W.F., Charles C. Thomas Publ., Springfield/Ill. (1960)

972. Rose, J.E.: Discharges of single fibers in the mammalian auditory nerve. In: Frequency Analysis and Periodicity Detection in Hearing. Eds.: Plomp, R. and

Smoorenburg, G.F., A.W. Sijthoff, Leiden 1970

973. Rose, J.E.: Electrical Activity of Single Auditory Nerve Fibers. In: Otophysiology. Advances in Oto-Rhino-Laryngology, Vol. 20. Eds.: Hawkins, J.E. Jr., Lawrence, M. and Work, W.P. S. Karger, Basel-München-Paris-London-New York-Sydney 1973

974. Rose, J.E.: Neural Correlates of Some Psychoacoustic Experiences. In: Neural Mechanisms in Behavior. A Texas Symposium. Ed.: McFadden, D., Springer-Verlag, New York-Heidelberg-Berlin 1980

975. Rose, J.E. and Woolsey, C.N.: The relations of thalamic connections, cellular structure, and evocable electrical activity in the auditory region of cat. J. comp. Neurol. 91, 441-466 (1949)

976. Rose, J.E. and Galambos, R.: Microelectrode studies on medial geniculate body of cat. I. Thalamic region activated by click stimuli. J. Neurophysiol. 15, 343-357 (1952)

977. Rose, J.E. and Woolsey, C.N.: Cortical connections and functional organization of thalamic auditory system of cat. In: Biological and biochemical bases of behavior. Eds.: Harlow, H.F. and Woolsey, C.N., University of Wisconsin Press, Madison 1958

978. Rose, J.E., Galambos, R. and Hughes, J.R.: Microelectrode studies of the cochlear nuclei of the cat. Johns Hopkins Hosp. Bull. 104, 211-251 (1959)

979. Rose, J.E., Greenwood, D.D., Goldberg, J.M. and Hind, J.E.: Some discharge characteristics of single neurons in the inferior colliculus of the cat. I. Tonotopical organization, relation of spike counts to tone intensity, and firing patterns of single elements. J. Neurophysiol. 26, 294-320 (1963)

980. Rose, J.E., Gross, N.B., Geisler, C.D. and Hind, J.E.: Some neural mechanisms in the inferior colliculus of the cat which may be relevant to localization of a sound source. J. Neurophysiol. 29, 288-314 (1966)

981. Rose, J.E., Brugge, J.F., Anderson, D.J. and Hind, J.E.: Phase-locked response to low-frequency tones in single auditory nerve fibers of the squirrel monkey. J. Neurophysiol. 30, 769-793 (1967)

982. Rose, J.E., Brugge, J.F., Anderson, D.J. and Hind, J.E.: Patterns of activity in single auditory nerve fibers of the squirrel monkey. In: Hearing Mechanisms in Vertebrates. A Ciba Foundation Symposium. Eds.: de Reuck, A.V.S. and Knight, J., J. & A. Churchill Ltd., London 1968

983. Rose, J.E., Brugge, J.F., Anderson, D.J. and Hind, J.E.: Some possible neural correlates of combination tones. J. Neurophysiol. 32, 402-423 (1969)

984. Rose, J.E., Hind, H.E., Anderson, D.J. and Brugge, J.F.: Some effects of stimulus intensity on response of auditory nerve fibers in the squirrel monkey. J. Neurophysiol. 34, 685-699 (1971)

985. Rose, J.E., Gibson, M.M., Kitzes, L.M. and Hind, J.E.: Studies of phase-locked cochlear output in cells of the anteroventral nucleus in the cochlear complex of the cat. In: Basic Mechanisms in Hearing. Ed.: Møller, A.R., Academic Press, New York and London 1973

986. Ross, M.D.: The Tectorial Membrane of the Rat. Amer. J. Anat. 139, 449-481 (1974)

987. Roth, W.T., Kopell, B.S. and Bertozzi, P.E.: The effect of attention on the average evoked response to speech sounds. Electroenceph. clin. Neurophysiol. 29, 38-46 (1970)

988. Rouiller, E., de Ribaupierre, Y. and de Ribaupierre, R.: Phase-locked responses to low frequency tones in the medial geniculate body. Hearing Research 1, 213-226 (1979)

989. Ruben, R.J.: Cochlear potentials as a diagnostic test in deafness. In: Sensorineural hearing processes and disorders. Ed.: Graham, A.B., Little, Brown and Cie, Boston 1967

990. Ruben, R.J. and Walker, A.E.: The eighth nerve action potential in Meniere's disease. Laryngoscope 73, 1456-1461 (1963)

991. Ruben, R.J., Bordley, J.E. and Lieberman, A.T.: Cochlear potentials in man. Laryngoscope 71, 1141-1164 (1961)

992. Ruben, R.J., Lieberman, A.T. and Bordley, J.E.: Some observations on cochlear

potentials and nerve action potentials in children. Laryngoscope *72*, 545-554 (1962)

993. Ruhm, H.B. and Jansen, J.W.: Rate of stimulus change and the evoked response: I. Signal risetime. J. Auditory Res. *3*, 211-216 (1969)

994. Rupert, A.L. and Moushegian, G.: Neuronal responses of kangaroo rat ventral nucleus to low-frequency tones. Expl. Neurol. *26*, 84-102 (1970)

995. Rupert, A., Moushegian, G. and Whitcomb, M.A.: Superior-olivary response patterns to monaural and binaural clicks. J. Acoust. Soc. Amer. *39*, 1069-1076 (1966)

996. Rupert, A.L., Caspary, D.M. and Moushegian, G.: Response characteristics of cochlear nucleus neurons to vowel sounds. Ann. Otol. *86*, 37-48 (1977)

997. Russel, I.J. and Sellick, P.M.: The tuning properties of cochlear hair cells. In: Psychophysics and Physiology of Hearing. Eds.: Evans, E.F., Wilson, J.P., Academic Press, London 1977

998. Russel, I.J., Sellick, P.M.: Intracellular studies of hair cells in the mammalian cochlea. J. Physiol. *284*, 261-290 (1978)

999. Rutherford, W.: A new theory of hearing. J. Anat. Physiol., London, *21*, 166-168 (1886)

1000. Ryan, A., Miller, J.: Effects of behavioral performance on single-unit firing patterns in inferior colliculus of the rhesus monkey. J. Neurophysiol. *40*, 943-956 (1977)

1001. Ryan, A. and Miller, J.: Single Unit Responses in the Inferior Colliculus of the Awake and Performing Rhesus Monkey. Exp. Brain Res. *32*, 389-407 (1978)

1002. Sachs, M.B.: Stimulus response relation for auditory nerve-fibers: two-tones stimuli. J. Acoust. Soc. Amer. *45*, 1025-1036 (1969)

1003. Sachs, M.B. and Kiang, N.Y.-S.: Two-tone inhibition in auditory nerve fibers. J. Acoust. Soc. Amer. *43*, 1120-1128 (1968)

1004. Sachs, M.B. and Abbas, P.J.: Rate versus level functions for auditory-nerve fibers in cats: tone-burst stimuli. J. Acoust. Soc. Amer. *56*, 1835-1847 (1974)

1005. Sachs, M.B., Young, E.D. and Lewis, R.H.: Discharge patterns of single fibers in the pigeon auditory nerve. Brain Res. *70*, 431-447 (1974)

1006. Sakai, H. and Woody, C.D.: Identification of Auditory Responsive Cells in Coronal-Pericruciate Cortex of Awake Cats. J. Neurophysiol. *44*, 223-231 (1980)

1007. Salomon, G. and Elberling, C.: Cochlear nerve potentials recorded from the ear canal in man. Acta Otolaryngol. (Stockh.) *71*, 319-325 (1971)

1008. Saul, L.J. and Davis, H.: Electrical phenomena of the auditory mechanism. Trans. Amer. Otol. Soc. *22*, 137-145 (1932)

1009. Schechter, P.B. and Murphy, E.H.: Response characteristics of single cells in squirrel monkey frontal cortex. Brain Res. *96*, 66-70 (1975)

1010. Scheuler, W. and Spreng, M.: Einfluß von Reizfolgefrequenz und Pausendauer auf das durch verschiedene Beschallung evozierte Rindenpotential des Menschen. Arch. Oto-Rhino-Laryng. *211*, 5-16 (1975)

1011. Schmiedt, R.A., Zwislocki, J.J. and Hamernik, R.P.: Effects of Hair Cell Lesions on Responses of Cochlear Nerve Fibers. I. Lesions, Tuning Curves, Two-Tone Inhibition, and Responses to Trapezoidal-Wave Patterns. J. Neurophysiol. *43*, 1367-1389 (1980)

1012. Schmiedt, R.A., Zwislocki, J.J. and Hamernik, R.P.: Effects of Hair Cell Lesions on Responses of Cochlear Nerve Fibers. II. Single- and Two-Tone Intensity Functions in Relation to Tuning Curves. J. Neurophysiol. *43*, 1390-1405 (1980)

1013. Schouten, J.F.: The perception of subjective tones. Proceedings Kon. Acad. Wetensch. (Neth.) *41*, 1086-1094 (1938)

1014. Schouten, J.F.: The residue, a new component in subjective sound analysis. Proc. Kon.Acad. Wetensch. (Neth.) *43*, 356-365 (1940)

1015. Schouten, J.F.: The residue and the mechanism of hearing. Proc.Kon.Acad. Wetensch. (Neth.) *43*, 991-999 (1940)

1016. Schouten, J.F.: De toonnoogtegewaarwording. Philips Technisch Tijdechr. *5*, 298-306 (1940)

1017. Schouten, J.F.: The Residue Revisited. In: Frequency Analysis and Periodicity Detection in Hearing. Eds.: Plomp, R. and Smoorenburg, G.F., A.W. Sijthoff, Leiden 1970

1018. Schuller, G.: Vocalization Influences Auditory Processing in Collicular Neurons of the CF-FM-Bat, Rhinolophus ferrumequinum. J. comp. Physiol. *132*, 39-46 (1979)

1019. Schuller, G.: Hearing Characteristics and Doppler Shift Compensation in South Indian CF-FM Bats. J. Comp. Physiol. *139*, 349-356 (1980)

1020. Schuller, G. and Pollak, G.: Disproportionate Frequency Representation in the Inferior Colliculus of Doppler-Compensating Greater Horseshoe Bats: Evidence for an Acoustic Fovea. J. comp. Physiol. *132*, 47-54 (1979)

1021. Schwartzkopff, J.: Structure and function of the ear and of the auditory brain areas in birds. In: Hearing Mechanisms in Vertebrates. A Ciba Foundation Symposium. Eds.: de Reuck, A.V.S. and Knight, J., J. & A. Churchill Ltd., London 1968

1022. Schwartzkopff, J.: Inner ear potentials in lower vertebrates: dependence on metabolism. In: Basic Mechanisms in Hearing. Ed.: Møller, A.R., Academic Press, New York and London 1973

1023. Schwartzkopff, J.: Physiologische und morphologische Grunlagen der zentralen Verarbeitung von Gehörinformation. Verh. Dtsch. Zool. Ges. 1976, 140-155 (Fischer, Stuttgart 1976)

1024. Schwartzkopff, J.: Comparative Physiology of Mechanoreception: Origin and Development of the Field of Research. J. comp. Physiol. *120*, 11-31 (1977)

1025. Seebeck, A.: Beobachtungen über einige Bedingungen der Entstehung von Tönen. Ann. Phys. Chem. *53*, 417-436 (1841)

1026. Seebeck, A.: Über die Sirene. Ann. Phys. Chem. *60*, 449-481 (1843)

1027. Sellick, P.M. and Russell, I.J.: Intracellular studies of cochlear hair cells: Filling the gap between basilar membrane mechanics and neural excitation. In: Evoked electrical activity in the auditory nervous system. Eds.: Naunton, R.F., Fernandez, C., Academic Press, New York 1978

1028. Sellick, P.M. and Russell, I.J.: Two-tone suppression in cochlear hair cells. Hearing Research *1*, 227-236 (1979)

1029. Sellick, P.M. and Russell, I.J.: The responses of inner hair cells to basilar membrane velocity during low frequency auditory stimulation in the guinea pig cochlea. Hearing Research *2*, 439-445 (1980)

1030. Semple, M.N. and Aitkin, L.M.: Representation of Sound Frequency and Laterality by Units in Central Nucleus of Cat Inferior Colliculus. J. Neurophysiol. *42*, 1626-1639 (1979)

1031. Shimizu, H., Konishi, T. and Nakamura, F.: An experimental study of adaptation and fatigue of cochlear microphonics. Acta Oto-Laryng. *47*, 358-363 (1957)

1032. Shnerson, A. and Pujol, R.: Age-related changes in the C57BL/6J mouse cochlea. I. Physiological Findings. Develop. Brain Res. *2*, 65-75 (1982)

1033. Shnerson, A., Devigne, C. and Pujol, R.: Age-related changes in the C57BL/6J mouse cochlea. II. Ultrastructural findings. Develop. Brain Res. *2*, 77-88 (1982)

1034. Shofer, R.J. and Nahvi, M.J.: Firing patterns induced by sound in single units of cerebellar cortex. Exp. Brain Res. *8*, 327-345 (1969)

1035. Siebert, W.M.: Models for the dynamic behavior of the cochlear partition. M.I.T. Research Laboratory of Electronics. Quarterly Progress Report *64*, 242-258 (1962)

1036. Siebert, W.M.: Ranke Revisited—A Simple Shortwave Cochlea Model. J. Acoust. Soc. Amer. *56*, 594-600 (1974)

1037. Simmons, F.B. and Linehan, J.A.: Observation on a single auditory nerve fiber over a six-week period. J. Neurophysiol. *31*, 799-805 (1968)

1038. Sinex, D.G. and Geisler, C.D.: Auditory-nerve fiber responses to frequency-modulated tones. Hearing Research *4*, 127-148 (1981)

1039. Skinner, P.H., Antinoro, F. and Shimota, J.: An evaluation of linear extrapolation to threshold in electroencephalic response audiometry. J. Aud. Res. *12*, 26-31 (1974)

1040. Skudrzyk, E.: Die Grundlagen der Akustik. Springer-Verlag, Wien 1954

1041. Skudrzyk, E.: The Foundation of Acoustics. Springer-Verlag, Wien-New York 1971

1042. Smith, C.A.: The Inner Ear: Its Embryological Development and Microstructure. In: The Nervous System, Vol. 3: Human Communication and Its Disorders. Ed.: Eagles, E.L., Raven Press, New York 1975

1043. Smith, C.A. and Sjostrand, F.S.: A synaptic structure in the hair cells of the guinea pig cochlea. J. Ultrastruct. Res. 5, 184-192 (1961)

1044. Smith, C.A. and Takasaka, T.: Auditory receptor organs of reptiles, birds and mammals. In: Contributions to Sensory Physiology, Vol. 5. Ed.: Neff, W.D., Academic Press, New York 1971

1045. Smith, C.A., Lowry, O.H. and Wu, M.-L.: The electrolytes of the labyrinthine fluids. Laryngoscope, St. Louis 64, 141-153 (1954)

1046. Smith, C.A., Davis, H., Deatherage, B.H. and Gessert, C.F.: DC potentials of the membraneous labyrinth. Am. J. Physiol. 193, 203-206 (1958)

1047. Smith, J.C., Marsh, J.T., Greenberg, S. and Brown, W.S.: Human Auditory Frequency-Following Responses to a Missing Fundamental. Science 201, 639-641 (1978)

1048. Smith, R.L.: Short-Term Adaptation in Single Auditory Nerve Fibers: Some Poststimulatory Effects. J. Neurophysiol. 40, 1098-1112 (1977)

1049. Smith, R.L.: Adaptation, saturation, and physiological masking in single auditory-nerve fibers. J. Acoust. Soc. Amer. 65, 166-178 (1979)

1050. Smith, R.L. and Zwislocki, J.J.: Responses of some neurones of the cochlear nucleus to tone intensity increments. J. Acoust. Soc. Amer. 50, 1520-1525 (1971)

1051. Smolders, J.W.T., Aertsen, A.M.H.J. and Johannesma, P.I.M.: Neural Representation of the Acoustic Biotope. A Comparison of the Response of Auditory Neurons to Tonal and Natural Stimuli in the Cat. Biol. Cybernetics 35, 11-20 (1979)

1052. Snider, R.S. and Stowell, A.: Receiving areas of the tactile, auditory and visual systems in the cerebellum. J. Neurophysiol. 7, 331-357 (1944)

1053. Sohmer, H.: The effect of contralateral olivo-cochlear bundle stimulation on the cochlear potentials evoked by acoustic stimuli of various frequencies and intensities. Acta oto-laryng. (Stockh.) 60, 59-70 (1965)

1054. Sohmer, H.: A comparison of the efferent effects of the homolateral and contralateral olivo-cochlear bundles. Acta Oto-Laryng. 62, 74-87 (1966)

1055. Sohmer, H. and Feinmesser, M.: Cochlear action potentials recorded from the external ear in man. Ann. Otol. 76, 427-435 (1967)

1056. Sohmer, H. and Feinmesser, M.: Routine use of electrocochleography (cochlear audiometry) on human subjects. Audiology 12, 167-173 (1973)

1057. Sohmer, H.S., Peake, W.T. and Weiss, T.F.: Intracochlear potential recorded with micropipets. I. Correlations with micropipet location. J. Acoust. Soc. Amer. 50, 572-586 (1971)

1058. Sohmer, H., Feinmesser, M., Bauberger-Tell, L., Lev, A. and David, S.: Routine use of cochlear audiometry in infants with uncertain diagnosis. Ann. Otol. 81, 72-75 (1972)

1059. Sokolich, W.G., Hamernik, R.P., Zwislocki, J.J. and Schmiedt, R.A.: Inferred response polarities of cochlear hair cells. J. Acoust. Soc. Amer. 59, 963-974 (1976)

1060. Sousa-Pinto, A.: Cortical Projections of the Medial Geniculate Body in the Cat. In: Advances in Anatomy, Embryology and Cell Biology, Vol. 48, Fasc. 2. Springer-Verlag, Berlin-Heidelberg-New York 1973

1061. Sousa-Pinto, A.: The structure of the first auditory cortex (A I) in the cat. I. Light microscopic observations on its organization. Arch. ital. de Biologie 111, 112-137 (1973)

1062. Sovijarvi, A.R.A. and Hyvarinen, J.: Auditory cortical neurons in the cat sensitive to the direction of sound source movement. Brain Res. 73, 455-471 (1974)

1063. Spoendlin, H.H.: The organization of the cochlear receptor. Vol. 13 of: Advances in Otorhino-Laryngology. S. Karger, Basel 1966

1064. Spoendlin, H.: The innervation of the organ of Corti. J. Laryng. Otol. 81, 717-738 (1967)

1065. Spoendlin, H.: Ultrastructure and peripheral innervation pattern of the receptor in relation to the first coding of the acoustic message. In: Hearing Mechanisms in Vertebrates. Eds.: de Reuck, A.V.S. and Knight, J., J. & A. Churchill Ltd., London 1968

1066. Spoendlin, H.: Innervation patterns in the organ of Corti of the cat. Acta Otolaryngol. 67, 239-254 (1969)

1067. Spoendlin, H.: Structural basis of peripheral frequency analysis. In: Frequency analysis and periodicity detection in hearing. Eds.: Plomp, R. and Smoorenburg, G.F., A.W. Sijthoff, Leiden 1970

1068. Spoendlin, H.: Degeneration behavior of the cochlear nerve. Arch.klin.exp.Ohr.-,Nas.-Kehlk.Heilk. 200, 275-291 (1971)

1069. Spoendlin, H.: Innervation densities of the cochlea. Acta Otolaryngol. 73, 235-248 (1972)

1070. Spoendlin, H.: Innervationsprinzipien der Cochlea. In: Funktion und Therapie des Innenohrs. Hals-, Nasen- und Ohrenheilkunde, Band 23. Hrsg.: Jakobi, H. and Lotz, P., Johann Ambrosius Barth, Leipzig 1973

1071. Spoendlin, H.: Neuroanatomy of the cochlea. In: Facts and Models in Hearing. Communication and Cybernetics, Vol. 8. Eds.: Zwicker, E. and Terhardt, E., Springer-Verlag, Berlin-Heidelberg-New York 1974

1072. Spoendlin, H.: Neuroanatomical Basis of Cochlear Coding Mechanisms. Audiology 14, 383-407 (1975)

1073. Spoendlin, H.: The afferent innervation of the cochlea. In: Evoked electrical activity in the auditory nervous system. Eds.: Naunton, R.F., Fernandez, C. Academic Press, New York 1978

1074. Spoendlin, H.: Neural connections of the outer haircell system. Acta Otolaryngol. 87, 381-387 (1979)

1075. Spreng, M.: Über die Messung der Frequenzgruppe und der Integrationszeit des menschlichen Gehörs durch vom Schall abhängige Hirnspannungen längs der Kopfhaut. Dissertation, Stuttgart 1967

1076. Spreng, M.: Problems in objective cerebral audiometry using short sound stimulation. Int. Audiol.-Audiol. Internationale 8, 424-429 (1969)

1077. Spreng, M.: Objektivierende Messungen am Schmerzsinn des Menschen. Habilitationsschrift, Erlangen 1970

1078. Spreng, M.: Small computers in evoked response audiometry (ERA). Arch. klin.exp. Ohr-, Nas- u. Kehlk.Heilk. 198, 50-70 (1971)

1079. Spreng, M.: Artefact recognition diazepam in electric response audiometry. Audiology 12, 137-149 (1973)

1080. Spreng, M.: Neuere Hinweise zu ERA und ECOG - aus physiologischer Sicht. Arch. Oto-Rhino-Laryng. 206, 191-215 (1974)

1081. Spreng, M.: Objective electrophysiological measurements of ear-characteristics, intelligibility of vowels and judgement of the stage of attention. Proceedings of the 31. Aerospace Medical Panel Meeting, Neapel 1974. AGARD publication, AGARD-CPP-152 A6, A6-10 (1974)

1082. Spreng, M.: Langsame Rindenpotentiale, objektive Audiometrie und Psychoakustik In: Physiologie des Gehörs. Hrsg.: Keidel, W.D. George Thieme Verlag, Stuttgart 1975

1083. Spreng, M.: Short sound stimulation and temporal integration model of evoked responses. Biennial Symposium of the International ERA Study Group. London 1975

1084. Spreng, M.: Remarks concerning the origin, the dependance on special stimulation parameters and some new applications of responses evoked by various acoustic stimulation. C.R.S. Meeting on Electrical Response Audiometry Evoked by Auditory Stimuli, Milano, April 1975

1085. Spreng, M.: Physiologische und psychophysikalische Gesichtspunkte zur Unbehaglichkeits- und Schmerzschwelle beim Hören. Zeitschrift fur Hörgerate-Akustik 14, 14-29 (1975)

1086. Spreng, M.: Grenzen der sensorischen Informationsverarbeitung des Menschen. Naturwissenschaft. Rundschau 29, 377-386 (1976)

1087. Spreng, M. and Keidel, W.D.: Human evoked cortical responses to auditory stimuli: Interaction, time course of adaptation, influence of stimuli parameters. In: Abstracts of free communications, films, and demonstrations, presented at the XXIInd International Congress of Physiological Sciences, Leyden. Int. Congr. Ser. 48, Excerpta Medica Foundation, Amsterdam 1962 Eds.: Duyff, J.W.

1088. Spreng, M. and Keidel, W.D.: Neue Möglichkeiten der Untersuchung menschlicher Informationsverarbeitung. Kybernetik *1*, 243-249 (1963)

1089. Spreng, M. and Keidel, W.D.: Objektive Audiometrie. Pflügers Archiv ges. Physiol. *281*, 82 (1964)

1090. Spreng, M. und Ichioka, M.: Langsame Rindenpotentiale bei Schmerzreizung am Menschen. Pflügers Arch. ges. Physiol. *279*, 121-132 (1964)

1091. Spreng, M. and Keidel, W.D.: Separierung von Cerebroaudiogramm (CAG), Neuroaudiogramm (NAG) und Otoaudiogramm (OAG) in der objektiven Audiometrie. Arch.Klin.exp.Ohr-, Nas- u. Kehlk.Heilk. *189*, 255-246 (1967)

1092. Spreng, M. and Keidel, W.D.: Recent status results and problems of objective audiometry in man. 2nd Part. J. franc. Oto-Rhino-Laryng. *19*, 55-60 (1970)

1093. Spreng, M. and Keidel, W.D.: Problems of simple averaging of electro-physiological recordings and the use of additional methods. In: Revue de Laryngologie, Suppl. 1971 Ed.: Portmann, G., Bordeaux

1094. Spreng, M. Bumm, P., Keidel, W.D. und Wiegand, H.P.: Elektrophysiologische Untersuchungen am peripheren Teil des menschlichen Ohres unter Benutzung geeigneter Rechnerprogramme. Pflügers Arch. *307*, R 134 (1969)

1095. Spychala, P., Rose, D.E. and Grier, J.B.: Comparison on the "On" and "Off" characteristics of the acoustically evoked response. Int. Audiology *8*, 416-423 (1969)

1096. Stange, G., Spreng, M. und Keidel, U.O.: Die Wirkung von Streptomycinsulfat auf Erregung und Adaptation der Haarzellen des Cortischen Organs. Pflügers Arch. ges. Physiol. *279*, 99-120 (1964)

1097. Stange, G., Holz, E., Terayama, Y. und Beck, Ch.: Korrelation morphologischer, biochemischer und elektrophysiologischer Untersuchungsergebnisse des akustischen Systems. Arch.klin.exp.Ohr-, Nas- u. Kehlk. Heilk. *186*, 229-246 (1966)

1098. Starr, A. and Britt, R.: Intracellular recordings from cat cochlear nucleus during tone stimulation. J. Neurophysiol. *33*, 137-147 (1970)

1099. Starr, A. and Britt, R.: Synaptic events in cochlear nucleus. In: Physiology of the Auditory System. Ed.: Sachs, M.B., National Educational Consultants, Inc. Baltimore/Maryland 1971

1100. Starr, A. and Hellerstein, D.: Distribution of Frequency Following Responses in Cat Cochlear Nucleus to Sinusoidal Acoustic Signals. Brain Res. *33*, 367-377

1101. Starr, A. and Don, M.: Responses of squirrel monkey (Samiri sciureus) medical geniculate units to binaural click stimuli. J. Neurophysiol. *35*, 501-517 (1972)

1102. Starr, A. and Achor, L.J.: Auditory Brain Stem Responses in Neurological Disease. Arch. Neurol. *32*, 761-768 (1975)

1103. Steele, C.R.: A possibility for sub-tectorial membrane fluid motion. In: Basic Mechanisms in Hearing. Ed.: Møller, A.R. Academic Press, New York and London 1973

1104. Steele, C.R.: Behavior of the Basilar Membrane with Pure-tone Excitation. J. Acoust. Soc. Amer. *55*, 148-162 (1974)

1105. Steele, C.R.: Cochlear mechanics. In: Handbook of Sensory Physiology, Vol. V/3: Auditory System. Eds.: Keidel, W.D. and Neff, W.D. Springer Verlag, Berlin-Heidelberg-New York 1976

1106. Stevens, K.N. and House, A.S.: Speech Perception. In: Foundations of Modern Auditory Theory, Vol. II. Ed.: Tobias, J.V. Academic Press, New York and London 1972

1107. Stevens, S.S., Davis, H. and Lurie, M.H.: The localization of pitch perception on the basilar membrane. J. Gen. Psychol. *13*, 297-315 (1935)

1108. Stopp, P.E.: "Afterpotential" in the cochlear response. Nature (Lond.) *215*, 1400 (1967)

1109. Stopp, P.E. and Comis, S.D.: Afferent and efferent innervation of the guinea-pig cochlea: A light microscopic and histochemical study. Neuroscience *3*, 1197-1206 (1978)

1110. Stotler, W.A.: An experimental study of the cells and connections of the superior olivary complex of the cat. J. comp. Neurol. *98*, 401-432 (1953)

1111. Strelioff, D. and Honrubia, V.: Neural Transduction in Xenopus laevis Lateral Line

System. J. Neurophysiol. *41*, 432-444 (1978)

1112. Strominger, N.L. and Oesterreich, R.E.: Localization of sound after section of the brachium of the inferior colliculus. J. comp. Neurol. *138*, 1-18 (1970)

1113. Strominger, N.L. and Strominger, A.I.: Ascending brain stem projections of the anteroventral cochlear nucleus in the rhesus monkey. J. comp. Neurol. *143*, 217-232 (1971)

1114. Strominger, N.L. and Bacsik, R.D.: The anteroventral cochlear nucleus in man and the rhesus monkey. Anat. Rec. *172*, 413 (1972)

1115. Suga, N.: Responses of cortical auditory neurones to frequency modulated sounds in echo-locating bats. Nature *206*, 890-891 (1965)

1116. Suga, N.: Functional properties of auditory neurons in the cortex of echo-locating bats. J. Physiol. *181*, 671-700 (1965)

1117. Suga, N.: Analysis of frequency-modulated and complex sounds by single auditory neurons of bats. J. Physiol. *198*, 51-80 (1968)

1118. Suga, N.: Classification of inferior collicular neurons of bats in terms of responses to pure tones, FM sounds and noise bursts. J. Physiol. *200*, 555-574 (1969)

1119. Suga, N.: Responses of Inferior Collicular Neurones of Bats to Tone Bursts with Different Rise Times. J. Physiol. *217*, 159-177 (1971)

1120. Suga, N.: Feature extraction in the auditory system of bats. In: Basic Mechanisms in Hearing. Ed.: Møller, A.R., Academic Press, New York and London 1973

1121. Suga, N.: Specialization of the auditory system for reception and processing of species-specific sounds. Fed. Proc. *37*, 2342-2354 (1978)

1122. Suga, N. and Schlegel, P.: Coding and processing in the auditory systems of FM-Signal-producing bats. J. Acoust. Soc. Amer. *54*, 174-190 (1973)

1123. Suga, N., O'Neill, W.E. and Manabe, T.: Cortical Neurons Sensitive to Combinations of Information-Bearing Elements of Biosonar Signals in the Mustache Bat. Science *200*, 778-781 (1978)

1124. Suga, N., O'Neill, W.E. and Manabe, T.: Harmonic-Sensitive Neurons in the Auditory Cortex of the Mustache Bat. Science *203*, 270-274 (1979)

1125. Summerfield, Q.: How a full account of segmental perception depends on prosody and vice versa. In: Structure and Process in Speech Perception. Communication and Cybernetics, Vol. 11 Eds: Cohen, A. and Nooteboom, S.G., Springer-Verlag, Berlin-Heidelberg-New York 1975

1126. Syka, J., Radionova, E.A. and Popelar, J.: Discharge Characteristics of Neuronal Pairs in the Rabbit Inferior Colliculus. Exp. Brain Res. *44*, 11-18 (1981)

1127. Symmes, D., Alexander, G.E. and Newman, J.D.: Neural processing of vocalizations and artificial stimuli in the medial geniculate body of squirrel monkey. Hearing Research *3*, 133-146 (1980)

1128. Takeuchi, A. and Takeuchi, N.: On the permeability of end-plate membrane during the action of transmitter. J. Physiol. (Lond.) *154*, 52-67 (1960)

1129. Tanaka, Y., Asanuma, A., Yanagisawa, K. and Katsuki, Y.: Electrical potentials of the subtectorial space in the guinea pig cochlea. Jap. J. Physiol. *27*, 539-549 (1977)

1130. Tarlov, E.C. and Moore, R.Y.: The tectothalamic connections in the brain of the rabbit. J. comp. Neurol. *126*, 403-421 (1966)

1131 Tasaki, I.: Nerve impulses in individual auditory nerve fibres of guinea pig. J. Neurophysiol. *17*, 97-122 (1954)

1132. Tasaki. I. and Fernandez, C.: Modifications of cochlear microphonics and action potentials by KCl solution and by direct currents. J. Neurophysiol. *15*, 497-512 (1952)

1133. Tasaki, I. and Spyropoulos, C.S.: Stria vascularis as source of endocochlear potential. J. Neurophysiol. *22*, 149-155 (1959)

1134. Tasaki. I., Davis, H. and Legouix, J.-P.: The space-time pattern of the cochlear microphonics (guinea pig) as recorded by differential electrodes. J. Acoust. Soc. Amer. *24*, 502-519 (1952)

1135. Tasaki, I., Davis, H. and Eldredge, D.H.: Exploration of cochlear potentials in guinea pig with a microelectrode. J. Acoust. Soc. Amer. *26*, 765-773 (1954)

1136 Teas, D.C., Eldredge, D.H. and Davis, H.: Cochlear responses to acoustic transients:

an interpretation of whole nerve action potentials. J. Acoust. Soc. Amer. *34*, 1438-1459 (1962)

1137. Ter Kuile, E.: Die Übertragung der Energie von der Grundmembran auf die Haarzellen. Pflügers Arch. ges. Physiol. *79*, 146-157 (1900)

1138. Thalmann, R., Comegys, T.H., Thalmann, I. and Webster, D.B.: Distribution of aspartate and glutamate in cochlear nucleus (CN) following destruction of organ of Corti (OC). J. Acoust. Soc. Am. *67*, S77 (1980)

1139. Thurlow, W.R., Gross, N.B., Kemp, E.H. and Lowry, K.: Microelectrode studies of neural activity of cat. I. Inferior colliculus. J. Neurophysiol. *14*, 289-304 (1951)

1140. Tomita, T.: Electrophysiological study of the mechanism subserving color coding in the fish retina. Cold Spr. Harb. Symp. quant. Biol. *30*, 559-566 (1965)

1141. Tomita, T., Kaneko, A., Murakami, M. and Pautler, E.L.: Spectral response curves of single cones in the carp. Vision Res. *7*, 519-531 (1967)

1142. Tonndorf, J.: Fluid motion in cochlear models. J. Acoust. Soc. Amer. *29*, 558-568 (1957)

1143. Tonndorf, J.: Harmonic distortion in cochlear models. J. Acoust. Soc. Amer. *30*, 929-937 (1959)

1144. Tonndorf, J.: Beats in cochlear models. J. Acoust. Soc. Amer. *31*, 608-619 (1959)

1145. Tonndorf, J.: Dimensional analysis of cochlear models. J. Acoust. Soc. Amer. *32*, 493-497 (1960)

1146. Tonndorf, J.: Response of cochlear models to aperiodic signals and to random noises. J. Acoust. Soc. Amer. *32*, 1344-1355 (1960)

1147. Tonndorf, J.: Shearing motion in scala media of cochlear models. J. Acoust. Soc. Amer. *32*, 238-244 (1960)

1148. Tonndorf, J.: Compressional bone conduction in cochlear models. J. Acoust. Soc. Amer. *34*, 1127-1131 (1962)

1149. Tonndorf, J: Time/Frequency analysis along the partition of cochlear models. J. Acoust. Soc. Amer. *34*, 1337-1350 (1962)

1150. Tonndorf, J.: Animal experiments in bone conduction. Ann. Otol. Rhinol. Laryng. *73*, 659-678 (1964)

1151. Tonndorf, J.: A new concept of bone conduction. Arch. Otolaryng. *87*, 595-600 (1968)

1152. Tonndorf, J.: Nonlinearities in cochlear hydrodynamics. J. Acoust. Soc. Amer. *45*, 304-305 (1969)

1153. Tonndorf, J.: Cochlear Mechanics and Hydro-dynamics. In: Foundations of Modern Auditory Theory, Vol. I. Ed: Tobias, J.V., Academic Press , New York and London 1970

1154. Tonndorf, J.: Nonlinearities in Cochlear Hydrodynamics. J. Acoust. Soc. Amer. *47*, 579-591 (1970)

1155. Tonndorf, J.: Bone conduction. In: Foundations of Modern Auditory Theory, Vol. II. Ed.: Tobias, J.V., Academic Press, New York and London 1972

1156. Tonndorf, J.: Cochlear Nonlinearities. In Basic Mechanisms in Hearing. Ed.: Møller, A.R., Academic Press, New York and London 1973

1157. Tonndorf, J.: Bone conduction. In: Auditory System. Handbook of Sensory Physiology, Vol. V/3. Eds.: Keidel, W.D. and Neff, W.D. Springer-Verlag, Berlin-Heidelberg-New York 1976

1158. Tonndorf, J. and Tabor, J.R.: Closure of the cochlear windows. Ann. Otol. Rhinol. Laryng. *71*, 5-29 (1962)

1159. Tonndorf, J., Campbell, R.A., Bernstien, L. and Reneau, J.P.: Quantitative evaluation of bone conduction components in cats. Acta Otolaryng. Suppl. *213*, 10-38 (1966)

1160. Tonndorf, J., Greenfield, E.C. and Kaufmann, R.S.: Bone conduction experiments in isolated middle ear specimens of cats. Acta Otolaryng. Suppl. *213*, 72-79 (1966)

1161. Toyoda, J. and Shapley, R.M.: The intracellularly recorded response in the scallop eye. Biol. Bull. *133*, 490 (1967)

1162. Toyoda, J., Nosaki, H. and Tomita, T.: Light-induced resistance changes in photoreceptors of Necturus and Gekko. Vision Res. *9*, 453-463 (1969)

1163. Trendelenburg, F.: Einführung in die Akustik. Springer-Verlag, Berlin-Heidelberg-Göttingen 1961

1164. Trincker, D.: Bestandspotentiale im Bogengangssystem des Meerschweinchens und ihre Änderungen bei experimentellen Cupula-Ablenkungen. Pflügers Arch. ges. Physiol. 264, 351-382 (1957)

1165. Trincker, D.: Neuere Untersuchungen zur Elektrophysiologie des Vestibular-Apparates. Naturwissenschaften 46, 344-350 (1959)

1166. Tsuchitani, C.: Functional Organization of Lateral Cell Groups of Cat Superior Olivary Complex. J. Neurophysiol. 40, 296-318 (1977)

1167. Tsuchitani, C. and Boudreau, J.C.: Single unit analysis of cat superior olive S segment with tonal stimuli. J. Neurophysiol. 29, 684-697 (1966)

1168. Tsuchitani, C. and Boudreau, J.C.: Stimulus level of dichotically presented tones and cat superior olive S-segment cell discharge. J. Acoust. Soc. Amer. 46, 979-988 (1969)

1169. Tyberghein, J.: Influence of some Streptomyces Antibiotics on the Cochlear Microphonics in the Guinea Pig. Acta oto-laryng. Suppl. 171 (1962)

1170. Vartanian, I.A.: On Mechanisms of Specialized Reactions of Central Auditory Neurons to Frequency-Modulated Sounds. Acustica 31, 305-310 (1974)

1171. Vater, M., Schlegel, P. and Zöller, H.: Comparative Auditory Neurophysiology of the Inferior Colliculus of Two Molossid Bats, Molossus ater and Molossus molossus. I. Gross Evoked Potentials and Single Unit Responses to Pure Tones. J. comp. Physiol. 131, 137-145 (1979)

1172. Vater, M. and Schlegel, P.: Comparative Auditory Neurophysiology of the Inferior Colliculus of Two Molossid Bats, Molossus ater and Molossus molossus. II. Single Unit Responses to Frequency-Modulated Signals and Signal and Noise Combinations. J. comp. Physiol. 131, 147-160 (1979)

1173. Vaughan, H.B.Jr. and Ritter, W.: The sources of auditory evoked responses recorded from the human scalp. Electroenceph. clin.Neurophysiol. 28, 360-367 (1970)

1174. Viergever, M.A.: Basilar membrane motion in a spiral-shaped cochlea. J. Acoust. Soc. Amer. 64, 1048-1053 (1978)

1175. Villablanca, J. and Schlag, J.: Cortical control of thalamic spindel wave. Exp. Neurol. 20, 432-442 (1968)

1176. Vinnikov, Y.A.: Sensory Reception. Cytology, Molecular Mechanisms and Evolution. Molecular Biology, Biochemistry and Biophysics 17. Springer-Verlag, Berlin-Heidelberg-New York 1974.

1177. Vinnikov, Y.A. und Titowa, L.K.: Der gegenwartige Stand der zytochemischen Theorie des Gehörs. In: Funktion und Therapie des Innenohrs. III. Internationales Symposium in Halle (Saale). Hals-, Nasen- und Ohrenheilkunde, Band 23. Hrsg.: Jakobi, H. und Lotz, P., Johann Ambrosius Barth, Leipzig 1973

1178, Voight, H.F. and Young, E.D.: Evidence of Inhibitory Interactions Between Neurons in Dorsal Cochlear Nucleus. J. Neurophysiol. 44, 76-96 (1980)

1179. Volkov, I.O.: The Cochleotopic Organization of the Cat Second Auditory Cortex. Neurophysiology 12, 18-27 (1980)

1180. Volkov, I.O. and Dembnovetsky, O.F.: The cochleotopic organization of the cat primary auditory cortex. Neurophysiology 11, 117-124 (1979)

1181. Wall, P.D.: Presynaptic Control of Impulses at the First Central Synapse in the Cutaneous Pathway. In: Progress in Brain Research. Vol. 12: Physiology of Spinal Neurons. Eds: Eccles, J.C. and Schade, J.P., Elsevier Publ. Comp., Amsterdam/London/New York 1964

1182. Walsh, B.T., Miller, J.B., Gacek, R.R. and Kiang, N.Y.-S.: Spontaneous activity in the eighth cranial nerve of the cat. Int. J. Neurosci. 3, 221-236 (1972)

1183. Walter, W.G., Cooper, R., Aldridge, V.J., McCallum, W.C. and Winter, A.L.: Contingent negative variation: An electric sign of sensorimotor association and expectancy in the human brain. Nature (Lond.) 203, 380-384 (1964)

1184. Wandhöfer, A. and Plattig, K.-H.: Stimulus-linked dc-shift and auditory evoked potentials in transcendental meditation (TM). Pflügers Arch. 343, R 79 (1973)

1185. Warr, W.B.: Fiber degeneration following lesions in the anterior ventral cochlear nucleus of the cat. Exp. Neurol. 14, 453-474 (1966)

1186.   Warr, W.B.: Fiber degeneration following lesions in the posteroventral cochlear nucleus of the cat. Exp. Neurol. *23*, 140-155 (1969)
1187.   Watanabe, T.: Fundamental study of the neural mechanism in cats subserving the feature extraction process of complex sounds. Jap. J. Physiol. *22*, 569-583 (1972)
1188.   Watanabe, T. and Katsuki, Y.: Response Patterns of Single Auditory Neurons of the Cat to Species-Specific Vocalization. Jap. J. Physiol. *24*, 135-156 (1974)
1189.   Webster, D.B.: Projection of the cochlea to the cochlear nuclei in Merriam's kangaroo rat. J. comp. Neurol. *143*, 323-340 (1971)
1190.   Webster, W.R. and Aitkin, L.M.: Evoked potential and single unit studies of neural mechanisms underlying the effects of repetitive stimulation in the auditory pathway. Electroenceph. clin. Neurophysiol. *31*, 581-592 (1971)
1191.   Weiss, T.F.: A model of the peripheral auditory system. Kybernetik *3*, 153-175 (1966)
1192.   Weiss, T.F., Peake, W.T. and Sohmer, H.S.: Intracochlear potential recorded with micropipets. II. Responses in the cochlear scalae to tones. J. Acoust. Soc. Amer. *50*, 587-601 (1971)
1193.   Weiss, T.F., Mulroy, M.J. and Altmann, D.W.: Intracellular responses to acoustic clicks in the inner ear of the alligator lizard. J. Acoust. Soc. Amer. *55*, 606-619 (1974)
1194.   Weiss, T.F., Peake, W.T., Ling. A.Jr. and Holten, T.: Which structures determine frequency selectivity and tonotopic organization of vertebrate nerve fibers? Evidence from the alligator lizard. In: Evoked electrical activity in the auditory nervous system. Eds.: Naunton, R.F., Fernandez, C. Academic Press, New York 1978
1195.   Wenthold, R.J.: Glutamic acid and aspartic acid in subdivisions of the cochlear nucleus after auditory nerve lesion. Brain Res. *143*, 544-548 (1978)
1196.   Wenthold, R.J.: Release of endogenous glutamate, aspartate and GABA from cochlear nucleus slices. Brain Res. *162*, 338-343 (1979)
1197.   Wenthold, R.J. and Morest, D.K.: Transmitter related enzymes in the guinea pig cochlear nucleus. Neurosci. Abstr. *2*, 28-30 (1976)
1198.   Wenthold, R.J. and Gulley, R.L.: Aspartic acid and glutamic acid levels in the cochlear nucleus after auditory nerve lesion. Brain Res. *138*, 111-123 (1977)
1199.   Wenthold, R.J. and Gulley, R.L.: Glutamic acid and aspartic acid in the cochlear nucleus of the waltzing guinea pig. Brain Res. *158*, 279-284 (1978)
1200.   Wepsic, J.G.: Multimodal sensory activation of cells in the magnocellular medial geniculate nucleus. Exp. Neurol. *15*, 299-318 (1966)
1201.   Werblin, F.S. and Dowling, J.E.: Organization of the retina of the mudpuppy, Necturus maculosus. II. Intracellular recording. J. Neurophysiol. *32*, 339-355 (1969)
1202.   Wersäll, J.: Problems and pitfalls in studies of cochlear hair cells pathology. In: Basic Mechanisms in Hearing. Ed.: Møller, A.R., Academic Press, New York and London 1973
1203.   Wersäll, J. and Flock, A.: Functional anatomy of the vestibular and lateral line organs. In: Contributions to Sensory Physiology, Vol. I. Ed.: Neff, W.D., Academic Press, Inc., New York 1965
1204.   Wersäll, J., Flock, A. and Lundquist, O.-G.: Structural basis for directional sensitivity in cochlear and vestibular sensory receptors. Cold Spr. Harb. Symp. quant. Biol. **30**, 115-145 (1965)
1205.   Westenberg, I.S. and Weinberger, N.M.: Evoked potential decrements in auditory cortex. II. Critical test for habituation. Electroenceph. clin. Neurophysiol. *40*, 365-369 (1976)
1206.   Westenberg, I.S., Paige, G., Golub, B. and Weinberger, N.M.: Evoked potential decrements in auditory cortex. I. Discrete-trial and continual stimulation. Electroenceph. clin. Neurophysiol. *40*, 337-355 (1976)
1207.   Wester, K.G., Irvine, D.R.F. and Thompson, R.F.: Acoustic tuning of single cells in middle suprasylvian cortex of cat. Brain Res. *76*, 493-502 (1974)
1208.   Wever, E.G.: Development of travelin-wave theories. J. Acoust. Soc. Amer. *34*, 1319-1324 (1962)
1209.   Wever, E.G. and Bray, C.W.: Action current in the auditory nerve in response to acoustical stimulation. Proc. nat. Acad. Sci. (Wash.) 16, 344-350 (1930)
1210.   Wever, E.G. and Smith, K.R.: The problem of stimulation deafness. J. Exp. Psychol.

34, 239-245 (1944)

1211. Wever, E.G. and Lawrence, M.: Patterns of injury produced by overstimulation of the ear. J. Acoust. Soc. Amer. *27,* 853-858 (1955)

1212. Whitfield, I.C.: The Auditory Pathway. Monographs of the Physiological Society, Number 17. Edward Arnold (Publ.) Ltd. London 1967

1213. Whitfield, I.C.: Comment on Honrubia, V. and Ward, P.H.: Temporal and spatial distribution of the CM and SP of the cochlea. In: Frequency Analysis and Periodicity Detection in Hearing. Eds.: Plomp, R. and Smoorenburg, G.F., A.W. Sijthoff, Leiden 1970

1214. Whitfield, I.C.: Auditory cortex: tonal, temporal, or topical? In: Physiology of the Auditory System. Ed.: Sachs, M.B. National Educational Consultants, Inc., Baltimore/Maryland 1971

1215. Whitfield, I.C.: Mechanisms of Sound Localization. Nature *233,* 95-97 (1971)

1216. Whitfield, I.C.: The Object of the Sensory Cortex. Brain Behav. Evol. *16,* 129-154 (1979)

1217. Whitfield, I.D.: Auditory cortex and the pitch of complex tones. J. Acoust. Soc. Amer. *67,* 644-647 (1980)

1218. Whitfield, I.C. and Evans, E.F.: Responses of auditory cortical neurons to stimuli of changing frequency. J. Neurophysiol. *28,* 655-672 (1965)

1219. Whitfield, I.C. and Ross, H.F.: Cochlear-microphonic and summating potentials and the outputs of individual hair-cell generators. J. Acoust. Soc. Amer. *38,* 126-131 (1965)

1220. Whitfield, I.C. and Purser, D.: Microelectrode study of the medial geniculate body in unanaesthetized free-moving cats. Brain Behav. Evol. *6,* 311-322 (1972)

1221. Whitfield, I.D., Diamond, I.T., Chiveralls, K. and Williamson, T.G.: Some Further Observations on the Effects of Unilateral Cortical Ablation on Sound Localization in the Cat. Exp. Brain. Res. *31,* 221-234 (1978)

1222. Whitlock, D.G. and Perl, E.R.: Central projections of the "spinothalamic" system in cat. Anat. Rec. *127,* 388 (1957)

1223. Whitlock, D.G. and Perl, E.R.: Afferent projections of ventrolateral funiculi to the thalamus of the cat. J. Neurophysiol. *22,* 133-148 (1959)

1224. Whitlock, D.G. and Perl, E.R.: Thalamic projections of spinothalamic pathways in monkey. Exp. Neurol. *3,* 240-255 (1961)

1225. Wickelgren, W.O.: Effect of acoustic habituation on click-evoked responses in cats. J. Neurophysiol. *31,* 777-784 (1968)

1226. Wiederhold, N.: Variations in the effects of electric stimulations of the crossed olivo-cochlear bundle on cat single auditory nerve-fiber-responses to tone burst. J. Acoust. Soc. Amer. *48,* 996-977 (1970)

1227. Wiederhold, M.L. and Peake, W.T.: Efferent inhibition of auditory-nerve responses: dependence on acoustic-stimulus parameters. J. Acoust. Soc. Amer. *40,* 1427-1430 ·(1966)

1228. Wiederhold, M.L. and Kiang, N.Y.-S.: Effects of electric stimulation of the crossed olivo-cochlear bundle on single auditory-fibers in the cat. J. Acoust. Soc. Amer. *48,* 950-965 (1970)

1229. Wien, M.: Ein Bedenken gegen die Helmholtz'sche Resonanztheorie des Hörens Festschr. A. Wüllner, Leipzig 1905

1230. Wigand, M.E.: Hearing and Equilibrium in Renal Failure. In: Auditory System. Handbook of Sensory Physiology, Vol. V/3. Eds.: Keidel, W.D. and Neff, W.D., Springer-Verlag, Berlin-Heidelberg-New York 1976

1231. Wigand, W.E. and Heidland, A.: Akute, reversible Hörverluste durch rasche, hochdosierte Furosemidinfusionen bei terminaler Niereninsuffizienz. Arch. klin. exp. Ohr- u. Kehlk.Heilk. *196,* 314-319 (1970)

1232. Wilson, J.P.: A sub-miniature capacitive probe for vibration measurements of the basilar membrane. J. Sound Vib. *30,* 483-493 (1973)

1233. Wilson, J.P.: Basilar membrane data and their relation to theories of frequency analysis. In: Facts and Models in Hearing. Communication and Cybernetics. Vol. 8. Eds.: Zwicker, E. and Terhardt, E., Springer-Verlag, Berlin-Heidelberg-New York

1974

1234. Wilson, J.P. and Johnstone, J.R.: Basilar membrane and middle-ear vibration in guinea pig measured by capacitive probe. J. Acoust. Soc. Amer. *57*, 705-723 (1975)

1235. Wilson, M.E. and Cragg, B.G.: Projections from the medial geniculate body to the cerebral cortex in cat. Brain Res. *13*, 462-475 (1969)

1236. Wilson, O.: In discussion to B.M. Johnstone and K. Taylor. Mechanical aspects of cochlear function. In: Frequency Analysis and Periodicity Detection in Hearing. Eds.: Plomp, R. and Smoorenburg, G.F. A.W. Sijthoff, Leiden 1970

1237. Winer, J.A., Diamond, I.T. and Raczkowski, D.: Subdivisions of the Auditory Cortex of the Cat: The Retrograde Transport of Horseradish Peroxidase to the Medial Geniculate Body and Posterior Thalamic Nuclei. J. comp. Neur. *176*, 387-418 (1977)

1238. Winter, P. Lautäußerungen im Kommunikationssystem von Totenkopfaffen. Naturwiss. Rundschau *5*, 185-190 (1968)

1239. Winter, P. and Funkenstein, H.H. The auditory cortex of the squirrel monkey: neuronal discharge patterns to auditory stimuli. Proc. 3rd int. Congr. Primat., Zürich, *2*, 14-28 (1970)

1240. Winter, P. and Funkenstein, H.H.: The Effect of Species-Specific Vocalization on the Discharge of Auditory Cortical Cells in the Awake Squirrel Monkey (Saimiri sciureus). Exp. Brain Res. *18*, 489-504 (1973)

1241. Wolfe, J.W.: Responses of the cerebellar auditory area to pure tone stimuli. Exp. Neurol. *36*, 295-309 (1972)

1242. Wollberg, Z. and Newman, J.D.: Auditory Cortex of Squirrel Monkey: Response Patterns of Single Cells to Species-Specific Vocalizations. Science *175*, 212-214 (1972)

1243. Wollberg, Z. and Sela, J.: Frontal cortex of the awake squirrel monkey: responses of single cells to visual and auditory stimuli. Brain Res. *198*, 216-220 (1980)

1244. Woolsey, C.N.: Organization of cortical auditory system: a review and a synthesis. In: Neural Mechanisms of the Auditory and Vestibular Systems. Eds.: Rasmussen, G.L. and Windle, W.F., Charles, C. Thomas, Springfield/Ill. 1960

1245. Woolsey, C.N.: Organization of the cortical auditory system. In: Sensory Communication. Ed.: Rosenblith, W.A., MIT Press, Cambridge, Mass. 1961

1246. Woolsey, C.N.: Tonotopic organization of the auditory cortex. In: Physiology of the Auditory System. Ed.: Sachs, M.B., National Educational Consultants, Inc. Baltimore/Maryland 1971

1247. Woolsey, C.N. and Walzl, E.M.: Topical projection of nerve fibers from local regions of the cochlea to the cerebral cortex of the cat. Amer. J. Physiol. *133*, 498-499 (1941)

1248. Woolsey, C.N. and Walzl, E.M.: Topical projection of nerve fibers from local regions of the cochlea to the cerebral cortex of the cat. Bull. Johns Hopk. Hosp. *71*, 315-344 (1942)

1249. Yoshie, N.: Auditory nerve action potential responses to clicks in man. Laryngoscope *78*, 198-215 (1968)

1250. Yoshie, N.: Clinical cochlear response audiometry by means of an average response computer: Non surgical technique and clinical use. Rev. Laryngol (Bordeaux) Supp. *92*, 646-672 (1971)

1251. Yoshie, N.: Diagnostic significance of the electrocochleogram in clinical audiometry. Audiology *12*, 504-539 (1973)

1252. Yoshie, N. and Ohashi, T.: Clinical use of cochlear nerve action potential responses in man for differential diagnosis of hearing loss. Acta Otolaryngol. (Stockh.) Suppl. *252*, 71-87 (1969)

1253. Yoshie, N. and Onashi, T.: Abnormal adaptation of human cochlear nerve action potential responses: Clinical observations by non-surgical recording. Rev. Laryngol. (Bordeaux) Suppl. *92*, 673-690 (1971)

1254. Yoshie, N., Ohashi, T. and Suzuki, T.: Non-surgical recording of auditory nerve action potentials in man. Laryngoscope *77*, 76-85 (1967)

1255. Young, E.D. and Brownell, W.E.: Responses to Tones and Notes of Single Cells in Dorsal Cochlear Nucleus of Unanesthetized Cats. J. Neurophysiol. *39*, 282-300

(1976)

1256. Zaretsky, M.D. and Konishi, M.: Tonotopic organization in the avian telencephalon. Brain Res. *111*, 167-171 (1976)

1257. Zöllner, F. and Stange, G.: Clinical Experiences with Evoked Responses Audiometry. In: Auditory System. Handbook of Sensory Physiology, Vol. V/3. Eds.: Keidel, W.D. and Neff, W.D., Springer-Verlag, Berlin-Heidelburg-New York 1976

1258. Zwicker, E.: Der ungerwöhnliche Amplitudengang der nichtlinearen Verzerrungen des Ohres. Acustica *5*, 67-74 (1955)

1259. Zwicker, E.: Ein hydromechanisches Ausschnittmodell des Innenohres zur Erforschung des adäquaten Reizes der Sinneszellen. Acustica *30*, 313-319 (1974)

1260. Zwicker, E.: Spaltweite und Spaltströmung in einem Ausschnittmodell des Innenohres. Acustica *31*, 47-49 (1974)

1261. Zwicker, E.: A "second filter" established within the scala-media. In: Facts and Models in Hearing. Communication and Cybernetics 8. Eds.: Zwicker, E. and Terhardt, E., Springer-Verlag, Berlin-Heidelberg-New York 1974

1262. Zwislocki. J.: Theorie der Schneckenmechanik. Acta Oto-Laryng., Suppl. *72*, (1948)

1263. Zwislocki, J. Theory of the acoustical action of the cochlea. J. Acoust. Soc. Amer. *22*, 778- (1950)

1264. Zwislocki, J.: Review of recent mathematical theories of cochlear dynamics. J. Acoust. Soc. Amer. *25*, 743-751 (1953)

1265. Zwislocki, J.: Wave motion on the cochlea caused by bone conduction. J. Acoust. Soc. Amer. *25*, 986-989 (1955)

1266. Zwislocki, J.: Analysis of some auditory characteristics. In: Handbook of Mathematical Psychology, Vol. III. Eds.: Luce, R.D., Buck, R.R. and Galanter, E., John Wiley and Sons, New York 1965

1267. Zwislocki, J.: A Possible Neuro-Mechanical Sound Analysis in the Cochlea. Acustica *31*, 354-359 (1974)

1268. Zwislocki, J.: Phase Opposition between Inner and Outer Hair Cells and Auditory Sound Analysis. Audiology *14*, 443-455 (1975)

1269. Zwislocki, J.J. and Sokolich, W.G.: Neuro-mechanical frequency analysis in the cochlea. In: Facts and Models in Hearing. Communication and Cybernetics, Vol. 8. Eds.: Zwicker, E. and Terhardt, E. Springer-Verlag, Berlin-Heidelberg-New York 1974

INDEX